Caring for Caregivers to Be

Caring for Caregivers to Be

A Comprehensive Approach to Developing Well-Being Programs for the Health Care Learner

EDITED BY

Jonathan A. Ripp

AND

Larissa R. Thomas

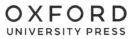

OXFORD
UNIVERSITY PRESS

OXFORD
UNIVERSITY PRESS

Oxford University Press is a department of the University of Oxford. It furthers
the University's objective of excellence in research, scholarship, and education
by publishing worldwide. Oxford is a registered trade mark of Oxford University
Press in the UK and certain other countries.

Published in the United States of America by Oxford University Press
198 Madison Avenue, New York, NY 10016, United States of America.

Library of Congress Cataloging-in-Publication Data

ISBN 978–0–19–765818–5

DOI: 10.1093/med/9780197658185.001.0001

Printed by Integrated Books International, United States of America

Contents

Foreword   vii
    Dennis S. Charney

Contributors   ix

Introduction   1
    Jonathan A. Ripp

SECTION I   **The Scope of Medical Student and Trainee Burnout**

1. Models of Well-Being: Developing a Conceptual Framework   9
    Larissa R. Thomas

2. On Measurement and Semantics: Metrics and Terminology   21
    Colin West

3. Taking the Pulse: Prevalence of Burnout   40
    Jordyn Feingold and Carly Kaplan

4. What's Causing the Problem?: Drivers of Well-Being   54
    Susan M. Orrange, Michael S. Adragna, and Ashley Jeanlus

5. What's at Stake?: Consequences of Burnout   82
    Ingrid Philibert and Lyuba Konopasek

SECTION II   **Design Considerations for a Comprehensive Well-Being Program**

6. Components of a Comprehensive Well-Being Program   107
    Jennifer G. Duncan, Michael Maguire, and Stuart J. Slavin

7. Individually Focused Well-Being Interventions   132
    Farah N. Hussain, Mary Elizabeth Yaden, and Oana Tomescu

8. System-Level Interventions   168
    *Mariah A. Quinn, Lauren Banaszak, Kathleen McFadden, and
    Kerri Palamara McGrath*

9. Raising Awareness and Ensuring Access to Mental Health Resources   196
    Carol A. Bernstein, Claire Haiman, and Laurel E. S. Mayer

10. Addressing and Meeting Regulatory Requirements   219
    Tara K. Cunningham and Michael Leitman

SECTION III   **Bringing It Home and Making the Case**

11. Diagnosing Your Institution's Readiness to Address Trainee Well-Being   243
    Larissa R. Thomas, Irina Kryzhanovskaya, and Saadia Akhtar

12. Making the Case for Institutional Commitment to Well-Being   257
    Elizabeth Harry, Katherine Morrison, and Elizabeth Lawrence

13. Preparing Your Pitch: Communications and Organizational Approaches   270
    Paul Chelminski and Mukta Panda

14. Initial Steps in Program Development   285
    Saadia Akhtar, Sakshi Dua, Paul Rosenfield, and Jonathan A. Ripp

SECTION IV   **Final Considerations**

15. Novel Technology and Discoveries: The Future of Physician Well-Being   305
    Keith A. Horvath and Anne J. Berry

16. Institutional Responses and the Role of the Chief Wellness Officer   322
    Jonathan A. Ripp, Sharon Kiely, and Amy Frieman

17. Advocating for Physician Well-Being at the Societal Level   334
    Christine A. Sinsky and Alexandra M. Ristow

18. Attending to Medical Student and GME Trainee Well-Being in the Midst
    of Crisis: The Example of the COVID-19 Pandemic   353
    *Jonathan DePierro, Lauren Peccoralo, Alicia Hurtado, Saadia Akhtar, and
    Jonathan A. Ripp*

Index   373

Foreword

To study and practice medicine is a great privilege, one that can deliver immense gratification to clinicians and physician-scientists and give deep purpose and meaning to their lives. Healing the ill or making a scientific discovery that leads to a cure are among the most noble achievements possible.

Yet gaining the knowledge and skill to accomplish these goals requires sacrifice. Medical students, residents, and fellows face intense academic competition, pressure to succeed, years of challenging study, sleep deprivation, and, at a relatively young age, exposure to cases of severe disease and tragic death. These experiences can trigger extreme anxiety, mental and physical exhaustion, burnout, and even posttraumatic stress disorder and depression.

After graduation, the practice of medicine presents still more stressors. Physician workloads have increased due to the demands of electronic medical recordkeeping and other administrative burdens, as well as financial pressure to see more patients but spend less time with them. Even so, clinicians still must be prepared, whenever a call comes, to help an ailing patient. They must confront a patient's impending death when the limits of medicine are reached and provide support to a grieving family. Physician-scientists must be able to handle repeated failures over years of work in the laboratory and remain motivated to keep driving toward solutions.

The COVID-19 pandemic has further intensified the stress on medical professionals as they have put their health at risk to treat patients and have witnessed colleagues succumb to the deadly virus. It is no surprise, then, that burnout and mental health disorders, including posttraumatic stress disorder, are highly prevalent among physicians as well as medical students. The situation is complicated by the fact that physicians are often resistant to receiving treatment because they typically view their role as being caregivers rather than recipients of care.

In this environment, it is essential not only that we care for our own by providing robust mental health support for physicians, but also that we prepare our students for the psychological challenges they will inevitably confront in the field of medicine. Medical students and graduate medical education trainees must learn to build their personal resilience. This is a capability that can be taught and enhanced over time through skills that include reframing stressful thoughts, developing a personal moral compass, facing one's fears, developing active coping skills, and training the brain to enhance emotional intelligence and moral integrity. These techniques should be included in the curriculum of every medical school and graduate school of biomedicine.

In 2018, when I appointed Dr. Ripp to be Senior Associate Dean for Well-Being and Resilience of the Icahn School of Medicine at Mount Sinai, he was one of the first physicians to hold such a title. Fortunately, today medical schools around the globe are recognizing their responsibility to promote the well-being of their students, residents, and fellows and are embracing a systems approach for wellness support and resilience training. This book will serve as a valuable resource for leaders at all medical schools in ensuring that their students and graduate medical education (GME) trainees are optimally supported by the system and culture at their institution and well prepared to manage the rigors of their course of study and the inevitable stressors they will face upon completing training.

Medical students and GME trainees are exceptional young men and women; they are smart, ambitious, compassionate, dedicated, and driven. But they are not superhuman. Even the most talented student is vulnerable to the pressures and heavy workload of medical school or biomedical graduate school, as well as residency or a research fellowship.

By elevating the resilience of medical students, residents, and fellows, educators will help them maintain their health through the rigors of their schooling and into their careers. This will increase their success in providing quality care and carrying out their research. It will have a positive impact on health care and on scientific discovery that can advance human health.

Prioritizing their well-being and building their resilience skills will also enable our students and residents to experience the personal growth that results from being a physician, appreciate the joy that should come from the diligent practice of medicine, and make it a special life mission.

Dennis S. Charney, MD
Anne and Joel Ehrenkranz Dean
Icahn School of Medicine at Mount Sinai
President for Academic Affairs
Mount Sinai Health System

Contributors

Michael S. Adragna, MD
Assistant Professor
Department of Psychiatry
University at Buffalo
Buffalo, NY, USA

Saadia Akhtar, MD
Associate Dean for Well-being and Resilience
for Graduate Medical Education
Department of Graduate Medical
Education and Department of
Emergency Medicine
Icahn School of Medicine at Mount Sinai
New York, NY, USA

Lauren Banaszak, MD
Clinical Fellow
Department of Medicine, Division
of Hematology, Oncology, and
Palliative Care
University of Wisconcin-Madison
Madison, WI, USA

Carol A. Bernstein, MD
Professor and Vice Chair for Faculty
Development and Wellbeing
Psychiatry and Behavioral Sciences
and Obstetrics and Gynecology and
Women's Health
Montefiore Medical Center/Albert Einstein
College of Medicine
Bronx, NY, USA

Anne J. Berry, MPP
Lead Specialist, Implementation Research
and Policy
Association of American Medical Colleges
Washington, DC, USA

Paul Chelminski, MD, MPH
Professor of Medicine
Department of Medicine
UNC Chapel Hill School of Medicine
Chapel Hill, NC, USA

Tara K. Cunningham, EdD, MS
Senior Associate Dean for Student Affairs
    and Associate Professor, Medical
    Education
Department of Medical Education
Icahn School of Medicine at Mount Sinai
New York, NY, USA

Jonathan Depierro, PhD
Associate Professor
Department of Psychiatry
Icahn School of Medicine at Mount Sinai
New York, NY, USA

Sakshi Dua, MBBS
Professor of Medicine and Professor of
    Medical Education
Department of Medicine and Medical
    Education
Icahn School of Medicine at Mount Sinai
New York, NY, USA

Jennifer G. Duncan, MD
Associate Professor and Director of Wellness
    for Graduate Medical Education
Department of Pediatrics
Washington University in St. Louis School of
    Medicine
St. Louis, MO, USA

Jordyn Feingold, MD
Resident Physician
Department of Psychiatry
Icahn School of Medicine at Mount Sinai
New York, NY, USA

Amy Frieman, MD, MBA
Chief Wellness Officer
Hackensack Meridian Health
Edison, NJ, USA

Claire Haiman, PsyD
Clinical Psychologist in Private Practice
Formerly of Columbia University Irving
    Medical Center
Brooklyn, NY, USA

Elizabeth Harry, MD
Senior Medical Director of Well-being,
    UCHealth
Assistant Dean of Faculty Well-being,
    University of Colorado, School of Medicine
Associate Professor of Medicine,
    Department of Medicine
Aurora, CO, USA

Keith A. Horvath, MD
Senior Director, Clinical Transformation
Health Care Affairs
Association of American Medical Colleges
Washington, DC, USA

Alicia Hurtado, MD
Associate Dean for Medical Student
    Wellbeing and Student Affairs
Department of Medical Education
Icahn School of Medicine at Mount Sinai
New York, NY, USA

Farah N. Hussain, MD
Assistant Professor of Clinical Medicine
Department of Medicine, Section of Hospital
    Medicine
Hospital of the University of Pennsylvania
Philadelphia, PA, USA

Ashley Jeanlus, MD
Resident Physician
Department of Obstetrics and Gynecology
University at Buffalo
Buffalo, NY, USA

Carly Kaplan
Medical Student
Icahn School of Medicine at Mount Sinai
New York City, NY, USA

Sharon Kiely, MD
Professor of Medicine
Department of Internal Medicine
Frank H Netter School of Medicine,
    Quinnipiac University
North Haven, CT, USA

Lyuba Konopasek, MD
Senior Associate Dean for Education,
  Professor of Medical Sciences
Department of Medical Sciences
Frank H. Netter MD School of Medicine at
  Quinnipiac University
Hamden, CT, USA

Irina Kryzhanovskaya, MD
Assistant Professor of Medicine
Department of Medicine, Division of
  General Internal Medicine
University of California, San Francisco
San Francisco, CA, USA

Elizabeth Lawrence, MD
Professor
Department of Internal Medicine—Chief
  Wellness Officer—Assistant Dean for
  Professional Wellbeing
University of New Mexico School of
  Medicine
Albuquerque, NM, USA

Michael Leitman, MD, FACS
Dean for Graduate Medical Education
Department of Medical Education
Icahn School of Medicine at Mount Sinai
New York, NY, USA

Kathleen McFadden
Instructor of Medicine
Harvard Medical School
Assistant Program Director, Newton-
  Wellesley Hospital
Boston, MA, USA

Katherine Morrison, MD
Associate Professor of Medicine
Department of Medicine
University of Colorado School of Medicine
Aurora, CO, USA

Michael Maguire, MD
Assistant Professor of Medicine & Pediatrics
  and Assistant Program Director, MedPeds
  Residency
ChristianaCare, Nemours Childrens Health
  & Sidney Kimmel Medical College at
  Thomas Jefferson University
Wilmington, DE, USA

Laurel E. S. Mayer, MD
Professor of Psychiatry at CUIMC/Director,
  NYP-House Staff Mental Health Service,
  Columbia Campus/CopeColumbia
  (Founder and Faculty)
Department of Psychiatry
Columbia University Irving Medical Center
  and the New York State Psychiatric
  Institute
New York, NY, USA

Susan M. Orrange, PhD
Assistant Dean for Education and Resident
  Services
Graduate Medical Education
Jacobs School of Medicine and Biomedical
  Sciences, University at Buffalo
Buffalo, NY, USA

Kerri Palamara McGrath, MD
Director, Center for Physician Well-being;
  Associate Professor of Medicine, Harvard
  Medical School
Department of Medicine
Massachusetts General Hospital; Harvard
  Medical School
Boston, MA, USA

Mukta Panda, MD, MACP, F-RCP London
Professor of Medicine, Assistant Dean for
  Well-Being and Medical Student Education
Department of Medical Education and
  Department of Internal Medicine
University of Tennessee College of Medicine
Chattanooga, TN, USA

Lauren Peccoralo, MD, MPH
Senior Associate Dean of Faculty Well-being and Development
Associate Professor
Department of Medicine
Icahn School of Medicine at Mount Sinai
New York, NY, USA

Ingrid Philibert, PhD, MA, MBA
Senior Director, Accreditation, Measurement and Educational Scholarship
Department of Medical Education
Frank H. Netter MD School of Medicine at Quinnipiac University
North Haven, CT, USA

Mariah A. Quinn, MD, MPH
Associate Professor of Medicine and Chief Wellness Officer (UW Health)
Department of Medicine
University of Wisconsin School of Medicine and Public Health
Madison, WI, USA

Jonathan A. Ripp, MD, MPH
Chief Wellness Officer
Professor of Medicine, Medical Education, Geriatrics and Palliative Medicine
Dean for Well-Being and Resilience Icahn School of Medicine at Mount Sinai
New York, NY, USA

Alexandra M. Ristow, MD
Lead Primary Care Practitioner
Patina Medical Group, PC
Cynwyd, PA, USA

Paul Rosenfield, MD
Associate Professor
Department of Psychiatry
Icahn School of Medicine at Mount Sinai
New York, NY, USA

Christine A. Sinsky, MD
Vice President
Professional Satisfaction
American Medical Association
Chicago, IL, USA

Stuart J. Slavin, MD, MEd
Senior Scholar for Well-Being
Department of Education
Accreditation Council for Graduate Medical Education
Chicago, IL, USA

Larissa R. Thomas, MD, MPH
Professor
Department of Medicine
University of California, San Francisco; Zuckerberg San Francisco General Hospital and Trauma Center
San Francisco, CA, USA

Oana Tomescu, MD, PhD
Associate Professor
Department of Medicine and Pediatrics
Perelman School of Medicine at the University of Pennsylvania; PennMedicine Health System; Children's Hospital of Philadelphia
Philadelphia, PA, USA

Colin West, MD, PhD
Professor of Medicine, Medical Education, and Biostatistics
Department of Medicine
Mayo Clinic
Rochester, MN, USA

Mary Elizabeth Yaden, MD
Department of Psychiatry and Behavioral Science
Johns Hopkins University
Baltimore, MD, USA

Introduction

Jonathan A. Ripp

Medicine as a profession has been considered a challenging career choice throughout the ages. And, across time, it has often been considered more than just a profession. For many, it is a "calling," a way of life, and those who do feel called to the work may derive greater meaning from it.[1] This level of commitment to career is in effect a contract with society in the interest of caring for the patient. Perhaps describing medicine as a calling is an appropriate characterization since the rewards of being a physician may be greater than the investment. Traditionally the return on this commitment has included prestige and position in society, financial remuneration, and significant meaning derived from one's career. Some have argued that while the societal position of the physician has declined[2] and relative compensation has been stagnant among steady and significant rises in the cost of education,[3] the potential to experience meaning from the work has remained high.[4] Nonetheless, there is significant current concern that the changing landscape of medicine has tipped the balance for the physician away from being able to experience the more meaning-*ful* aspects of work (such as patient interaction) toward an increasing burden of more meaning-*less* demands. (e.g., clerical work, documentation, billing, etc.). Furthermore, there has developed an understanding that the well-being of the health professional workforce is a necessary component of an optimally functioning health care system.[5]

So Why Now a Book on Learner Well-Being?

The tension between the calling of the healing professions and the personal toll on the individual physician has likely been a perennial issue across the ages. The field of health professional student and trainee well-being, which perhaps began as a small niche subject, has blossomed into a priority topic for many schools of medicine and health care organizations. The evolution of this area of study over the past nearly two decades has been dramatic. Early on, like-minded researchers and educators would gather in small groups to discuss their interests. At one point in time, there was one group that, perhaps not knowing how best to refer to itself, was dubbed the "Resident Burnout Research Interest Group"—maybe not the most catchy or appealing moniker. Participants with varied and heterogeneous interests formed these initial learning communities. In more recent years, there have been large international meetings dedicated to the topic of physician well-being; for example, there is the International Conference on Physician Health[6] and the American Conference on Physician Health.[7] In addition, the major undergraduate medical education (UME) and graduate medical education (GME) accrediting bodies and professional organizations have created task force committees and dedicated large meetings to the topic, such as the Accreditation Council on GME's (ACGME) Symposia on Physician Health[8] and the collaborative effort between the ACGME and Association of American Medical Colleges (AAMC) yielding the National Academy of Medicine's (NAM) Action Collaborative on Clinician Well-Being.[9] This book itself is largely co-authored by members of the Collaborative for Healing and Renewal in Medicine (CHARM), a collection of medical educators, well-being researchers, academic leaders, and administrators all sharing a common desire to help disseminate knowledge and develop products to aid in the advancement of clinician well-being.

So why, now, has the attention to physician well-being gained such momentum and visibility, so much so that we are dedicating a book to the subject? There are some important historical considerations to keep in mind which in part explain the current spotlight of attention.

While mention of modern medicine's current transformation as a driver of change seems almost cliché, in truth this metamorphosis has been going on for some time. It can be traced back at least in part to the Flexner Report of 1910, which many attribute as the spark leading modern medicine down a pathway that has embraced science and technology.[10] From that time and along this trajectory, the art of medicine, and in turn the meaning associated with medical practice, has perhaps in part been subsumed by science.

Quite a number of years later, in 1984, the famed Libby Zion case drew particular attention to the hazards—or at least the potential hazards—of overwork. The circumstances surrounding Libby Zion's tragic death highlighted a host of deficiencies within the physician training environment of the time.[11] This event began to focus some much-needed attention on several areas, including the imposition of limitations on the demands placed on physicians-in-training. Notably, these concerns were initially directed mainly at physician trainees, without much consideration of the physician who was already in practice. Much of this attention focused on duty-hour limitations, which led to a series of regulations on resident duty hours, at first limited to the state level, specifically New York state where the Libby Zion case was heard. National guidelines overseen by the ACGME followed, emerging in 2003, with a series of revisions in later years.

More recently, a greater attention to tragic events, such as student and GME trainee suicide, has further elevated the urgency to proactively address and regulate the learning and work environments, especially given the concern that there may be a link between the stressors within these environments and such tragic outcomes.[12] From inside the medical literature and beyond, the issue of student and GME trainee suicide has become significantly visible.[13] Some would argue that particular attention to tragedy was one of the final motivating factors that led to significant regulatory change. In many ways, it was tragedy that sparked the launching of the ACGME Symposia in Physician Well-being.[8] Related to and as an outcome of these symposia came the ACGME Common Program Section VI Requirements.[14] These regulatory requirements effectively mandated that attention be placed on the well-being of GME trainees with a scope of focus well beyond the original attention to work hours alone. At present, and as a result of these regulations, all accredited training programs must provide accommodation, programming, and curricula dedicated to well-being. These well-being requirements are assessed through the ACGME regulatory review process.

Concurrent with these important historical events has been a dramatic growth in the literature examining the prevalence, drivers, and consequences related to student and GME trainee well-being. As an example, a PubMed literature search looking for publications using the term "Resident Burnout" prior to 2000 shows no more than 10 citations annually. In 2020 alone, there were 371 citations found when conducting the same search. Not only has the volume of citations grown, but so, too, has the quality. This point is perhaps best exemplified by the publication of several well-conducted large survey-based studies, including a number of systematic reviews now available to provide direction on how best to support student and GME trainee populations. One singularly notable publication, the availability of which speaks to the breadth and depth of current clinician well-being data, is the NAM Consensus Study, "Systems Approaches to Improve Patient Care by Supporting Clinician Well-Being." This important work synthesizes the available literature and provides a series of important recommendations intended to guide the field forward.[15]

As the medical sciences have advanced over the past 100-plus years, the growth of information and available diagnostic and therapeutic modalities has been simply astounding. Whereas resident physicians, named as such because they originally resided or lived in the hospital, had relatively few data points to track in the care of a patient, they had fewer still diagnostic and therapeutic options. Now the amount of information that is available and the expansive and ever-evolving testing and treatment landscape is simply too much for an individual to possess. External resources and a growing partnership with artificial intelligence platforms are increasingly entering standard practice. Nonetheless, the student or GME trainee remains, at least presently, at a moment in time where the need to have access to and awareness of an enormous amount of patient data for synthesis and translation into clinical decision-making places enormous demands on them, which are constrained by limitations of time and cognitive load.

How these demands are received is almost certainly affected by each generation of medical students and resident physicians. As the field of medicine has evolved, so, too, have the attitudes and beliefs of its future physicians.[16] There may have been a time when total commitment to one's career at the exclusion of all else was an accepted mantra. While there is no doubt that current students and GME trainees work as hard as their predecessors, they almost certainly place a greater priority on work–life integration. There is also a growing acceptance and priority placed on the importance of self-care. A good example is the growth and normalization of mindfulness as a mainstream resource to support one's well-being and resilience. When Michael Krasner's seminal paper looking at the impact of mindfulness training on clinician well-being came out in the *Journal of the American Medical Association*[17] in 2007, the landscape was quite different in terms of the presence of mindfulness resources. Now mindfulness is ubiquitous and considered standard and mainstream. There are mindfulness apps and courses, and numerous experts abound. Some additional changes with the times are reflected in the acceptance, or lack thereof, of unprofessional behavior. In the past, it may be fair to say that there was a certain tolerance of what we now consider unacceptable behavior, often committed by the head of the medical hierarchy—the physician leader. While such behavior has by no means been eliminated in the health professional workplace and much remains to be done to create an equitable work environment, mistreatment and unprofessional behavior is now appropriately being called out and targeted more than ever. A number of institutions have established effective mechanisms to work toward mitigating or eliminating unprofessional work cultures. Importantly, this now extends to a heightened attention in addressing and eliminating discrimination and racism in the medical learning environment.

In summary, these considerations taken in total have brought the health professions to a point in time where the importance of addressing learner and GME trainee well-being has become a moral imperative. It simply can't be ignored. And despite the host of negative drivers that have helped launch this attention and maintain the momentum needed to prioritize UME and GME well-being, we are developing a framework that moves away from preventing a negative outcome and toward the enabling of our future physicians to thrive and flourish.

How This Book Is Organized

This book is organized into four sections. Section I is intended to provide the background that captures the current state of the literature in describing the scope of the problem and what is at stake as it relates to medical student and GME trainee and well-being. Section II includes content that is intended to inform the reader who may be in the "design phase" of their own program, looking to understand the pieces that make up a comprehensive portfolio of well-being offerings. Section III is meant to aid the reader who is looking to examine at what stage of well-being promotion their home learning or work environment currently is at where it may need to be. This section's content can aid the individual who is in the position of trying to make the case for greater commitment to well-being initiatives. Finally, Section IV entertains some additional considerations for the reader to help unify the preceding content.

Many of the chapters include a "Putting It Into Practice" segment for the purposes of directing the reader to practical tips and tools for application toward program development. In addition, there are many figures and summary sections intended for quick reference, with the hope that this book will serve as a user-friendly reference guide for readers to return to from time to time.

Promoting medical student and trainee well-being should be seen as a journey. Those of us who take on a role in this space often face many challenges and opportunities along the way. Though there are times when the drivers that erode well-being appear insurmountable, the explosion of interest and the dramatic cultural shift toward caring for the caregiver provides good reason for solace and optimism along the way. We hope this book conveys that sentiment.

References

1. Jager AJ, Tutty MA, Kao AC. Association between physician burnout and identification with medicine as a calling. *Mayo Clin Proc.* 2017 Mar;92(3):415–422.
2. Lipworth W, Little M, Markham P, Gordon J, Kerridge I. Doctors on status and respect: A qualitative study. *J Bioeth Inq.* 2013;10(2):205–217.
3. Hughes, JF. Is it better to be a doctor now than it was 50 years ago? *Physician Sense.* April 28, 2021. Accessed May 23, 2022. https://www.mdlinx.com/article/is-it-better-to-be-a-doctor-now-than-it-was-50-years-ago/1rM6t8WzbSTfGQqgmBT5hD
4. West CP, Dyrbye LN, Rabatin JT, et al. Intervention to promote physician well-being, job satisfaction, and professionalism: a randomized clinical trial. *JAMA Intern Med.* 2014;174(4):527–533.
5. Bodenheimer T, Sinsky C. From triple to quadruple aim: care of the patient requires care of the provider. *Ann Fam Med.* 2014;12(6):573–576.
6. International Conference on Physician Health™ | American Medical Association (ama-assn.org). 1995–2022. Accessed May 23, 2022. https://www.ama-assn.org/practice-management/physician-health/international-conference-physician-health
7. American Conference on Physician Health 2021 | ACPH 2021: ACPH (physician-wellbeing-conference.org). 1995–2022. Accessed May 23,2022. https://www.physician-wellbeing-conference.org/
8. Accreditation Council for Graduate Medical Education. The 2017 ACGME Symposium on Physician Well-being. 2017. Accessed May 23, 2022. https://www.acgme.org/globalassets/PDFs/Symposium/2017ACGMESymposiumonPhysicianWell-BeingBrochure.pdf
9. Clinician Resilience and Well-being | National Academy of Medicine. 2022. Accessed May 23, 2022. https://nam.edu/initiatives/clinician-resilience-and-well-being/
10. Duffy TP. The Flexner Report: 100 years later. *Yale J Biol Med.* 2011;84(3):269–276
11. Asch DA, Parker RM. The Libby Zion case: one step forward or two steps backward? *N Engl J Med.* 1988;318(12):771–775.
12. Yaghmour NA, Brigham TP, Richter T, et al. Causes of death of residents in ACGME-accredited programs 2000 through 2014: implications for the learning environment. *Acad Med.* 2017;92(7):976–983.
13. Muller D. Kathryn. *N Engl J Med.* 2017;376(12):1101–1103.

14. Accreditation Council for Graduate Medical Education. ACGME Common Program Requirements Section VI with background and intent. January 2017. Accessed May 23, 2022. https://www.acgme. org/globalassets/PFAssets/ProgramRequirements/CPRs_Section-VI_with-Background-and-Intent_ 2017-01.pdf

15. National Academy of Medicine. *Taking Action Against Clinician Burnout: A Systems Approach to Professional Well-being.* National Academies Press; 2019.

16. Smith LG. Medical professionalism and the generation gap. *Am J Med.* 2005;118(4):439–442.

17. Krasner MS, Epstein RM, Beckman H, et al. Association of an educational program in mindful communication with burnout, empathy, and attitudes among primary care physicians. *JAMA.* 2009;302(12):1284–1293.

The Scope of Medical Student and Trainee Burnout

Models of Well-Being
Developing a Conceptual Framework

Larissa R. Thomas

Introduction

A shared mental model for how to conceptualize well-being is foundational to approaching and addressing well-being challenges. Such a framework helps to guide priorities and ensure that the entire organization is speaking the same language when discussing well-being. As with other major thought discourses, conceptual models of clinician well-being have evolved as studies on drivers and interventions have emerged. Most commonly used models for approaching well-being now include considerations of a shared responsibility and interaction between individuals and the systems in which they work. In this chapter, we describe why selecting a model for well-being is an important step in organizational change. We include a summary of the evolution of thought on models for well-being, describe several common models used for understanding drivers and intervention frameworks, and address the value of commitments to aspirational states.

Choosing a Model: Why and How
Why a Model?

Selecting a model for well-being that an organization will use consistently is an essential component of a comprehensive approach to supporting clinician and learner well-being. Well-being can be considered a complex adaptive problem; that is, a problem in which the causes are interactive, dynamic, and multiple and the potential interventions are undertaken in an interconnected and changing environment. Such problems are situated within complex systems (such as health care) in which feedback and impacts are nonlinear, the environment and human behavior are interconnected, and interventions often have unintended impacts on parts of the systems distal from the initial target.[1] Well-being as a complex problem therefore requires a framework through which to strategically and holistically approach and evaluate interventions, which by the nature of the system must be multifaceted and allow for complexity and adaptation. Use of a model ensures that everyone is "speaking the same language" throughout the organization in terms of what well-being means and what priorities are valued. Because the spectrum of potential interventions that fall under the umbrella of well-being can, at times, feel infinite, models help to define the scope of well-being initiatives that fall under the purview of the well-being team and justify prioritizing certain interventions over others in order to advance strategic goals. This alignment of interventions within a model can help to maintain focus and identify ongoing gaps that require further interventions.

Considerations in Model Selection

Several considerations come into play in selecting a model of well-being for an organization:

- *Simplicity*: Models for approaching well-being interventions range from simple to detailed and complex. While more detailed models can be useful for illustrating nuances of a problem, for wider communication outside of the well-being community, simpler models often lend themselves more easily to memorable talking points. So an organization may choose to have a simple model as its branding or communication model and add more details or submodels within the work plan of the well-being team, for example.
- *Flexibility and adaptability*: Ideally, a model will be specific enough to help guide strategic directions but not so specific that it will require rigidity in implementation. A model should allow an organization enough flexibility to pivot to meet emerging needs of the community while providing enough specificity to keep organizational change on track toward an aspirational state.
- *Alignment with organizational values and processes*: Those working in well-being will often meet with greater success when they can find values or process alignment with tools their organizations already use. While a model may not have a direct corollary with health systems improvements models, illustrating the intersection of well-being with health systems aims will help to demonstrate that addressing well-being is in the interest of the organization as a whole. For example, many organizations espouse the Institute for Healthcare Improvement triple aim for simultaneously improving care experience, high-value care, and population health. Subsequently, an influential piece published by Bodenheimer and Sinsky advocated to include well-being as the fourth aim of a Quadruple Aim to improve health care.[2] A well-being model that illustrates how to achieve this component of health systems improvement can therefore illustrate strategic alignment of well-being goals with overall organizational strategy.

- *Durability*: While the nature of models is that they may evolve over time as new literature emerges, well-being leaders should seek to adopt a model that is likely to have longevity. Models that are specific to a certain discipline or specialty or a contemporary challenge (e.g., the electronic health record, the COVID-19 pandemic) may be important tools for an organization for specific scenarios (response to the pandemic, addressing needs of a specific stakeholder group) but are less suited for long-term organizational strategy. Conversely, models for strategic approaches to well-being include durable principles (such as the importance of leadership support) that remain useful during times of crisis.
- *Avoiding zero-sum traps*: A chosen model should avoid emphasizing the well-being of one group at the expense of another, or addressing one well-being need to the exclusion of others. While in practice different groups and priorities may need to be addressed in depth at certain points in time, the overall model should seek to "lift all boats" in an effort to address well-being as a multifaceted challenge within the entire organization.

Process for Choosing a Model

The decision about which model to use does not have to involve an extensive process. Depending on the stage of the well-being work, well-being leaders may already have a top candidate model to present to their collaborators, or the group may decide to review different models and get input from others before confirming the model. Most important is that everyone is in alignment about what model their group or institution is using for strategic well-being initiatives going forward.

Evolution of Understanding About Well-Being in Medicine

From Absence of Disease to Holistic Promotion of Physical and Mental Health

For much of modern history, the aspirational state of health was often considered avoiding or recovering from disease. The publication of the World Health Organization constitution in 1948, bold for its time, was a turning point in defining health as "a state of complete physical, mental, and social well-being and not merely the absence of disease or infirmity."[3] Well-being, therefore, was conceived of as an active state of thriving, rather than a passive state of existence. This concept aligned with the well-known and oft-referenced *hierarchy of needs* developed by Maslow in 1943, a developmental psychology framework that describes shared needs that must be met for each human to move from a deficiency state (physiologic needs, safety, belonging, and esteem) to reaching their full potential through self-actualization.[4]

Despite much progress in the ensuing decades toward health promotion in the general community, research on the role and responsibility of the workplace in supporting well-being beyond basic health and safety regulations began to emerge only in the latter

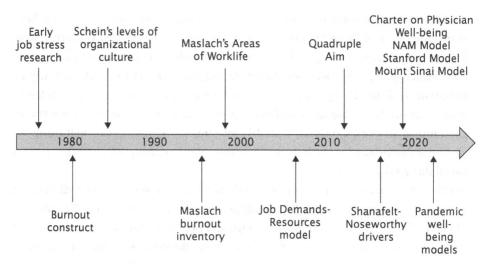

FIGURE 1.1 Timeline of important contributions to current models of well-being.

half of the 20th century. Beginning in the 1970s, the field of organizational psychology began to define the drivers of burnout and well-being in the workplace in general. Near the turn of the 21st century, with burnout increasingly recognized as a problem within health care, research began to define models for understanding burnout in medicine. In the late 2000s, research increasingly determined that medicine-specific drivers of well-being involved a predominance of system factors. Finally, within the past decade, robust models have emerged that synthesize a holistic approach to addressing well-being in the health system. This section describes how theories from organizational psychology and health systems improvement have contributed to current understanding, with the resulting emergence of some of the most commonly used models for well-being. Figure 1.1 shows the timeline depicting the evolution of major theories and models for clinician well-being. While models for well-being in clinicians have primarily been developed based on studies of practicing physicians, these models are generally thought to be applicable to the experience of students and graduate medical education (GME) trainees as well, with the important caveat that the learning environment is a unique factor in well-being in medical training.

The Influence of the Workplace on Well-Being: Lessons from Organizational Psychology and Systems Science

Organizational psychologists have been studying the connection between the workplace and worker well-being long before the well-being of the health care workforce rose to the forefront of collective consciousness. Early research in the 1970s and 1980s focused on descriptive or qualitative studies of individual experience, with additional studies characterizing the role of the workplace in job stress and early descriptions of burnout.[5]

Subsequent research led by Maslach and Leiter in the 1980s and 1990s, which focused on the physical manifestations and consequences of job stress, led to the development of what is now used as the most common definition of burnout. In this definition, burnout manifests in three components: emotional exhaustion, cynicism or depersonalization, and feelings of inefficacy or decreased personal accomplishment.[6] This definition helped to elevate awareness that the impact of workplace well-being goes beyond the simple presence or absence of stress, with not only significant physical and psychological consequences, but also implications for the health and sustainability of the workforce as a whole.[5] Importantly, this definition described burnout as an occupational syndrome, not an individual's deficiency.

Maslach and Leiter's research on areas of work life (see Table 1.1) helped to further define specific dimensions of the workplace that contribute either to well-being (when optimized) or burnout (when lacking): workload, control, rewards, community, fairness, and values.[7] Thus, a more nuanced and holistic explanatory model for the interaction between the system and the individual began to emerge, one characterized by factors that create a mismatch between ideals of a job and the everyday realities of work expected to be done. The greater this mismatch, the more likely burnout is to develop.[5] Not surprisingly then, burnout was found to exist across occupations, but with higher risk in people-oriented professions that tend to draw highly caring and altruistic people such as social work, education, and health care.

The Job Demands-Resources model also emerged as a simple explanatory model for job stress and burnout that involves a supply–demand mismatch in an individual's job. In this model, all jobs can be evaluated in terms of demands that include physical, cognitive, emotional, and time-related needs and resources including adequate time, financial support, material needs, space, and personnel. When the demands of the job exceed resources, job stress or burnout results; workplaces can therefore enhance well-being by either increasing resources or decreasing demands to achieve equilibrium.[8] Advantages of this model include its simplicity and its use in helping an individual to define specific needs in their own job and identify changes that could optimize well-being. The disadvantage of

TABLE 1.1 Comparison of Maslach and Shanafelt-Noseworthy well-being drivers

Maslach's areas of work life	Shanafelt-Noseworthy drivers of well-being in health care organizations
Workload	Workload/demands
Control	Control and flexibility
Rewards	Meaning
Community	Community at work
Fairness	Efficiency/resources
Values	Organizational culture/values
	Work–life integration

Adapted from Leiter MP, Maslach C. Six areas of worklife: A model of the organizational context of burnout. *J Health Hum Serv Adm.* 1999;21(4):472–489 and Shanafelt TD, Noseworthy JH. Executive leadership and physician well-being: Nine organizational strategies to promote engagement and reduce burnout. *Mayo Clin Proc.* 2017;92(1):129–146.

this model is that it could lead to oversimplification of the complex problem of well-being in health care, in which an individual's job intersects with other members of the health care team in addition to patient care. In complex systems, particularly when resources are limited across an organization, addressing an individual's job demands and resources in isolation could lead to collateral impacts (a zero-sum game mentality, see Chapter 11).

Finally, a word about organizational culture as it relates to models for well-being. Similar to burnout research, research on organizational culture first emerged in the organizational psychology and anthropology fields. *Culture* is frequently referenced as essential to identity and meaning within a group, but is difficult to define and cannot readily be measured quantitatively. Edgar Schein's work on organizational culture beginning in the 1970s and 1980s identifies three levels of organizational culture: artifacts and behaviors (tangible or evident elements of culture), espoused values (the organization's purported or published values), and tacit assumptions ("truths" or unwritten rules that are implicitly understood and influence behavior).[9] This model for organizational culture was groundbreaking in establishing the role of values alignment between leadership and the workforce and the danger of a mismatch between espoused or purported values and the "lived" values that workers see on the ground. Note that many tools to "measure" culture more accurately are assessing the organizational *climate*; that is, the way that people *perceive* the workplace rather than an objective/ethnographic description of the workplace.[10] Both concepts have a role in understanding whether the espoused values and mission of an organization are lived in practice.

The "Quadruple Aim": Clinician Well-Being and Health Systems Improvement

In the early 2000s, patient safety and quality improvement movements developed in health care in recognition that errors and quality of care are interdependent on many systems factors, rather than solely resulting from one individual's actions. This sea change in thinking from a focus solely on individuals to addressing systems was captured in the Institute for Healthcare Improvement's framework known as the "Triple Aim": simultaneously optimizing population health, care experience, and high-value care to improve health care systems.[11] In 2014, Bodenheimer and Sinsky advanced a new framework with clinician well-being as the fourth arm of a "quadruple aim" for health systems improvement, emphasizing that clinicians are best able to provide high-quality care when they are, themselves, well.[2] This influential perspective is built on prior well-being efforts and research to emphasize the importance of well-being as a crucial issue for the health care system.

Models for Approaching Organizational Well-Being

Currently, the most commonly used models for approaching well-being for clinicians within health care organizations include an emphasis on the shared role and interaction of the system and the individual in promoting well-being. The system has a responsibility to address system-level drivers of well-being and to provide opportunities for individuals to address their needs and do meaningful work; individuals also have a role in organizational culture and in developing skills and practices that promote their own self-care so that they can care for others. Several of the most commonly used models for well-being are described below.

Shanafelt-Noseworthy (Mayo) Model

Along with the increasing emphasis on burnout and well-being as systems issues, new frameworks synthesized prior work by Maslach with research on drivers of well-being specific to the field of medicine. In 2017, Shanafelt and Noseworthy identified seven drivers of well-being in health care organizations: workload/demands, control/flexibility, meaning in work, efficiency/resources, community at work, organizational culture/values, and work–life integration.[12] Building on the Maslach areas of work life (see Table 1.1), these drivers in medicine lead to burnout when not optimized and, conversely, promote engagement, the "positive antithesis" of burnout, when enhanced. As is further discussed in future chapters, others have built on this model to emphasize the unique influence of mistreatment and the learning environment on GME trainee well-being, in comparison to practicing physicians.[13]

National Academy of Medicine Model

An important turning point for the well-being movement was the launch of the National Academy of Medicine (NAM) Action Collaborative for Clinician Well-Being.[14] In the vein of prior transformational efforts such as the "To Err is Human" report, which launched the patient safety movement, this collaborative further elevated well-being as a defining challenge of our time. The NAM model for factors contributing to clinician well-being seeks to broaden understanding of individual and system drivers that would be applicable across professions and career stages and to connect resulting effects on clinician well-being with effects on the clinician–patient relationship and patient well-being.

Stanford Model

Appealing in its simplicity and comprehensiveness, the Stanford Model for Professional Fulfillment is used by many organizations and includes three domains that interact: culture of well-being, efficiency of practice, and individual resilience.[15] The approach to a culture of well-being draws on concepts by Schein, with an aim of realigning mismatches between artifacts (observed behaviors or practices) and espoused values (ideals).[16] Addressing efficiency of practice includes attention to many of the previously described organizational drivers such as job resources, manageable workload, teamwork, and control and flexibility. An emphasis on individual resilience recognizes that individuals have inherent resilience yet need the time and resources to develop skills and practices to sustain self-care.

Mount Sinai Model

The Mount Sinai Model is another frequently used model. Similarly to the Stanford Model, the Sinai model emphasizes culture and workplace efficiency, but includes physical health in the personal factors/resilience domain and adds mental health support as a fourth domain to which organizations need to devote targeted efforts and resources.[17] The addition of mental health highlights the special attention that is necessary beyond support for self-care in order to destigmatize and improve access to mental health supports for depression and other needs.

Charter on Physician-Well-Being (Social-Ecological Model)

The Charter on Physician Well-being was developed and published in 2018 with collaborative input from members of multiple national organizations and professional societies, and is widely considered as a model for an aspirational state of well-being in medicine. The four principles of the charter emphasize the role of well-being in providing effective patient care, the interrelation of well-being of all members of the health care team, the importance of viewing well-being as a quality marker, and the shared responsibility of systems and individuals.[18] The Charter's section on key commitments uses a social-ecological model, a common approach used in preventive and public health interventions. Social-ecological models help to illustrate the interplay between the individual and different levels and factors in the individual's environment or ecosystem.[19] Such models help to highlight that challenges that have effects on individuals often require simultaneous interventions in the community and society at large in order to maximally impact individuals. The Charter identifies 8 key commitments at the societal, organizational, and interpersonal/individual levels to support well-being (see Figure 1.2).[18] These

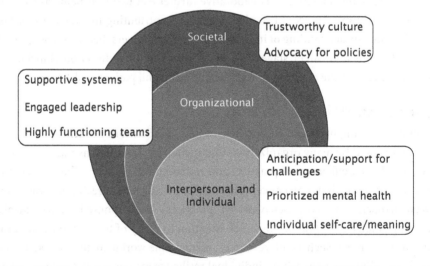

FIGURE 1.2 The three levels of commitments from the Charter on Physician Well-Being. Adapted from Thomas LR, Ripp JA, West CP. Charter on Physician Well-being. *JAMA*. 2018;319(15):1541–1542.

commitments generally parallel the Stanford and Sinai models: the societal level commitments support a culture of well-being, the organizational commitments are similar to the practice efficiency domains, and the interpersonal/individual commitments emphasize self-care and mental health support.

Models to Meet Specific Needs

While the above organizational models are some of the most commonly used schemas for a long-term strategic approach to address clinician well-being in health care organizations, some additional models are useful for specific situations, such as response to disasters and other traumatic events (e.g., the COVID-19 pandemic). Many of these models draw from the crisis management literature and include attention to the identification of needs, clear and consistent communication, and provision of basic resources and psychological first aid.[20]

Model for Addressing Well-Being Needs During Pandemics/Disasters

Developed at the height of the first surge of the COVID-19 pandemic, this model emphasizes five domains of most importance during the pandemic: hear me (get input via leader rounds, town halls), protect me (reduce risk of infection or bodily harm), prepare me (provide training to support competent care), support me (identify and support family needs, physical needs, and mental health needs), and care for me (provide quarantine/isolation housing, paid time off, and access to health care).[21] These principles could also be applicable for supporting health care worker well-being in other disaster scenarios, such as during wars or natural disasters. While the specific tactics that are deployed differ from the longer-term approach to well-being, this approach still has alignment with the basic tenets of the organizational well-being models described in the previous section.

Stress Continuum Model for Individual Support

The stress continuum model was initially developed to normalize military combat stress and identify individuals who need additional support or may need to be relieved of combat responsibilities. It has since been used as a practical intervention model for other high-stress occupations including health care. This model places stress on a four-zone continuum from "ready" (green) to "ill" (red) and, for each zone, describes features, suggested interventions, and parties responsible for supporting the stressed individual. This model helps to illustrate the dynamic nature of occupational stress and targeted supports that may be needed or useful for individuals at different stages of the continuum.[22]

Organizational Commitment Statements

In addition to choosing a model to guide strategic interventions, organizations may also choose to tangibly demonstrate institutional commitment to an aspirational state or ideal of well-being. Such statements, "sign-ons," or recognitions, when aligned with a strategic implementation model, can help to provide benchmarks that challenge organizations to move past the status quo. Such visible statements, described further in Chapter 14, also hold organizations accountable to their workforce to continually strive to enhance well-being efforts. Additionally, such efforts may capitalize on the competitive nature and pursuit of excellence that is prominent in health care organizations, helping to generate a critical mass that encourages others to adopt or enhance their own organizational approaches to address well-being. Importantly, to enhance trust in the organization and values alignment to support a culture of well-being, commitment statements need to be backed up by timely organizational action to support well-being. Some examples of sign-on or commitments statements are included below.

National Academy of Medicine Commitment Statement

The NAM Collaborative on Clinician Well-Being and Resilience has encouraged organizations to create and share concise commitment statements in support of clinician well-being, which are published on the NAM website.[23] In visibly demonstrating support for well-being, such statements also serve as institutional mission statements for well-being.

American Medical Association Health System Recognition

The American Medical Association launched its Joy in Medicine recognition system in 2019, to spur organizational change in well-being and recognize high-performing organizations.[24] This program includes a requirement to sign on to the Charter on Physician Well-Being, deploy a well-being assessment tool, and meet prespecified thresholds in different competency areas in order to be eligible for recognition. With recognition levels at the bronze, silver, and gold tiers, this program aligns with other common performance improvement recognition programs and therefore can help to elevate well-being as an institutional priority on par with other system-wide initiatives.

Conclusion

This chapter has explored the evolution of models describing well-being in physicians, including students and GME trainees, toward a holistic understanding of well-being. Today's models incorporate an understanding of well-being as a complex problem that requires interventions to address systems and the culture of medicine while supporting individuals. The rest of this book will refer to many of these models in building a shared understanding of the problem, its consequences, and how to develop comprehensive interventions to support medical students and GME trainees.

Summary Points

- With roots in organizational psychology and systems science, current approaches to well-being emphasize the shared responsibility of systems and individuals in supporting well-being, rather than focusing solely on individual well-being and resilience.
- Well-being as a complex problem requires a framework to strategically and holistically approach and evaluate multifaceted interventions. Ideal models will combine simplicity, flexibility, alignment with organizational values, and durability, while avoiding zero-sum traps that pit one group against another.
- Several published frameworks can serve as a starting point for broad organizational approaches to well-being, including the Stanford model, the National Academy of Medicine model, the Mount Sinai model, and the Charter on Physician Well-being.

Putting It into Practice

- Does your organization have a model for well-being? If so, does the current model best meet the needs of the organizations? If not, begin to evaluate some of the models described here and consider selecting a model for your organization.
- Consider additional situations for which adjunctive models for well-being described here may be useful to address specific situations in your organization.
- Consider making a visible commitment to well-being through an organizational sign-on or commitment statement.

References

1. Sterman JD. Learning from evidence in a complex world. *Am J Public Health*. 2006;96(3):505–514.
2. Bodenheimer T, Sinsky C. From triple to quadruple aim: care of the patient requires care of the provider. *Ann Fam Med*. 2014;12(6):573–576.
3. Constitution of the World Health Organization. 2022. Accessed May 9, 2022. https://www.who.int/about/governance/constitution
4. Maslow AH. A theory of human motivation. *Psychol Rev*. 1943;50(4):370–396.
5. Maslach C, Leiter MP. Understanding the burnout experience: recent research and its implications for psychiatry. *World Psychiatry*. 2016;15(2):103–111.
6. Maslach C, Jackson SE. The measurement of experienced burnout. *J Organ Behav*. 1981;2(2):99–113. doi:10.1002/job.4030020205
7. Leiter MP, Maslach C. Six areas of worklife: a model of the organizational context of burnout. *J Health Hum Serv Adm*. 1999;21(4):472–489.
8. Demerouti E, Bakker AB, Nachreiner F, Schaufeli WB. The job demands-resources model of burnout. *J Appl Psychol*. 2001;86(3):499–512. doi:10.1037/0021-9010.86.3.499
9. Schein EH, Schein P. *Organizational Culture and Leadership*, 5th edition. Wiley; 2016.
10. Denison DR. What is the difference between organizational culture and organizational climate? A native's point of view on a decade of paradigm wars. *Acad Manage Rev*. 1996;21(3):619–654. doi:10.5465/amr.1996.9702100310
11. Berwick DM, Nolan TW, Whittington J. The triple aim: care, health, and cost. *Health Aff (Millwood)*. 2008;27(3):759–769.

12. Shanafelt TD, Noseworthy JH. Executive leadership and physician well-being: nine organizational strategies to promote engagement and reduce burnout. *Mayo Clin Proc.* 2017;92(1):129–146.

13. Zhang LM, Cheung EO, Eng JS, et al. Development of a conceptual model for understanding the learning environment and surgical resident well-being. *Am J Surg.* 2021;221(2):323–330.

14. Dzau VJ, Kirch DG, Nasca TJ. To care is human: collectively confronting the clinician-burnout crisis. *N Engl J Med.* 2018;378(4):312–314. doi:10.1056/NEJMp1715127

15. The Stanford Model of Professional Fulfillment. WellMD & WellPhD. 2022. Accessed May 22, 2022. https://wellmd.stanford.edu/about/model-external.html

16. Shanafelt TD, Schein E, Minor LB, Trockel M, Schein P, Kirch D. Healing the professional culture of medicine. *Mayo Clin Proc.* 2019;94(8):1556–1566.

17. The Office of Well-Being and Resilience | Icahn School of Medicine. Icahn School of Medicine at Mount Sinai. 2022. Accessed May 22, 2022. https://icahn.mssm.edu/about/well-being

18. Thomas LR, Ripp JA, West CP. Charter on physician well-being. *JAMA.* 2018;319(15):1541–1542.

19. Bronfenbrenner U. Toward an experimental ecology of human development. *Am Psychol.* 1977;32(7):513–531.

20. Center for the Study of Traumatic Stress. Sustaining the well-being of healthcare personnel during coronavirus and other infectious disease outbreaks. Center for the Study of Traumatic Stress. 2022. Accessed May 22, 2022. https://www.cstsonline.org/assets/media/documents/CSTS_FS_Sustaining_WellBeing_Healthcare_Personnel_during_Infectious_Disease_Outbreaks.pdf

21. Shanafelt T, Ripp J, Trockel M. Understanding and addressing sources of anxiety among health care professionals during the COVID-19 pandemic. *JAMA.* 2020;323(21):2133–2134.

22. Nash W, Steenkamp M, Conoscenti L, Litz B. The stress continuum model: a military organizational approach to resilience and recovery. In: Southwick SM, Litz BT, Charney D, Friedman M, eds. *Resilience and Mental Health: Challenges Across the Lifespan.* Cambridge University Press; 2011:238–252.

23. Commitment Statements on Clinician Well-Being. National Academy of Medicine. 2022. Accessed May 22, 2022. https://nam.edu/initiatives/clinician-resilience-and-well-being/commitment-statements-clinician-well-being/

24. Joy in Medicine Health System Recognition Program. American Medical Association. 1995–2022. Accessed May 9, 2022. https://www.ama-assn.org/practice-management/sustainability/joy-medicine-health-system-recognition-program

2

On Measurement and Semantics

Metrics and Terminology

Colin West

Measures of Well-Being

Before reviewing specific measures, it is important to develop a broad understanding of the characteristics of what makes for a "good" measure. Instrument *validity*, the "degree to which evidence and theory support the interpretations of test scores entailed by the proposed uses of tests,"[1] provides confidence in the use of a metric to assess its target *construct*, the concept or characteristic an instrument is intended to measure. Validity relates to a specific interpretation of an instrument rather than the instrument itself, and validity is not binary.[2] Evidence in support of instrument validity derives from several distinct sources which should be considered together: content, response process, internal structure, relationships with other variables, and consequences.[3] These sources are summarized in Table 2.1. Importantly, a single source of validity evidence should not be considered adequate to provide strong support for instrument validity.

Instrument Validity Domains

Historical Validity Paradigms

Historical classifications of validity have often separated validity into content, criterion, and construct categories.[4] Under this scheme, *content* validity refers to how completely a measure represents the construct it is intended to measure. *Criterion* validity refers to the performance of the measure in assessing its target construct in comparison with an established standard either concurrently used or in predictive models. *Construct* validity refers

TABLE 2.1 Sources of validity evidence for well-being assessment instruments

Evidence source	Description	Burnout example
Content	The content of the measure fully represents the relevant construct.	The Maslach Burnout Inventory[6] (MBI) was developed to capture the syndrome elements of work-related emotional exhaustion, depersonalization, and sense of reduced personal accomplishment.
Response process	Responders think about and act on items in alignment with the intended construct.	The MBI underwent multiple rounds of evaluations in different samples. Item selection evolved over 8 years of interview and questionnaire evaluations by a team of psychologists.
Internal structure	Items align with the dimensions underlying the overall construct and demonstrate reliability.	Factor and confirmatory data analysis across multiple samples supports the 3 dimensions assessed within the MBI, with satisfactory subscale reliability and internal consistency.
Relationships with other variables	The metric's scores correlate appropriately with related measures.	The MBI has demonstrated consistent correlations with self-reported work-related feelings, externally reported work experiences, and other job-related outcomes, without duplicating constructs such as clinical depression.
Consequences	The instrument's scores and changes in response to interventions have impact beyond related constructs.	The MBI has been demonstrated to closely relate to perceived medical errors, job turnover, racial biases, and many other important outcomes in medical training and practice, with improvements in these outcomes when interventions improve burnout.

to how well an instrument measures the construct it is intended to measure. Currently, construct validity is considered the most essential and overarching validity concept, with content and criterion validity represented as key elements in support of construct validity.[5]

Content Validity

Instrument content refers to the text, items, format, and themes of the elements appearing on an instrument. Validity evidence from this domain is provided when the content of a measure fully represents the relevant construct. This requires assessment of the alignment of an instrument's content with a clearly defined target construct. Content validity is supported by engaging experts in the instrument development process, question-writing itself, and the construct under study, but, regardless of this, expertise requires careful analysis of how well the instrument maps to its intended purpose.

Response Process Validity

This source of evidence to support validity considers how those who complete an instrument think about and act on its items as they consider their responses. Response process validity can involve the responders themselves and others connected with the assessment such as observers and raters. Response process validity is supported by specific evaluation of these thought processes and actions, training of responders and raters to ensure their engagement with the measure is in accordance with the intended assessment, and clarity of instruction materials for responders and raters.

Internal Structure Validity

Internal structure validity involves how well the relationships among test items align with the construct being measured. Metrics assessing unidimensional constructs would be expected to be broadly homogeneous across items (since they are measuring the same thing), whereas measures of multidimensional constructs should separate across the anticipated construct domains. Factor analysis of items (finding relationships among a group of items) should align with the dimensionality of the underlying construct. Within construct domains, items should demonstrate reliability (i.e., the reproducibility of results across different administrations and assessment when other factors remain the same). Evidence of reliability may come from internal consistency across items comprising each factor included in the instrument, stability of metric responses over time assuming other factors have not changed, and interrater agreement in assessments.

Relationships with Other Variables Validity

Evidence of associations of a metric's scores with instruments measuring similar (positive associations expected) or distinct (absent or negative associations expected) constructs provides support for instrument validity. These associations may be evaluated concurrently or as part of predictive models.

Consequences Validity

Consequences validity evidence refers to connections between the instrument's scores and scoring structure and impacts beyond simply associations with other variables involving related constructs. This requires evaluation of how the measure is used to influence outcomes and whether these uses introduce unintended biases or consequences. Consequences validity evidence can also be provided by evidence that interventions affecting the relevant construct result in changes in important outcomes.

Domains of Well-Being

Current Models

Comprehensive well-being models are difficult to develop because the term "well-being" is itself so broad. The *Oxford English Dictionary* defines well-being with reference to a person or community as "The state of being healthy, happy, or prosperous; moral, psychological, or physical welfare (of a person or community)."[7] Applying this expansive state to medical students and graduate medical education (GME) trainees, and in particular considering focused measurement instruments for well-being, is extremely challenging. It is therefore understandable that assessment of health care learner and professional well-being tends to focus on specific domains within the larger construct. Commonly assessed domains are discussed in subsequent section of this chapter, but first we review three prominent models outlining dimensions of well-being in medicine that were introduced in Chapter 1.

The National Academy of Medicine (NAM) model[8] for factors affecting clinician well-being is intended to apply across all health care professions, specialties, settings, and career stages. It also emphasizes the interrelationship between physician well-being and the well-being of our patients, families, communities, and health care systems. This critical observation has been cited as a guiding principle in other work, including the Charter on Physician Well-Being.[9] The NAM model highlights contributions to well-being from seven sources, each of which relates to clinician well-being, patient well-being, and the clinician–patient relationship. The seven sources include five external factors (learning and practice environment, organizational factors, rules and regulations, society and culture, and health care responsibilities) and two individual factors (personal factors and skills and abilities). Each of these sources is expanded further within the NAM model, with an explicit note that the external factors have primacy.

The learning and practice environment contributes to well-being through its promotion (or lack thereof) of autonomy, collaboration (versus competition), efficient support mechanisms (such as electronic medical records and other health information technology), mentorship, workplace safety, and emphasis on what learners and practicing physicians need to thrive and flourish in their roles. Organizational contributors include organizational mission and values, how authentically these are experienced by students and employees, and how well aligned they are with individual values. Balancing of job demands with resources to successfully meet those demands is a crucial organizational factor affecting well-being, in accordance with the Job Demands-Resources model of workplace well-being.[10,11] Rules and regulations can be barriers to well-being when they are not clearly connected with the core values of the medical profession, and in particular when they add layers of bureaucracy and documentation requirements without improving patient care or the physician work experience. Societal and cultural contributors include evolving alignment and discordance between societal expectations and tenets of medical professionalism. In addition, cultures of bias, discrimination, and racism adversely affect well-being. Stigmatization of help-seeking, especially for mental health support, is yet another cultural factor hindering progress toward learner and physician well-being. Finally, health care responsibilities must be clear as graduated responsibility develops over the course of training and physician careers. These may differ across job roles and specialties, but support for practice, research, and education roles should align with what is expected for each individual.

Individual factors also contribute to well-being in the NAM model. Personal factors include personality traits, stress management skills, and resilience. Holistic self-care across physical, mental, spiritual, financial, and other aspects of well-being is important. Fostering positive relationships both inside and outside of the learning and work environments benefits well-being. Perhaps most importantly, students and practicing physicians alike should strive to align their lives with the "MVPs of well-being": meaning, values, and purpose. Skills and abilities promote well-being by increasing self-confidence, facilitating relationships with patients and colleagues, enhancing interdisciplinary team dynamics, and optimizing patient and health care system outcomes.

A second common model is the Stanford Model of Professional Fulfillment.[12] This model does not organize itself specifically around well-being per se, but around professional fulfillment, which is closely related to workplace well-being. Contributing dimensions include a culture of wellness, efficiency of practice, and personal resilience. The culture of wellness dimension involves the work and learning environment that supports personal and professional growth, mutual respect and compassion, and shared values. Efficiency of practice is supported by involvement of physicians in the design of clinical processes and workflows, identification and mitigation of work and work processes that distract learners and physicians from their primary roles in health care, and realistic workloads. The personal resilience dimension is facilitated by support for self-care, systems for health care maintenance and crisis intervention, peer support, and efforts that acknowledge personal needs outside of the workplace.

A third foundational model comes from Mayo Clinic.[13] This model, also known as the Shanafelt-Noseworthy Model focuses on drivers such as workload and job demands, control and flexibility, work-life integration, social support and community and work, organizational culture and values, efficiency and resources, and meaning in work as central factors in physician well-being. In the Mayo model, each of these factors is influenced at the individual, work unit, organizational, and national levels, yielding the concept of well-being as a "shared responsibility" of individual physicians and the environments within which they learn and work.

Discussion of Domains

As noted previously, well-being is a very wide-ranging construct. It may include physical, emotional, psychological, and economic well-being, along with global or specific areas of satisfaction. The focus here is on aspects of well-being commonly aligned with the frameworks presented in the previous section. This remains a broad umbrella, but important domains include stress, quality of life, fatigue, mental health (including depression and suicide risk), burnout, engagement, professional fulfillment, meaning, and joy. These domains correlate and overlap with each other to varying degrees but are individually distinct. We will briefly describe each of these domains before presenting a summary of selected evidence-based instruments for their measurement.

Stress refers to the human response to any source of strain. Although commonly viewed as a negative experience, it is important to note that stress is not inherently harmful. In fact, some degree of stress is necessary to promote growth and sustain engagement.

The key is to match the degree of stress with the support necessary to prevent that stress from becoming overwhelming, in alignment with the Job Demands-Resources model of workplace well-being.

Quality of life is a broad term encompassing subjective assessment of satisfaction with life experiences. As for well-being, this can include experiences in essentially any dimension of life. Therefore, quality of life can be assessed both overall and for more specific areas such as mental, physical, emotional, and spiritual, as relevant to an individual.

Fatigue describes feelings of tiredness and lack of energy and may include or be separate from sleepiness. These issues may be caused by insufficient sleep, overwork, and other daily health behaviors; by medical issues such as obstructive sleep apnea, hypothyroidism, anemia, and depression; or by chronic stress and other challenges to well-being.

Mental health includes overall psychological and emotional well-being. For this discussion, illnesses such as depression and anxiety are of particular importance. In addition, thoughts of self-harm, including suicide, can lead to devastating consequences and are all too common among medical students, GME trainees, and health care professionals.

Burnout is a work-related syndrome involving dimensions of emotional exhaustion, depersonalization, and a sense of reduced personal accomplishment.[6] For health care professionals, emotional exhaustion means feeling emotionally drained and having nothing left to give patients from an emotional perspective. Depersonalization denotes feelings of treating patients as objects rather than human beings, becoming hardened emotionally, and feeling more callous toward patients and their experiences. A sense of reduced personal accomplishment includes feelings of ineffectiveness in helping patients with their problems or positively influencing their lives and perceiving a lack of value from work-related activities, such as patient care or professional achievements.

Engagement refers in general terms to involvement and commitment in the work environment. Although sometimes thought of as simply the opposite end of a workplace well-being continuum from burnout, engagement is a separate construct. It includes dimensions of energy or vigor, dedication, and absorption at work.[14]

Professional fulfillment refers to the degree of intrinsic positive reward an individual derives from their work. As described previously, this domain of well-being aligns with workplace satisfaction, self-worth, and self-efficacy. Meaning in work addresses the question of why we engage in the work we have chosen. It includes the perceived purpose and significance of our work and how much our work is seen as a calling. As suggested by this language, meaning in work is closely related to professional fulfillment.

Joy in the workplace commonly refers to a combination of contributors to well-being, including satisfaction, happiness, and engagement. This stands in distinction to many of joy's everyday dictionary synonyms, such as delight or bliss, with its meaning in medicine typically connected less to overtly celebratory feelings and more to deeper emotions aligned with a sense of fulfillment.

Evidence-Based Instruments

Each of the described domains of well-being and associated definitions is amenable to measurement, with some domains having better developed sets of instruments than others. This section highlights selected instruments with evidence in support of their application to assessment of their intended aspect of well-being. Common features of useful measures in addition to the previously described validity evidence domains include relevance to diverse health care professional groups and stakeholders, simplicity in both implementation and response, and sensitivity to change over relevant time periods.[15] Additional descriptions and recommendations have been published by the National Academy of Medicine Action Collaborative in Clinician Well-Being and Resilience.[16]

Stress

There are stress instruments to evaluate innumerable different aspects and severities of the stress construct. Perhaps the most commonly used tool in health care professionals is the Perceived Stress Scale (PSS)[17] consisting of 10 items scored from 0 to 4 on an experience frequency scale ranging from "never" to "very often" over the past month. These items assess general feelings of stress, responses to life events, and ability to cope with stressors. The PSS has been used in numerous studies of nurses, physicians, and learners across medical disciplines.

Quality of Life

Quality of life measures range from very simple single-item assessments to lengthy evaluations encompassing many areas of lived experience. Single-item linear analog scale assessments (LASA) exist for overall quality of life and individual dimensions such as quality of physical, emotional, spiritual, and intellectual aspects of life. These have been used extensively in cancer research, with subsequent extensions into other research areas including health care professional well-being.[18-22] They most commonly involve 0–10 scales on which respondents select their current degree of quality of life in the relevant domain. Another instrument is the Professional Quality of Life (ProQOL) Scale, a 30-item tool evaluating multiple dimensions of well-being under an overall umbrella of quality of life.[23] Each item is responded to with the frequency of the relevant feeling over the past 30 days, on a 5-point scale from "never" to "very often." The ProQOL has been studied and applied extensively in health care professional groups. Similarly, the Short Form Survey has been studied and deployed widely.[24] This self-reported health-related quality-of-life measure can be administered in complete form as the SF-36, but shorter SF-12 and SF-8 versions also exist. The items are of varying types and have varying scales and response options, so scoring requires adherence to specific procedures and criteria.

Fatigue

Care should be taken to distinguish fatigue (a chronic, limiting sense of tiredness or weariness) from sleepiness (characterized by a pre-sleep sense with difficulty staying alert and slowed reaction times). Fatigue can be assessed using single-item LASA items asking respondents about satisfaction with their fatigue level or by more involved instruments. For example, the Brief Fatigue Inventory[25] consists of 9 items, each rated on a 0–10 severity scale. Patient-Reported Outcomes Measurement Information System (PROMIS)[26] fatigue measures range from 4 to 13 items, with scoring against normative standards. Common sleepiness measures include the Epworth Sleepiness Scale,[27] which is comprised of 8 items each scored from 0 to 3 to denote increased risk of dozing associated with specific activities, and the Pittsburgh Sleep Quality Index,[28] a more complex 19-item instrument involving multiple domains of sleep quality.

Mental Health

As a domain of well-being, mental health encompasses an incredibly broad range of issues. This discussion focuses on depression and suicide risk, two of the areas of greatest concern for graduate medical trainees. The Patient Health Questionnaire has 9-item[29] and 2-item[30] forms (PHQ-9 and PHQ-2, respectively) to screen for depression. The PHQ-2 asks about the frequency of having little interest or pleasure in doing things and feeling down, depressed, or hopeless in the past 2 weeks on a 0–3 scale for each item. The PRIME-MD[31] instrument asks these same questions but with an even simpler yes–no response scale. The PHQ-9 extends these items to evaluate a more comprehensive set of depression symptoms and includes an item on frequency of thoughts of self-harm. There are also PROMIS scales for depression,[26] including a 28-item tool assessing symptoms in the prior 7 days. Short forms with 4, 6, and 8 items are also available, and each of the PROMIS instruments is scored against normative standards as for other PROMIS measures.

Suicidal ideation can be queried directly, but it is important to note that any assessment of active suicidal thoughts requires an immediate action plan. This necessity makes surveys of active suicidal risk challenging. To avoid this issue, it is common for surveys to ask about suicidal ideation over a prior time period, such as the past 12 months, without asking about clinically actionable current symptoms. Investigators should discuss parameters for these lines of investigation with their local Institutional Review Board and research oversight groups to ensure compliance with regulatory requirements.

Burnout

Measures of burnout have been summarized in detail by the National Academy of Medicine.[16] The Maslach Burnout Inventory[6,32] (MBI) is widely regarded as the gold standard for burnout measurement. For health care professionals, the most applicable version of the MBI is the MBI-Human Services Survey (MBI-HSS). This instrument includes 9 items in the emotional exhaustion domain, 5 in the depersonalization domain, and 8 in the personal accomplishment domain. These are each scored on a 7-point frequency scale ranging from experiencing the relevant job-related feelings "never" to "every day." Scores within each domain are determined separately; there is no single "burnout score". Normative data allow determination of relatively higher or lower scores within each domain, but there is no absolute threshold for dichotomizing these results. That said, common thresholds have been associated with clinically and educationally important outcomes and therefore do have meaning. In addition, one approach to describing an overall burnout experience has been to consider higher levels of emotional exhaustion, depersonalization, or both as indicative of an impactful level of overall burnout. This approach to using threshold levels for high overall burnout has also been linked to important consequences in physicians[33] but was not part of the MBI's development. An area of developing research interest is in patterns seen across the burnout domains, so-called *latent profiles*.[34] For example, different profiles may differentially associate with distinct outcome patterns. Analysis of profiles may allow more detailed understanding of the combined impact of an individual's burnout scores, currently made difficult by the separate nature of the three domains within the MBI.

Several adaptations of the MBI have been reported. First, McManus and colleagues examined an abbreviated MBI consisting of 3 items drawn from each of the three burnout domains.[35,36] Preliminary evidence suggested useful instrument performance, but robust validity evaluations have not been completed. Even simpler single-item adaptations have also been demonstrated to perform well relative to their full domain counterparts,[37,38] although these cannot be viewed as replacements for the full MBI. When these single items are applied, a threshold of feelings "once a week" or more has been associated with impactful consequences. It is important to note that modifications of the MBI items cannot be assumed to retain the validity characteristics of the original MBI's content and should not be assumed to be interpretable or credible measures. The MBI is also a proprietary instrument owned and licensed by a private company, and use requires appropriate contract parameters with associated costs.

Alternative instruments have been developed to address potential limitations identified in critiques of the MBI. The 16-item Oldenburg Burnout Inventory[39,40] (OLBI) includes exhaustion and disengagement from work domains, with both positively and negatively worded items, unlike the MBI. Each item is scored on a 4-point scale ranging from "strongly agree" to "strongly disagree," and the domains are scored separately. The 19-item Copenhagen Burnout Inventory[41] also contains positively and negatively worded items across three domains assessing overall physical and psychological fatigue, work-related fatigue, and patient-related burnout. Each dimension is scored separately after a recoding process.

Finally, the Stanford Professional Fulfillment Index[42] (PFI) was developed to evaluate both burnout and professional fulfillment among physicians. The burnout dimensions evaluate work exhaustion (4 items) and interpersonal disengagement (6 items) feelings over the past two weeks, scored on a 5-point scale from "not at all" to "extremely." Total scoring is converted to a 0–100 range, and both continuous and dichotomized overall scoring is described. Although these tools have evidence to support their use, normative data are lacking and their overall validity evidence base is less robust than that of the MBI at this time.

Perhaps the simplest approach to burnout measurement involves a single item asking about the respondent's assessment of the severity of their burnout. This approach, applied as part of the Mini Z tool,[43,44] has demonstrated moderate correlations with the emotional exhaustion domain of the MBI, but does not correlate well with the depersonalization or personal accomplishment domains.[45-48]

Engagement

The Utrecht Work Engagement Scale[49] (UWES) is the most widely tested and utilized instrument for the assessment of engagement at work. It includes 6 items on vigor, 5 items on dedication, and 6 items on absorption, each scored on a 7-point frequency scale analogous to that of the MBI. An abbreviated version consisting of only 3 items in each domain also exists.[50]

Professional Fulfillment, Satisfaction, and Meaning

Feeling fulfilled and satisfied at work is often assessed on workplace surveys by directly asking about level of job satisfaction. A more robust approach with similar goals is to use the Physician Job Satisfaction Scale[51] consisting of 12 items scored on a 5-point scale ranging from "strongly disagree" to "strongly agree." Subdomains include global job satisfaction (5 items), global career satisfaction (4 items), and global specialty satisfaction (3 items), each of which may be applied individually. The Psychological Empowerment at Work Scale[52] is a 12-item tool covering four domains, including meaning at work. The meaning domain contains 3 items, each scored on a 7-point scale from "very strongly disagree" to "very strongly agree." Additionally, there is a Patient-reported Outcomes Measurement Information Systems (PROMIS) scale for meaning and purpose,[26] including a comprehensive 37-item tool. Short forms with 4, 6, and 8 items are also available.

As noted previously, the Stanford PFI was developed to evaluate both burnout and professional fulfillment among physicians.[42] The professional fulfillment domain includes 6 items scored on a 5-point scale from "not at all true" to "completely true" with reference to the past 2 weeks and total scoring converted to a 0–100 range. Both continuous and dichotomized overall scoring is described.

Joy

Measurement instruments specific to joy are not well developed to date, with many metrics oriented to other aspects of well-being previously described. The Institute for Healthcare Improvement has published resources to guide joy improvement efforts as part of its Joy in Work initiative, including recommendations for measuring joy.[53] Importantly, these recommendations suggest assessment of both system-level measures (e.g., organizational satisfaction, burnout, and turnover) and local-level measures (e.g., "pulse checks" within work units). None of the suggested metrics, however, is built directly around a construct of joy. This issue is a common challenge affecting joy instruments as they are often developed to be synonymous with happiness, satisfaction, or other distinct constructs. The development of robust joy measures with strong evidence to support their validity is a key need for well-being research.

In addition to instruments for specific domains of well-being, measures of composite well-being have been increasingly developed in recent years. These include the aforementioned Mini Z[43,44,54] and Stanford PFI[42] tools, as well as the Well-Being Index[55] developed at Mayo Clinic. The Mini Z includes questions on job satisfaction, workplace stress, burnout (emotional exhaustion in particular), and work environment factors. As previously described, the Stanford PFI includes questions on both burnout and professional fulfillment, assessing the degree of intrinsic positive reward individuals derive from their work. The Mayo Well-Being Index includes questions on meaning in work, burnout, fatigue, and mental health. With available normative data, the Well-Being Index allows individuals to calibrate their well-being relative to their professional peers nationally as well as to colleagues locally. Table 2.2 displays a summary of selected instruments across domains.

TABLE 2.2 Selected evidence-based instruments for domains of well-being

Domain	Instrument	Description
Stress	Perceived Stress Scale	10 items, 5-point frequency scale, publicly available
Depression	PHQ-2	2 items, 4-point frequency scale, publicly available
	PHQ-9	9 items, 4-point frequency scale, publicly available
	PRIME-MD	2 items, binary response options, publicly available
Burnout	Copenhagen Burnout Inventory	19 items across 3 subscales, 5-level response options, publicly available
	Maslach Burnout Inventory (MBI)	22 items across 3 subscales, 7-point frequency scale, proprietary
	MBI Single Items	2 items across emotional exhaustion and depersonalization subscales, 7-point frequency scale, proprietary
	Oldenburg Burnout Inventory	16 items across 2 subscales, 4-point scale from strongly agree to strongly disagree, publicly available
Engagement	Utrecht Work Engagement Scale	17 items across 3 subscales, 7-point frequency scale, publicly available
Job satisfaction	Physician Job Satisfaction Scale	12 items across 3 subscales, 5-point scale from strongly disagree to strongly agree, publicly available
Meaning from work	Psychological Empowerment at Work Scale	12 items across 4 subscales (including meaning), 7-point scale from very strongly disagree to very strongly agree, publicly available
Cross-domain tools	Mini-Z	Single burnout item correlating with emotional exhaustion subscale of MBI plus 9 other work-related assessment items, publicly available
	Stanford Professional Fulfillment Index	16 items across professional fulfillment and burnout (both work exhaustion and interpersonal disengagement) subscales, 5-level response options, publicly available
	Well-Being Index	7 or 9 items, binary response options, publicly available

It should be noted that each of these measures shares common limitations. Differences across demographic categories are incompletely understood, and, because the drivers of such differences are typically multifactorial and complex, observed differences should not simply be ascribed to the demographic factor alone. For example, burnout is commonly found to be more severe among women,[33] but because women are also more likely to pursue medical specialties within which other drivers of burnout are more prevalent, increased burnout among women is more likely to be a function of these other drivers rather than due to an inherent feature of female health care professionals.[56] Similarly, differences across diverse job roles and health care systems are not fully understood even where national data exist. Beyond these cautions regarding data interpretation, there are key gaps in available data on well-being for underrepresented and marginalized communities, including minoritized races and ethnicities, the full spectrum of gender identities and sexual orientations, and populations with varied socioeconomic statuses.

Optimal Survey Design

Because well-being is a diverse concept, no single instrument can adequately address its entirety. When the focus of assessment is specific to one domain of well-being (e.g., burnout), single instruments are reasonable and appropriate. For surveys with broader goals, multiple instruments will be necessary, increasing survey length and forcing investigators to carefully think through their options in evaluating the different domains of interest. Common to both scenarios is the need to apply (and develop, if instruments do not already exist) robust survey items and design. The following sections briefly introduce these topics. For additional detail, numerous published papers and textbooks provide more information on survey design and methodology, including the brief summary text from Phillips et al.[57-59]

Item Development

When existing instruments are available, these are often preferable for convenience. However, the previously discussed elements in support of validity should be carefully reviewed, as many instruments used in the literature actually do not have strong levels of such support despite their common applications. It is also important to remember that validity evidence for an existing instrument does not technically extend to altered versions of that instrument. In practice, prior validity evidence is often accepted as applicable when modifications are minor, but major changes to instrument structure or the targeted population may require reassessment of validity evidence. In reviewing existing items or developing novel ones, there are additional key considerations, including basic relevance to the domain of interest.

It is crucial that items be clearly understood in the intended manner. Terms in the items should have broadly known definitions, or the intended definitions should be provided. Having multiple individuals (including content experts, typical respondents, and survey design experts) review items for different and unanticipated perspectives can be very helpful in avoiding these issues. Lists of common cognitive inconsistencies in survey items are available to guide developers away from these problems.[59] These include "double-barreled items" that ask about two or more concepts within the same item, response options that are not mutually exclusive, mismatches between items and associated responses, and leading questions that suggest a preferred response.[60]

Question Types

Survey items can be open- or closed-ended. The former typically involves some form of free-text response. As with any qualitative inquiry, the depth and focus of these responses may vary, so clear directions to survey respondents are necessary if a specific focus is desired. Closed-ended questions can include a limited set of possible responses in categories, numerical choices such as numbers of events or frequencies, or expressions of degrees of agreement with a statement (e.g., Likert scales). Regardless of the question type, the previously described attention to question clarity is critical to survey success and interpretability.

Maximizing Response Rate

Perhaps the most important contributor to response rate is respondent interest in the survey topic. This can be maximized and sustained by ensuring that survey items are well-written and clear and that survey length is as short as possible to address the intended topic. Estimated time to complete a survey should be reported honestly. Fundamentally, respect for respondents' time and effort is central.

Surveys can be distributed across multiple different media, and a multipronged approach with multiple waves may help maximize response.[59,61,62] It is important to keep in mind that evaluation of representativeness requires an understanding of the eligible respondent pool, however, and response rate calculations require a clearly defined denominator of potential respondents. Surveys shared via social media, for example, often do not meet these criteria, making interpretation of results more challenging. Paper surveys typically generate the highest response rates but can be the most difficult to distribute to broad target respondent populations. Incentives can be helpful in increasing response rates, but the amount and nature of the most effective incentives for survey response remain unclear.[63]

Aligning Data Analysis Plans with Survey Items

Translating survey responses into conclusions, or "understanding the story the data are telling," is essential. Partnering with analytics experts such as formally trained statisticians and qualitative researchers is advisable whenever possible. Data analysis plans should be developed as part of the project protocol before any data are actually collected.

Qualitative data, such as from free-text responses, should be connected to appropriate qualitative analysis methods. Quantitative data should similarly be linked with specific methodological choices. For example, noncontinuous data (e.g., Likert scale responses) require specific analysis methods for such categorical data rather than the commonly used strategy of extending strategies for analyses designed for continuous data, unless justified by certain criteria (e.g., such strategies often rely on the assumption that data are normally distributed). Similarly, for a given instrument, the full range of responses should generally be analyzed unless specific meaning can be assigned to collapsed categories. Because instruments are developed and validated as a whole, individual items from a validated instrument should not be extracted and analyzed as stand-alone measures unless those items have also been specifically studied for use independently from the full instrument. Analysis of single-item assessments from the Maslach Burnout Inventory illustrate this point: frequencies of feeling at least weekly have been reported as indicative of important degrees of burnout domain symptoms, an approach that is only justified because that threshold has been specifically studied and found to associate with important outcomes.[33,37,38] Therefore, those single items can now be used separately from the full MBI in accordance with how they have been studied.

Studies interested in changes in well-being over time (prospective analyses rather than cross-sectional studies) raise unique considerations as multiple assessments from the same individuals need to be correlated, thus requiring special analytical methods. Data resulting from repeated measures for the same individuals cannot be analyzed as independent responses, and the need to correlate these responses has implications for respondent identifiability, as discussed in the following section.

Human Subjects Protection Issues

Survey studies require the same attention to risk as any other research effort. For example, common considerations include individual identifiability and potential for coerced participation.[64,65] Participants should expect their responses to be private, and a solid practice is to employ data analysts outside of the participants' peers or have evaluators strip data of identifying information. For linked data across time, some form of participant identification is necessary to correctly connect individuals' responses across surveys (although, e.g., these may be self-selected unique identifiers that participants use with each administration). Ideally, such studies will involve central management of surveys and identifiers, but, regardless of the approach, participant confidentiality is paramount.

In well-being research, there are also risks associated with exploration of sensitive topics such as depression and suicidality. Questions about diagnosable mental health issues or active suicidal ideation require active monitoring for an immediate response plan if respondents are identifiable. An alternative is to ask screening rather than diagnostic questions and questions about a history of certain experiences without clear disclosure of active symptoms. For example, the PRIME-MD screening instrument for depressive symptoms may not necessitate an active referral for psychiatric assessment if it returns positive. Even in this case, however, investigators are advised to include a summary sheet of available resources for mental health support and related resources as a service to participants.

Words Matter: Getting the Message Right . . . or Wrong

As well-being has become a larger focus in medicine, the distinctions and relationships among terms and constructs related to well-being have become easily blurred. Well-being is not simply the absence of burnout, and burnout is only one aspect of distress. As important as each dimension of well-being and distress is, recognizing that each is part of a larger whole is crucial.[66] This section briefly notes several specific areas of need with respect to clear discussion or future study.

First, well-being is a holistic state. The World Health Organization asserts that "Health is a state of complete physical, mental, and social well-being and not merely the absence of disease or infirmity."[67] Similarly, well-being is more than the absence of distress, and mental health is more than the absence of mental disorders. Accordingly, for example, improving burnout is a worthy goal but should not be the only goal. Rather, a broad approach to promote learning and working environments within which health care professionals can truly flourish and thrive is necessary to support well-being.

Second, terms describing specific aspects of well-being and distress should be used precisely and measured individually. For example, burnout and depression are related but distinct experiences.[6] This is perhaps most easily evidenced by the fact that an individual can experience burnout without being depressed or can experience depression without burnout.[33] This simple fact renders nonsensical assertions that burnout is just another name for a form of depression. These constructs are related and typically positively correlated, but burnout is not simply "depression at work." It is important that burnout be clearly defined as a work-related phenomenon experienced by the individual but rooted in the workplace itself, as conceptualized by Maslach and others.[6] This definition emphasizes that burnout is not a victim-blaming term, as is often posited by the less well-informed, but actually highlights the role of the workplace if the term is understood properly. This is no different from someone exposed to contaminated water being described as having lead poisoning: we fundamentally understand that the source of the lead poisoning is the problem, not the suffering victim. If this is misunderstood, the problem is with our understanding of the language, not the language itself.

Similarly, the term "moral injury," which has increased in prominence in well-being publications, has a specific definition distinct from burnout and other aspects of distress involving the distress that results from having to transgress one's moral values,[68,69] although working and learning environments that generate moral injury will likely generate burnout as well. Conflating these and other terms within the "well-being tent" or using them interchangeably confuses the issues and can make it more difficult to advance our understanding of the drivers and solutions to these problems so that effective solutions to promote well-being can be developed and implemented.

Finally, there remains much we do not adequately understand about well-being and related constructs. Although measurement tools for these constructs generally exist, there is ongoing debate about which tools are best. Furthermore, measurement in specific groups (e.g., by job role, gender identity, race, ethnicity, and any other characteristic potentially affecting individual experiences and interactions with larger systems) has been explored to a surprisingly small degree. As an example, it is widely reported that certain aspects of burnout are more prevalent among women than men in health professions. However, when additional factors such as specialty[56] or workplace mistreatment and discrimination experiences[70] are examined, gender differences resolve, suggesting that such difference are driven by environmental disparities rather than intrinsic individual characteristics. To optimize well-being for all of our learners and colleagues, we must continue to deepen our understanding of these aspects of individual experiences in the larger health care systems within which we learn and work.

Summary Points

- Well-being is a broad and often imprecisely defined concept connected with a multitude of specific terms, each with its own metrics.
- Selecting a metric for assessment should include consideration of evidence supporting the validity of the metric for its intended use.
- Well-being assessments benefit from attention to optimal item and overall survey design.

Putting It into Practice

When measuring well-being, the following tips may be helpful:

- Be clear about which dimensions of well-being you wish to assess.
- Select metrics with more robust validity evidence when possible.
- Employ recommended survey design and deployment strategies to promote both item validity and overall survey response.

References

1. American Educational Research Association, American Psychological Association, National Council on Measurement in Education. *Standards for Educational and Psychological Testing*. American Educational Research Association; 1999.
2. Downing SM. Validity: on the meaningful interpretation of assessment data. *Med Educ*. 2003;37:830–837.
3. Messick S. Validity. In: Linn RL, ed. *Educational Measurement*, 3rd Ed. American Council on Education and Macmillan; 1989:13–103.
4. American Psychological Association. *Standards for Educational and Psychological Tests and Manuals*. American Psychological Association; 1966.
5. Cook DA, Beckman TJ. Current concepts in validity and reliability for psychometric instruments: theory and application. *Am J Med*. 2006;119:166.e7–166.e16.

6. Maslach C, Jackson SE, Leiter MP. *Maslach Burnout Inventory Manual*. 3rd ed. Consulting Psychologists Press; 1996.

7. Oxford English Dictionary. "Well-being." Accessed December 3, 2021. https://www.oed.com/viewdictionaryentry/Entry/227050.

8. National Academies of Sciences, Engineering, and Medicine. *Taking Action Against Clinician Burnout: A Systems Approach to Professional Well-Being*. The National Academies Press; 2019. https://doi.org/10.17226/25521.

9. Thomas LR, Ripp JA, West CP. Charter on physician well-being. *JAMA*. 2018;319:1541–1542.

10. Demerouti E, Bakker AB, Nachreiner F, Schaufeli WB. The job demands-resources model of burnout. *J Appl Psychol*. 2001;86:499–512.

11. Bakker AB, Demerouti E. The job demands-resources model: state of the art. *J Manag Psychol*. 2007;22:309–328.

12. Stanford Medicine. The Stanford Model of Professional Fulfillment. 2016. Accessed December 3, 2021. https://wellmd.stanford.edu/about/model-external.html.

13. Shanafelt TD, Noseworthy JH. Executive leadership and physician well-being: nine organizational strategies to promote engagement and reduce burnout. *Mayo Clin Proc*. 2016;92:129–146.

14. Bakker AB, Leiter MP, eds. *Work Engagement: A Handbook of Essential Theory and Research*. Psychology Press; 2010.

15. Dyrbye LN, Meyers D, Ripp J, Dalal N, Bird SB, Sen S. A pragmatic approach for organizations to measure health care professional well-being. Discussion Paper. *NAM Perspectives*. National Academy of Medicine; 2018. https://doi.org/10.31478/201810b.

16. National Academy of Medicine. Valid and reliable instruments to measure burnout, well-being, and other work-related dimensions. Accessed December 3, 2021. https://nam.edu/valid-reliable-survey-instruments-measure-burnout-well-work-related-dimensions/.

17. Cohen S, Kamarck T, Mermelstein R. A global measure of perceived stress. *J Health Soc Behav*. 1983;24:385–396.

18. Spitzer WO, Dobson AJ, Hall J, et al. Measuring the quality of life of cancer patients: a concise QL-index for use by physicians. *J Chronic Dis*. 1981;34:585–597.

19. Grunberg SM, Groshen S, Steingass S, Zaretsky S, Meyerowitz B. Comparison of conditional quality of life terminology and visual analogue scale measurements. *Qual Life Res*. 1996;5:65–72.

20. Gudex C, Dolan P, Kind P, Williams A. Health state valuations from the general public using the visual analogue scale. *Qual Life Res*. 1996;5:521–531.

21. Shanafelt TD, Novotny P, Johnson ME, et al. The well-being and personal wellness promotion strategies of medical oncologists in the North Central Cancer Treatment Group. *Oncology*. 2005;68:23–32.

22. Rummans TA, Clark MM, Sloan JA, et al. Impacting quality of life for patients with advanced cancer with a structured multidisciplinary intervention: a randomized controlled trial. *J Clin Oncol*. 2006;24:635–642.

23. Stamm BH. *The Concise ProQOL Manual*, 2nd ed. ProQOL.org; 2010.

24. RAND Health Care. RAND medical outcomes study: Measures of quality of life core survey from RAND Health Care. 1994–2022. Accessed December 3, 2021. https://www.rand.org/health-care/surveys_tools/mos.html.

25. MD Anderson Cancer Center. The Brief Fatigue Inventory. 2022. Accessed December 3, 2021. https://www.mdanderson.org/research/departments-labs-institutes/departments-divisions/symptom-research/symptom-assessment-tools/brief-fatigue-inventory.html.

26. HealthMeasures. PROMIS (Patient-Reported Outcomes Measurement Information System). 2022. Accessed December 3, 2021. https://www.healthmeasures.net/explore-measurement-systems/promis

27. The Epworth Sleepiness Scale. 2015. Accessed December 3, 2021. https://epworthsleepinessscale.com/

28. Buysse DJ, Reynolds CF, Monk TH, Berman SR, Kupfer DJ. The Pittsburgh Sleep Quality Index (PSQI): a new instrument for psychiatric research and practice. *Psychiatry Res*. 1989;28:193–213.

29. Spitzer RL, Kroenke K, Williams JB. Validation and utility of a self-report version of PRIME-MD: the PHQ primary care study. Primary Care Evaluation of Mental Disorders. Patient Health Questionnaire. *JAMA*. 1999;282:1737–1744.

30. Kroenke K, Spitzer RL, Williams JB. The Patient Health Questionnaire-2: validity of a two-item depression screener. *Med Care*. Nov 2003;41:1284–1292.

31. Spitzer RL, Williams JB, Kroenke K, et al. Utility of a new procedure for diagnosing mental disorders in primary care: the PRIME-MD 1000 study. *JAMA*. 1994;272:1749–1756.

32. Maslach C, Jackson SE, Leiter MP. *Maslach Burnout Inventory Manual*. 4th ed. Mind Garden, Inc.; 2016.

33. West CP, Dyrbye LN, Shanafelt TD. Physician burnout: contributors, consequences and solutions. *J Intern Med*. 2018;283:516–529.

34. Leiter MP, Maslach C. Latent burnout profiles: a new approach to understanding the burnout experience. *Burn Res*. 2016;3:89–100.

35. McManus IC, Winder BC, Gordon D. The causal links between stress and burnout in a longitudinal study of UK doctors. *Lancet*. 2002;359:2089–2090.

36. McManus IC, Keeling A, Paice E. Stress, burnout and doctors' attitudes to work are determined by personality and learning style: a twelve year longitudinal study of UK medical graduates. *BMC Med*. 2004;2:29.

37. West CP, Dyrbye LN, Sloan JA, Shanafelt TD. Single item measures of emotional exhaustion and depersonalization are useful for assessing burnout in medical professionals. *J Gen Intern Med*. 2009;24:1318–1321.

38. West CP, Dyrbye LN, Satele DV, Sloan JA, Shanafelt TD. Concurrent validity of single-item measures of emotional exhaustion and depersonalization in burnout assessment. *J Gen Intern Med*. 2012;27:1445–1452.

39. Demerouti E, Bakker AB, Vardakou I, Kantas A. The convergent validity of two burnout instruments: a multitrait-multimethod analysis. *Eur J Psychol Assess*. 2002;18:296–307.

40. Halbesleben JR, Demerouti E. The construct validity of an alternative measure of burnout: investigating the English translation of the Oldenburg Burnout Inventory. *Work Stress*. 2005;19:208–220.

41. Kristensen TS, Borritz M, Villadsen E, Christensen KB. The Copenhagen Burnout Inventory: a new tool for the assessment of burnout. *Work Stress*. 2005;19:192–207.

42. Trockel M, Bohman B, Lesure E, et al. A brief instrument to assess both burnout and professional fulfillment in physicians: reliability and validity, including correlation with self-reported medical errors, in a sample of resident and practicing physicians. *Acad Psychiatry*. 2018;42:11–24.

43. McMurray JE, Linzer M, Konrad TR, Douglas J, Shugerman R, Nelson K. The work lives of women physicians: results from the Physician Work Life Study. The SGIM Career Satisfaction Study Group. *J Gen Intern Med*. 2000;15:372–380.

44. Williams ES, Manwell LB, Konrad TR, Linzer M. The relationship of organizational culture, stress, satisfaction, and burnout with physician-reported error and suboptimal patient care: results from the MEMO study. *Health Care Manag Rev*. 2007;32:203–212.

45. Rohland BM, Kruse GR, Rohrer JE. Validation of a single-item measure of burnout against the Maslach Burnout Inventory among physicians. *Stress Health*. 2004;20:75–79.

46. Hansen V, Girgis A. Can a single question effectively screen for burnout in Australian cancer care workers? *BMC Health Serv Res*. 2010;10:341.

47. Dolan, ED, Mohr D, Lempa M, et al. Using a single item to measure burnout in primary care staff: a psychometric evaluation. *J Gen Intern Med*. 2014;30:582–587.

48. Waddimba AC, Scribani M, Nieves MA, Krupa N, May JJ, Jenkins P. Validation of single-item screening measures for provider burnout in a rural health care network. *Eval Health Prof*. 2016;39:215–225.

49. Schaufeli W, Bakker A. Utrecht Work Engagement Scale (UWES) Preliminary Manual. Dec 2014. Accessed December 3, 2021. https://www.wilmarschaufeli.nl/publications/Schaufeli/Test%20Manuals/Test_manual_UWES_English.pdf

50. Schaufeli WB, Bakker AB, Salanova M. The measurement of work engagement with a short questionnaire: a cross-national study. *Educ Psychol Meas*. 2006;66:701–716.

51. Williams ES, Konrad TR, Linzer M, et al. Refining the measurement of physician job satisfaction: results from the Physician Worklife Survey. SGIM Career Satisfaction Study Group. *Med Care*. 1999;37:1140–1154.

52. Spreitzer GM. Psychological empowerment in the workplace: dimensions, measurement, and validation. *Acad Manage J*. 1995;38:1442–1465.

53. Perlo J, Balik B, Swensen S, Kabcenell A, Landsman J, Feeley D. *IHI Framework for Improving Joy in Work*. IHI White Paper. Institute for Healthcare Improvement; 2017.

54. Institute for Professional Worklife. Mini Z Survey. 2020. Accessed December 3, 2021. https://www.professionalworklife.com/mini-z-survey

55. Well-Being Index. 2021. Accessed December 3, 2021. https://www.mywellbeingindex.org/

56. Marshall AL, Dyrbye LN, Shanafelt TD, et al. Disparities in burnout and satisfaction with work-life integration in U.S. physicians by gender and practice setting. *Acad Med*. 2020;95:1435–1443.

57. Artino AR Jr, La Rochelle JS, Dezee KJ, Gehlbach H. Developing questionnaires for educational research: AMEE Guide No. 87. *Med Teach*. 2014;36:463–474.

58. Gehlbach H, Artino AR Jr. The survey checklist (manifesto). *Acad Med*. 2018;93:360–366.

59. Phillips AW, Durning SJ, Artino AR Jr. *Survey Methods for Medical and Health Professions Education: A Six-Step Approach*. Elsevier; 2022.

60. Artino AR Jr, Gehlbach H, Durning SJ. AM Last Page: avoiding five common pitfalls of survey design. *Acad Med*. 2011;86:1327.

61. Cho YI, Johnson TP, VanGeest JB. Enhancing surveys of health care professionals: a meta-analysis of techniques to improve response. *Eval Health Prof*. 2013;6:382–407.

62. Phillips AW Reddsy S, Durning SJ. Improving response rates and evaluating nonresponse bias in surveys: AMEE Guide No. 102. *Med Teach*. 2016;38:217–228.

63. Cook DA, Wittich CM, Daniels WL, West CP, Harris AM, Beebe TJ. Incentive and reminder strategies to improve response rate for online physician surveys: a randomized experiment. *J Med Internet Res*. 2016;18:e244.

64. Sullivan GM. Education research and human subject protection: crossing the IRB quagmire. *J Grad Med Educ*. 2011;3:1–4.

65. Boileau E, Patenaude J, St-Onge C. Twelve tips to avoid ethical pitfalls when recruiting students as subjects in medical education research. *Med Teach*. 2018;40:20–25.

66. Keyes CLM. The mental health continuum: from languishing to flourishing in life. *J Health Soc Behav*. 2002;43:207–222.

67. World Health Organization. Health and well-being. 2022. Accessed December 3, 2021. https://www.who.int/data/gho/data/major-themes/health-and-well-being.

68. Litz, BT, Stein, N, Delaney, E, et al. Moral injury and moral repair in war veterans: a preliminary model and intervention strategy. *Clin Psychol Rev*. 2009;29:695–706.

69. Williamson V, Stevelink S, Greenberg N. Occupational moral injury and mental health: Systematic review and meta-analysis. *Br J Psychiatry*. 2018;212:339–346.

70. Dyrbye LN, West CP, Sinsky C, et al. Mistreatment and discrimination by patients, families, and visitors and physician burnout: a national cross-sectional study. *JAMA Netw Open*. 2022;5(5):e2213080.

3

Taking the Pulse

Prevalence of Burnout

Jordyn Feingold and Carly Kaplan

Introduction
What Is Burnout?

The term "burnout" was coined in the medical literature in 1974, by psychologist Herbert J. Freudenberger, who characterized the emotional exhaustion of individuals in the "helping professions." He observed the phenomenon in medical staff suffering from stress and anxiety resulting from caregiving activities at work and "excessive demands on energy, strength, or resources."[1] While this term didn't formally appear in the literature until Freudenberger introduced it, discussions of distress, mental illness, and suicidal ideation among medical students date back to the 1950s.[2] In the early 1980s, Christina Maslach and Susan Jackson concretized this concept, defining burnout as a multifaceted syndrome of emotional exhaustion, depersonalization or detachment, and a low sense of personal accomplishment resulting from chronic work-related stress.[3] In 1981, Maslach and Jackson published the first instrument to assess burnout, the 22-item Maslach Burnout Inventory (MBI), which since then has been widely used and adapted.[4] Today, many consider it the gold standard by which to evaluate burnout among health care workers.

Explorations of burnout within the medical literature have exploded in the past two decades. Burnout is now primarily considered a systems issue[5,6] that likely begins in medical school or earlier[7-9] and often worsens during residency training,[10] with some medical school and residency programs reporting a burnout prevalence as high as 75%.[11,12] Indeed, medical student, resident, and clinical fellow burnout do not exist in a vacuum or independently from one another. Rather, complex interrelationships likely exist between burnout in medical students and resident physicians, both through the natural educational trajectories of learners within the health care system and by virtue of the shared work environment. For example, the burnout and attitudes of residents may influence the development of burnout in medical students who interact extensively with these residents in their clinical years. Some studies report that medical students have a higher odds of burnout when their interns and residents are seen as cynical.[13]

Unlike mental illnesses such as major depressive disorder, burnout is an occupational phenomenon—driven by factors within the work environment—and not a medical condition.[14] While the individual's manifestations of burnout can resemble depression (e.g., fatigue, low sense of self-worth or self-efficacy), burnout is specifically related to workplace, whereas major depressive disorder persists in many dimensions of one's life. It is important to distinguish the two because the evidence-based interventions to address burnout and depression differ. Burnout itself is likely correlated with depression and is independently related to substance use, relationship difficulties, and suicidal ideation[8,15] While this chapter focuses primarily on the prevalence of burnout among medical students, residents, and clinical fellows, we also include a brief discussion of related mental health challenges facing this population. Chapter 9 describes the distinctions between burnout and depression as well as their association in further detail.

Burnout Among Health Care Professionals

Burnout is clearly higher among physicians than other workers in the United States, and it is estimated that up to 50% of practicing physicians experience at least one symptom of burnout.[16,17] A national study of burnout in a sample of more than 7,000 US doctors compared to a probability-based sample of the general US population in 2011 found that doctors had a 36% increased odds of burnout compared to those with a high school diploma. In the same study, those with bachelor's degrees, master's degrees, or other professional doctorate degrees (other than MDs or DOs) had the lowest risk of burnout. In particular, physicians working on the front lines of patient care (e.g., general internal medicine, emergency medicine, family medicine) seem to be at the highest risk for burnout, though it is not entirely clear whether this pattern is mirrored among students and graduate medical education (GME) trainees.[16] Recent data would suggest that the proportion of physicians experiencing burnout remains high, indicative of a systemic problem.

Consequences of Burnout for Medical Students and Residents

In addition to the adverse mental health and relationship outcomes mentioned above, burnout among medical students and residents is associated with unethical and unprofessional behaviors, such as academic dishonesty, and lower-quality patient care, such as a reduced likelihood to report medical errors.[15] For example, research shows that anesthesia residents with burnout or depression are less likely to read about the next day's surgery cases or visit a patient prior to their surgery.[18] Medicine residents with burnout are more likely to self-report discharging patients prematurely,[19] and pediatrics residents with burnout have been shown to make six times as many medication errors as their peers.[20] These consequences of burnout will be further elaborated in Chapter 5.

Depression and Suicidality Among Medical Professionals and Trainees

In a national survey of medical students, residents and fellows, and early career physicians (those in practice for 5 or fewer years) conducted in 2011–2012, after controlling for relationship status, sex, age, and career stage, being a resident or clinical fellow was associated with an increased odds of burnout and being a medical student was associated with an increased odds of depressive symptoms. Compared to population control samples, students, residents/fellows, and early career physicians were significantly more likely to be burned out, but not to have suicidal ideation. Medical students and residents were also more likely to have symptoms of depression.[23]

Most reviews and meta-analyses have indicated that practicing medical physicians have an increased risk for suicide compared with their aged-matched peers. Data through the 1980s showed that male and female physicians had a 40% and 230% higher risk of suicide, respectively, compared with gender- and age-matched counterparts in the general population.[21,22] Suicidal ideation has been shown to impact up to 11.2% of medical students,[8] though it is not entirely clear whether this rate differs significantly from the age-matched population of college graduates.[23] While resident physicians specifically have not been shown to be at increased risk for suicide, studies show that depression affects 22–35% of resident physicians, compared with 17% of the general population.[24] Among medical students, a 2016 meta-analysis revealed a 28% global prevalence of depression.[25] Regardless of potential trends in prevalence of suicide, the burden of depression among medical students and GME trainees clearly highlights a population needing targeted availability of resources to support mental health.

Those entering the profession of medicine have significant stressors depending on the stage of training and its intersection with individual circumstances, as shown in Figure 3.1. In the remainder of this chapter, we outline the prevalence of medical student and resident burnout, synthesizing findings from the available literature and scoping this problem within each population. Although we will mention certain factors correlated with burnout to contextualize the prevalence, more robust descriptions of the measurement tools to assess burnout were discussed in Chapter 2, and drivers and consequences of burnout will be addressed in Chapters 4 and 5, respectively.

Burnout in Undergraduate Medical Education

Prevalence Estimates Among Medical Students in the United States

While burnout is not a novel concept within the clinical career trajectory of health care professionals, the emergence of studies specifically evaluating burnout among medical

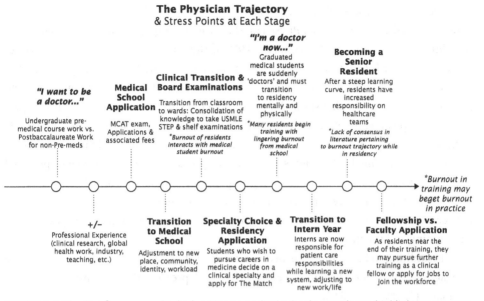

FIGURE 3.1 Timeline from premedical education to medical school to residency, highlighting common stress points that have been shown in the literature to contribute to burnout.

students is a relatively recent development. Until 2006, there were no studies that assessed the prevalence of burnout in North American medical students. At that time, Liselotte Dyrbye and colleagues conducted a systematic review that examined the prevalence of "distress" among medical students, including measures of depression, anxiety, and general mental health, finding that medical students, particularly those in the later years of training, had greater depression severity than more junior students and non-student populations.[26] They also found that medical students had significantly more severe anxiety than age-matched samples within the general population.

While classically thought of as a workplace-related construct, burnout is also quite common in the medical educational space, including during the preclinical years of medical school. In the following discussion about burnout among medical students, it may therefore be helpful to think of the school-based learning environment itself as the workplace in which burnout develops. The early 2000s represented the beginning of a reckoning with medical student burnout, with some of the first American multi-institutional studies reporting a prevalence of 45% among 1,098 students at three Minnesota medical institutions in 2006 and 47% among 3,080 students from multiple institutions across five states.[27,28] Both of these studies used the 22-item MBI to evaluate burnout. By 2013, an international systematic review of burnout in medical schools included four additional US-based studies published between 2006 and 2011.[29] This review revealed that burnout prevalence among medical students ranged from 45% to 75%.[30]

A more recent national survey of burnout among medical students in the United States was conducted between 2011 and 2012 by Dyrbye and colleagues.[23] This study included 4,402 medical students, generally representative of all medical students from the American Medical Association's Physician Master File, geographically distributed across the United States. Among this cohort, 55.9% of the students met criteria for burnout based on the MBI-22, compared to 35.7% in the age-matched general population. The subdimensions of burnout were also reported, with 44.6% of medical students screening positive for emotional exhaustion, 37.9% for depersonalization, and 35.8% for low personal accomplishment. While emotional exhaustion in medical school was comparable to that of residents and fellows, and depersonalization was comparable to that of early-career physicians, medical students had a higher prevalence of a low sense of personal accomplishment than any other studied group (35.8% compared with 22.0% and 18.2% in residents and early-career physicians, respectively). These findings may shed light on how certain symptoms of burnout can manifest more strongly at different stages of medical training and practice.

In addition to being more burned out, medical students in this national study were also significantly more likely to screen positive for depression than age-matched college graduates (58.0% vs. 47.5%).

Burnout in Premedical Students

Based on the prevalence of burnout and distress among medical students, one might reasonably wonder whether those who pursue a degree as a medical doctor are in some way predisposed to burnout or perhaps are already more burned out than their peers before even beginning medical school. Indeed, researchers have asked this question to assess burnout and distress in premedical students—those undergraduate college students preparing for application to medical school—with some conflicting results.

Comparing premedical students with other college-aged students during their undergraduate careers, one single institution study found that college students on a premedical track experienced greater depression severity, as measured by the Patient Health Questionnaire, (PHQ-9) and a higher degree of emotional exhaustion, assessed with the MBI-SS, (Student Survey) than their counterparts not on premedical tracks.[31] However, premedical students also had a greater sense of personal efficacy than did the surveyed students not on premedical tracks.

When looking at newly matriculating medical students (those who have completed their premedical training and have been accepted into medical school), data from 938 students across six medical schools showed that the matriculating medical students actually had a significantly *lower* prevalence of burnout than their counterparts in the general population (27.3% vs. 37.3%).[32] Furthermore, only 26.2% of these medical students-to-be demonstrated symptoms of depression compared with 42.4% of their age- and education-matched counterparts from the general population. These findings persisted with multivariable analysis accounting for demographic factors like age, race/ethnicity, sex, and relationship status.

However, once in medical school, many students experience burnout and a downward trajectory in their mental health analogous to that which they may have begun to experience as premedical undergraduates. Interestingly, one study found that taking a gap year between college and the beginning of medical school was associated with a significant decrease in burnout among medical students at one institution.[33] Thus, perhaps these findings reflect a transient period of reduced burnout prior to the start of medical school, and importantly, the population entering medical school does not appear to be inherently burned out at the beginning. Further investigation into the origins of burnout among premedical students and interventions aimed at this population is warranted.

Burnout Among Medical Students Globally

Burnout in medical education has also garnered attention in other countries. A 2017 meta-analysis of Chinese medical students found the prevalence of moderate or greater burnout to be more than 40% in most studies.[34] This analysis included 33 individual studies, the majority of which measured burnout using various versions of the MBI or the Lian Rong Survey (LRS).[35] Higher levels of burnout were found in more senior students, consistent with data from the United States and other international samples.[27]

Meta-analyses of medical students have found a high degree of heterogeneity across studies and countries, making it difficult to estimate a definitive global prevalence of medical student burnout. However, one global meta-analysis from 2019 (including studies from the United States, Mexico, the United Kingdom, Australia, Brazil, Saudi Arabia, Lebanon, Spain, New Zealand, Israel, Pakistan, Romania, South Korea, Netherlands, and the Caribbean Islands) estimated the international burnout prevalence to be 44.2% (95% confidence interval [CI], 33.4–55.0%) of medical students.[36] This analysis included a total of 24 studies, nine of which included subscale measurements of burnout. Prevalence of emotional exhaustion was estimated to be 40.8% (95% CI, 32.8–48.9%), depersonalization was estimated to be 35.1% (95% CI, 27.2–43.0%), and low sense of personal accomplishment was estimated to be 27.4% (95% CI, 20.5–34.3%), a pattern consistent with the aforementioned US-based study. [27]

Another global meta-analysis from 2019 also found markedly wide ranges of burnout prevalence—from 7% to 75.2%—using different versions of the MBI.[11] This wide range may very well stem from the diversity of medical educational trajectories across countries, including differences in typical age of matriculation, medical school curriculum, cost of attendance and financial strain on students, and overarching structures of medical systems within a country. For this reason, further discussion of the drivers of and solutions to address burnout discussed throughout this book will primarily focus on factors specific to medical training in the United States and the US health care system.

One commonality across international studies and those in the United States is that senior medical students have a greater severity and higher prevalence of burnout than junior students, likely reflecting the shift from the preclinical classroom to the clinical environment that typically occurs at the end of the second or beginning of the third year of medical school. More specific attention to the differential drivers of burnout at each stage of medical school will appear in Chapter 4. When developing interventions to ameliorate burnout, it will thus be important to understand these different context-specific drivers.

Overall, the prevalence of burnout among medical students is quite high, hovering around 50% across studies, and it remains consistently higher than age-matched cohorts in the general population. Quite possibly, the origins of medical student burnout begin in competitive premedical undergraduate programs, and prevalence is likely to grow over the course of medical school. Additionally, compared to residents and early-career physicians, medical students have a lower sense of personal accomplishment. The personal accomplishment dimension is not included in abbreviated burnout measures but is an important consideration to keep in mind for medical students who, by circumstance, are the least experienced members of their clinical teams. As we describe in the next section, consequences of burnout often stay with students as they emerge from medical school to proceed on with their residency training.

Burnout in Graduate Medical Education

Prevalence Estimates Among Residents in the United States

Physicians within their GME training (e.g., residents and clinical fellows) are clearly at particular risk for burnout, with rates comparable to those of attending physicians and higher than other US workers in the general population.[17] Resident physicians are learners within the health care system but are also employees who are tasked with very significant patient care duties and therefore must navigate simultaneously high responsibility while having low levels of control and autonomy.[37-39] Additionally, residents are frequently subject to sleep deprivation and have dramatically lower salaries than attending-level physicians.[38]

Studies show that residents start residency with high levels of burnout. A 2015 narrative review of burnout in medical school and residency highlights that, once in residency, the prevalence of high emotional exhaustion continues to be comparable to that found during medical school (44–50%); however, the prevalence of high depersonalization (32–38%) and overall burnout (60%) increases.[14,40] Research regarding the trajectory of burnout symptoms across years of residency is inconsistent, with some studies showing that burnout increases throughout each subsequent year of residency, some showing equal prevalence across years, and others showing a lower risk of developing burnout following the intern year.[14]

The aforementioned national survey of burnout among medical students, residents/ fellows, and early-career clinicians in the United States from 2011 to 2012 by Dyrbye and colleagues included data from 1,701 residents and fellows.[23] Among this cohort, 50.7% of the residents/fellows met criteria for burnout based on the MBI-22 (based on high scores on emotional exhaustion and depersonalization subscales), compared to 31.4% in an age-matched population of college graduates. The subdimensions of burnout were also reported, with 44.4% of residents/fellows screening positive for high emotional exhaustion, 50.7% for high depersonalization, and 22.0% for low sense of personal accomplishment.

A 2018 study was the first to prospectively evaluate rates of burnout symptoms among resident physicians by clinical specialty and medical school–related factors.[41] This prospective cohort study examined burnout in a nationally representative cohort of 3,588 second-year residents from 20 specialties, followed since their fourth year of medical school, from 49 allopathic medical institutions in the United States. Symptoms of burnout were measured using the abbreviated 2-item MBI. Burnout symptoms at least weekly occurred in 45.2% (95% CI, 43.6–46.8%) of this population. Prevalence within specialities ranged from as low as 29.6% in dermatology to 63.8% in urology programs. Symptoms of emotional exhaustion at least weekly were reported by 35.6% (99% CI, 34.0–37.2%) of respondents, and symptoms of high depersonalization at least weekly were reported by 34.9% (99% CI, 33.3–36.5%). After controlling for demographic characteristics, debt, board scores, levels of anxiety, empathy, and social support in medical school, the presence of burnout was associated with a higher relative risk of career and specialty choice regret. Controlling for the same factors, training in the specialties of urology, neurology, emergency medicine, ophthalmology, and general surgery were associated with a higher relative risk of burnout in the second year of residency relative to training in internal medicine as the reference group. Training in dermatology was associated with a lower relative risk of burnout compared to training in internal medicine.

In addition to specialty, identifying as female in this cohort was associated with a higher relative risk of burnout. Higher anxiety scores and lower empathy scores during the fourth year of medical school were also associated with a higher relative risk of burnout in residency, suggesting that factors in medical school may contribute to the development of burnout in the next phase of training.

Resident Burnout Globally

Moving beyond exclusively US-based studies, we report findings of three global systematic reviews and meta-analyses of resident burnout. Importantly, these results reflect aggregations of studies of residents in training programs across the world, which likely have significantly distinct educational and training cultures and practices. As such, these conclusions should be interpreted with this in mind.

A 2007 study by Prins and colleagues was the first meta-analysis to explore the prevalence of medical resident burnout in multiple countries.[39] This analysis included 19 studies published between 1986 and 2005 from eight countries; a majority of these were conducted in the United States, with four conducted in Europe, two in Africa, and one in Israel. Heterogeneity in the burnout scales and cutoff scores used to diagnose burnout across these studies makes it very challenging to compare studies with one another and, in turn, to draw explicit conclusions about the extent of burnout among postgraduate medical trainees worldwide. For example, while prevalence of burnout ostensibly ranged from 17.6% in a study of obstetrics and gynecology (OBGYN) residents in Texas to 76.0% in a study of internal medicine residents in Washington state, these studies defined burnout using different criteria, with 17.6% likely an underestimation of burnout and 76% likely an overestimation. Despite these methodological shortcomings, this study was a step forward in putting the issue of resident burnout on the map and exposing the need for more systematic designs of resident burnout research using consistent measurement instruments.

A 2018 meta-analysis examined the prevalence of overall burnout and its subdimensions in residents from different medical specialties globally.[38] This analysis benefited from being able to use more consistent burnout metrics and cutoff criteria. Specifically, all studies analyzed in this meta-analysis relied on the 22-item MBI; the subdimensions cutoff points were defined as low emotional exhaustion ≤18, high emotional exhaustion ≥27; low depersonalization ≤5, high depersonalization ≥10; and high personal accomplishment ≥40, low personal accomplishment ≤33; overall high burnout risk was defined as high depersonalization and/or emotional exhaustion. The 26 included studies were published between 2007 and 2017 and involved 4,664 residents from North America, South America, Europe, Australia, and Asia. Specialties included radiation oncology ($n = 45$ residents, 1 study from Turkey), otolaryngology ($n = 599$; 1 study from Saudi Arabia, 1 from the United States), OBGYN ($n = 473$; 5 studies across the United States, Spain, Canada, and France), pediatrics ($n = 77$; 1 study from the United States, 1 from Brazil), orthopedics ($n = 78$; 1 study from the United States), plastic surgery ($n = 52$; 1 study from France), general surgery ($n = 797$; 1 study from the United States, 1 from Pakistan), urgency/emergency medicine ($n = 165$; 1 study from Iran), family medicine ($n = 168$; 1 study from the United States), internal medicine ($n = 306$; 5 studies from across the United States, Candara, and Hungary), radiology ($n = 266$; 1 study from the United States), anesthesiology ($n = 1,417$; 1 study from the United States), neurology ($n = 116$; 1 study from Greece), and cardiology ($n = 105$; 1 study from Argentina).

The overall burnout prevalence in this analysis was found to be 35.1% (95% CI, 26.8–43.5%). Single-specialty studies were divided into three groups based on levels of overall burnout symptoms. A "high-prevalence group," with a burnout prevalence rate of 42.5%, included general surgery, anesthesiology, OBGYN, and orthopedics. The "moderate-prevalence" group with a burnout rate of 29.4% included internal medicine, plastic surgery, and pediatrics. The "low-prevalence" group, with a burnout rate of 23.5%, included otolaryngology and neurology. However, these differences were not found to be statistically significant by meta-regression, and several specialties were not included in this analysis.

When examining the subdimensions of burnout, emotional exhaustion, depersonalization, low sense of personal accomplishment, the prevalence of high depersonalization for all specialties in this study was 43.6% (95% CI, 38.4–48.9%). The highest levels of depersonalization were found in cardiology (a fellowship in the United States, but defined as a residency in one study of cardiology residents in Argentina), otolaryngology, and OBGYN programs. Those with the lowest depersonalization were plastic surgery, radiology, and family medicine. Prevalence of high emotional exhaustion was 38.9% (95% CI, 31.8–46.0%) across studies, with general surgery, otolaryngology, and radiation oncology having the highest prevalence of emotional exhaustion. The lowest emotional exhaustion was found in plastic surgery and family medicine. Prevalence of low personal accomplishment was 34.3% (95% CI, 21.3–47.2%). The lowest personal accomplishment scores (i.e., those with the lowest sense of personal accomplishment) were found within internal medicine, plastic surgery, and emergency medicine training programs. The highest personal accomplishment scores were found within radiation oncology and cardiology.

In summary, within this overall sample, surgical/urgency specialties (general surgery, anesthesiology, OBGYN, and orthopedics) were found to have the highest prevalence of burnout. General surgery was also associated with the highest relative risk of burnout in the US-based 2018 prospective cohort study.[41] Residencies in otolaryngology, plastic surgery, and neurology, found in this study to be associated with lower burnout, have also been previously shown to be at lower risk, although neurology residents had among the highest prevalences of burnout (61.6%) in the US-based prospective cohort study. The single study of neurology residents in this analysis was from Greece.

An even larger 2019 meta-analysis also examined prevalence rates of burnout among medical residents across countries, although this study provided less information about scales and cutoff scores used to diagnose burnout.[42] This study involved 22,778 residents across 47 studies from 2004 to 2018. Thirty-seven studies were from North and South America, three studies were from Europe, five from Asia, one from Africa, and one from Australia. The overall prevalence in this analysis was 51.0% (95% CI, 45.0–57.0%). Residents in radiology, neurology, and general surgery had the highest prevalence of burnout, a picture more consistent with studies of residents in the United States. More than 50% of residents experienced burnout in internal medicine, orthopedics, dermatology, OBGYN, and neurosurgery. The lowest burnout prevalence was found in psychiatry, oncology, and family medicine. However, none of these differences was found to be statistically significant.

In subgroup analyses examining differences by geographic region, burnout was higher in Asian (57.2%) and North American countries (51.6%), compared with European countries (27.7%), though these differences were also not statistically significant. Year of publication was not a significant moderator, suggesting a relatively constant prevalence of burnout over time.

In sum, this study revealed a global prevalence of resident burnout hovering around 50%—markedly higher than the smaller, more methodologically rigorous 2018 study[38]—and comparable prevalence rates between medical and surgical subspecialties. Interestingly, in this analysis, mean age and the proportion of males were significant moderators of burnout, revealing that older male residents suffered more than younger female residents. This finding is counter to the US-based cohort study and a majority of the burnout literature among physicians that shows females to be at higher relative risk for overall burnout. However, only a small portion of the studies included in this meta-analysis reported age and sex variables, and thus this finding could be subject to ecological fallacy.

Together, these studies reveal that burnout is not a single-specialty problem or one experienced only by residents in the United States. Rather, all residents and fellows are likely at risk for burnout in ways that vary by context, not just by specialty, but also by how these specialties are practiced in various training programs in different countries. These differences may explain why differences in burnout prevalence across specialties do not reach statistical significance; aggregating prevalence by specialty and country may neutralize some of the meaningful context-specific drivers of burnout, making it challenging to draw explicit conclusions about high-risk groups. Future efforts for greater consistency and rigor related to the measurement and cutoff criteria for burnout, as well as more robust systems for tracking burnout by specialty, would enhance our ability to draw conclusions about true burnout prevalence in residency training.

Conclusion

In this chapter we have summarized the existing literature on prevalence of burnout in the undergraduate medical education and GME context, with a focus on medical student and resident populations. Given the large amount of heterogeneity in studies on burnout, partially attributable to different metrics and cutoff scores used to "diagnose" burnout, there is a need for more consistent and rigorous methods to evaluate and compare burnout across studies and populations. Ultimately, understanding the burnout within a given population can be critical in helping institutions mobilize resources to support the well-being of groups at heightened risk. The literature to date demonstrates that burnout is a persistent and significant problem in medical training both in the United States and around the world. Later chapters will delve into consequences of burnout, and individual and system interventions to address it.

Summary Points

- Burnout likely begins in medical school—or earlier—and increases during residency. Medical students, residents, and clinical fellows in the United States experience burnout at significantly higher rates than age-matched college graduates in the general population.
- Although a lack of standardization in metrics and cutoff scores makes it very challenging to get accurate prevalence data and compare studies head-to-head, many studies report a prevalence of burnout among medical students, residents, and clinical fellows of approximately 50%.

- More standardized and rigorous methodology is needed across studies to enable meaningful comparisons of burnout prevalence by populations.

Putting It into Practice

- "Taking the pulse" of burnout in one's own institution or program will likely be a helpful first step to both demonstrate a need for change and also to have the baseline data needed to document change as it occurs.
- Leaders should be up-front with medical students and trainees about the general prevalence of burnout in medical training, using local data when available to contextualize trends. While burnout is very common, it is not inevitable, and building awareness can help with early detection and intervention to prevent downstream consequences.
- Leaders should normalize that burnout is a systems issue—not a sign of individual weakness or a personal failure. While burnout is distinct from depression, if signs of either are emerging, trainees should have access to resources available to them for evidence-based treatments.

References

1. Freudenberger HJ. Staff burn-out. *Journal of Social Issues*. 1974;30(1):159–165.
2. Saslow G. Psychiatric problems of medical students. *J Med Educ*. 1956;31(1):27–33.
3. Maslach C, Schaufeli WB, Leiter MP. Job burnout. *Annu Rev Psychol*. 2001;52:397–422.
4. Maslach C, Jackson SE. The measurement of experienced burnout. *Journal of Organizational Behavior*. 1981;2(2):99–113.
5. Shanafelt TD, Noseworthy JH. Executive leadership and physician well-being: nine organizational strategies to promote engagement and reduce burnout. *Mayo Clin Proc*. 2017;92(1):129–146.
6. Williams ES, Konrad TR, Linzer M, et al. Physician, practice, and patient characteristics related to primary care physician physical and mental health: results from the Physician Worklife Study. *Health Serv Res*. 2002;37(1):119–141.
7. Dyrbye LN, Power DV, Massie FS, et al. Factors associated with resilience to and recovery from burnout: a prospective, multi-institutional study of US medical students. *Med Educ*. 2010;44(10):1016–1026.
8. Dyrbye LN, Thomas MR, Massie FS, et al. Burnout and suicidal ideation among U.S. medical students. *Ann Intern Med*. 2008;149(5):334–341.
9. Dyrbye LN, Thomas MR, Power DV, et al. Burnout and serious thoughts of dropping out of medical school: a multi-institutional study. *Acad Med*. 2010;85(1):94–102.
10. Ishak WW, Lederer S, Mandili C, et al. Burnout during residency training: a literature review. *J Grad Med Educ*. 2009;1(2):236–242.
11. Erschens R, Keifenheim KE, Herrmann-Werner A, et al. Professional burnout among medical students: systematic literature review and meta-analysis. *Med Teach*. 2019;41(2):172–183.
12. Martini S, Arfken CL, Churchill A, Balon R. Burnout comparison among residents in different medical specialties. *Acad Psychiatry*. 2004;28(3):240–242.
13. Dyrbye LN, Thomas MR, Harper W, et al. The learning environment and medical student burnout: a multicentre study. *Med Educ*. 2009;43(3):274–282.
14. Dyrbye L, Shanafelt T. A narrative review on burnout experienced by medical students and residents. *Med Educ*. 2016;50(1):132–149.

15. Dyrbye LN, Massie FS, Eacker A, et al. Relationship between burnout and professional conduct and attitudes among US medical students. *JAMA*. 2010;304(11):1173–1180.
16. Shanafelt TD, Boone S, Tan L, et al. Burnout and satisfaction with work-life balance among US physicians relative to the general US population. *Arch Intern Med*. 2012;172(18):1377–1385.
17. Shanafelt TD, Hasan O, Dyrbye LN, et al. Changes in burnout and satisfaction with work-life balance in physicians and the general US working population between 2011 and 2014. *Mayo Clin Proc*. 2015;90(12):1600–1613.
18. de Oliveira GS, Jr., Chang R, Fitzgerald PC, et al. The prevalence of burnout and depression and their association with adherence to safety and practice standards: a survey of United States anesthesiology trainees. *Anesth Analg*. 2013;117(1):182–193.
19. Shanafelt TD, Bradley KA, Wipf JE, Back AL. Burnout and self-reported patient care in an internal medicine residency program. *Ann Intern Med*. 2002;136(5):358–367.
20. Fahrenkopf AM, Sectish TC, Barger LK, et al. Rates of medication errors among depressed and burnt out residents: prospective cohort study. *BMJ*. 2008;336(7642):488–491.
21. Dutheil F, Aubert C, Pereira B, et al. Suicide among physicians and health-care workers: a systematic review and meta-analysis. *PLoS One*. 2019;14(12):e0226361.
22. Schernhammer ES, Colditz GA. Suicide rates among physicians: a quantitative and gender assessment (meta-analysis). *Am J Psychiatry*. 2004;161(12):2295–2302.
23. Dyrbye LN, West CP, Satele D, et al. Burnout among U.S. medical students, residents, and early career physicians relative to the general U.S. population. *Acad Med*. 2014;89(3):443–451.
24. Collier VU, McCue JD, Markus A, Smith L. Stress in medical residency: status quo after a decade of reform? *Ann Intern Med*. 2002;136(5):384–390.
25. Puthran R, Zhang MW, Tam WW, Ho RC. Prevalence of depression amongst medical students: a meta-analysis. *Med Educ*. 2016;50(4):456–468.
26. Dyrbye LN, Thomas MR, Shanafelt TD. Systematic review of depression, anxiety, and other indicators of psychological distress among U.S. and Canadian medical students. *Acad Med*. 2006;81(4):354–373.
27. Dyrbye LN, Thomas MR, Huntington JL, et al. Personal life events and medical student burnout: a multicenter study. *Acad Med*. 2006;81(4):374–384.
28. Dyrbye LN, Thomas MR, Eacker A, et al. Race, ethnicity, and medical student well-being in the United States. *Arch Intern Med*. 2007;167(19):2103–2109.
29. Ishak W, Nikravesh R, Lederer S, Perry R, Ogunyemi D, Bernstein C. Burnout in medical students: a systematic review. *Clin Teach*. 2013;10(4):242–245.
30. Willcock SM, Daly MG, Tennant CC, Allard BJ. Burnout and psychiatric morbidity in new medical graduates. *Med J Australia*. 2004;181(7):357–360.
31. Fang DZ, Young CB, Golshan S, Moutier C, Zisook S. Burnout in premedical undergraduate students. *Acad Psychiatry*. 2012;36(1):11–16.
32. Brazeau CM, Shanafelt T, Durning SJ, et al. Distress among matriculating medical students relative to the general population. *Acad Med*. 2014;89(11):1520–1525.
33. Guang SA, Eltorai AEM, Durand WM, Daniels AH. Medical student burnout: impact of the gap year in burnout prevention. *Work*. 2020;66(3):611–616.
34. Chunming WM, Harrison R, MacIntyre R, Travaglia J, Balasooriya C. Burnout in medical students: a systematic review of experiences in Chinese medical schools. *BMC Med Educ*. 2017;17(1):217.
35. Boni R, Paiva CE, de Oliveira MA, Lucchetti G, Fregnani J, Paiva BSR. Burnout among medical students during the first years of undergraduate school: prevalence and associated factors. *PLoS One*. 2018;13(3):e0191746.
36. Frajerman A, Morvan Y, Krebs MO, Gorwood P, Chaumette B. Burnout in medical students before residency: a systematic review and meta-analysis. *Eur Psychiatry*. 2019;55:36–42.
37. Lockley SW, Cronin JW, Evans EE, et al. Effect of reducing interns' weekly work hours on sleep and attentional failures. *N Engl J Med*. 2004;351(18):1829–1837.
38. Rodrigues H, Cobucci R, Oliveira A, et al. Burnout syndrome among medical residents: a systematic review and meta-analysis. *PLoS One*. 2018;13(11):e0206840.

39. Prins JT, Gazendam-Donofrio SM, Tubben BJ, van der Heijden FM, van de Wiel HB, Hoekstra-Weebers JE. Burnout in medical residents: a review. *Med Educ*. 2007;41(8):788–800.
40. Dyrbye LN, Moutier C, Durning SJ, et al. The problems program directors inherit: medical student distress at the time of graduation. *Med Teach*. 2011;33(9):756–758.
41. Dyrbye LN, Burke SE, Hardeman RR, et al. Association of clinical specialty with symptoms of burnout and career choice regret among US resident physicians. *JAMA*. 2018;320(11):1114–1130.
42. Low ZX, Yeo KA, Sharma VK, et al. Prevalence of burnout in medical and surgical residents: a meta-analysis. *Int J Environ Res Public Health*. 2019;16(9):1479.

4

What's Causing the Problem?

Drivers of Well-Being

Susan M. Orrange, Michael S. Adragna, and Ashley Jeanlus

Introduction

The medical community first began to understand what drives well-being in students and GME trainees as we explored what drives burnout in these groups. Numerous drivers of burnout have been examined in students and GME trainees. Some are related to the individual, such as attention to self-care, social support, coping mechanisms, and personality traits. While such factors are important in student and GME trainee burnout, the current literature suggests that systemic factors may be more prominent drivers of burnout. These systemic factors include demands placed on individuals by institutions, such as work and clinical demands, and the institutional diversity climate. Systemic factors also include resources provided to individuals by institutions that can reduce burnout and improve well-being, such as curricular support, institutional support of self-care, a learning-oriented focus, scheduling control and flexibility, clear expectations, and a supportive team. With many of these potential drivers, the available research cannot determine directionality. Numerous studies are cross-sectional or qualitative and point to significant correlations, associations, and relationships. Since the literature on this topic is still emerging, these associations will be considered as potential drivers in this chapter.

Working to mitigate student and GME trainee burnout by considering all of these potential individual and system-level drivers will hopefully promote medical student and resident well-being. Understanding and exploring these drivers can guide our work as educators to create changes that positively impact the well-being of our future physicians and enable them to be at their best while caring for patients. In fact, some would argue that physician, GME trainee, and student well-being are critical to the success of our health care system and that the two are inextricably linked together.[1]

Drivers of Well-Being in Medical Students

As stated in the previous chapter, burnout is common in medical students.[2] While many authors have explored the role of "burnout," relatively less attention and research have been dedicated to examining the other end of the spectrum, which might be characterized as engagement, well-being, or satisfaction. Much remains to be understood about what drives well-being (i.e., "Why are some students well?"). We summarize the literature here, beginning with institutional-level factors, followed by individual behaviors that may promote well-being and decrease burnout.

Where Students Start

Prior to beginning medical school, matriculating medical students begin with similar or better mental health, measured by less burnout, less depression, and better quality of life across multiple dimensions compared with their age-matched peers.[3] Some students will be more likely to maintain relative well-being, while others are at greater risk for burnout.[4,5] One contributor to this difference may be variable childhood exposures. In one study, a survey measuring adverse childhood experiences (ACEs) administered to a third-year medical school class found that the student responses were similar to those from a group sampled from a US primary care setting.[4] The ACE Scale assesses a variety of exposures to childhood emotional, physical, and sexual abuse, as well as household dysfunction.[6] High scores are associated with increases in alcohol and drug use disorders, depression, and suicide attempts.[6] Medical students have a prevalence of history of ACEs similar to that of the population in general,[7] yet they remarkably begin medical school with a greater degree of well-being than peers similar in age and educational attainment. The fact that medical students have similar exposure to childhood trauma yet arrive at medical school with greater well-being suggests they may have *greater* resiliency, as demonstrated by having better well-being despite overcoming similar hurdles to their similarly aged peers.

Institutional Drivers of Well-Being in Medical Students

Medical students (and residents, as detailed later in this chapter) have been shown to develop a higher prevalence of burnout than age-matched college graduates in other fields despite arriving with better well-being than their peers.[8] Current work is focused on understanding the stressors, or demands, faced by students in the medical learning environment. Specific factors that make up a "stressful" climate for medical students can include a poor learning environment; inadequate support from faculty, medical school staff, and peers; the perception that education of medical students is not a priority for faculty and staff; disorganized clinical rotations; poor supervision; cynical residents; little variety of medical problems encountered; mistreatment; and type of grading schema.[9,10] Furthermore, recent work has demonstrated an association between a negative learning environment, including mistreatment specifically, and later development of exhaustion, disengagement, and career regret.[11] Later, we explore various ways that institutions can provide resources to medical students to support their well-being at the institutional level.

Support for Learning: Pass-Fail Grading and Other Curricular Changes

Medical schools are realizing the importance of creating an environment that supports student learning and academic success in order to promote student well-being. Most students come to medical school with superb academic records, yet half will rank in the bottom half of their class. One survey of burnout in 249 medical students found their most common stressor was grades, but did not explore an association between the emotional consequences of disappointing grades and burnout.[12]

To reduce stress and support learning, some medical schools have begun to grade students on a pass–fail basis. Changing grading systems to pass–fail has become perhaps the most straightforward system-level curricular intervention studied with regard to burnout. Beginning with the medical school class of 2006, Mayo Medical School shifted from a five-tier grading system to a pass–fail system for the preclinical years and found improved measures of stress and cohesion, respectively, on the Perceived Stress Scale and Perceived Cohesion Scale, without adverse impacts on USMLE scores.[13] A large comparison of first- and second-year students from seven institutions revealed that those graded in pass–fail curricula had lower stress, less emotional exhaustion, and less depersonalization than students graded with three or more tiers.[14]

Two schools studied pass–fail grading and curricular reform efforts on a longer-term scale. The University of Virginia changed to a pass–fail grading schema and found similarly promising results in preclinical students: improved well-being on the Dupuy General Well-Being Schedule, with no change in attendance, USMLE scores, clerkship performance, or residency placement. However, benefits to well-being were no longer evident 2 years later.[15] In addition to instituting a pass–fail grading system, Washington University School of Medicine undertook a full-scale curriculum modification with the express purpose of trying to achieve greater student well-being.[16] After gathering information on anxiety and stress in students, the medical school made multiple curricular changes: institution of a pass–fail grading system, a 10% reduction in preclinical course hours, the addition of elective courses, and, finally, establishing "learning communities" for students and faculty with similar interests. They bolstered these changes with education on resilience and mindfulness and made further modifications to the grading system and first-year courses. Ultimately, these changes were associated with significant reductions in reported depression, anxiety, and stress and an increase in community cohesion, as measured by the Perceived Cohesion Scale.[17] Furthermore, mean scores on the Step 1 exam increased, indicating that these efforts may have also provided support for learning as measured on a standardized test score. However, as with the University of Virginia efforts, later work at Washington University revealed that the gains were not maintained through the clinical years of medical school, suggesting that the clinical environment quickly exerts negative influences on medical student well-being.[18]

Schedule Control and Flexibility

In recognition of known drivers of burnout, providing students with some additional control and flexibility in their schedules is beginning to be recognized by medical schools as important to student well-being. Research has found preclinical students with burnout were most likely to feel that they lacked control over their schedule and to feel unprepared to become interns.[19] As described above, Washington University addressed this by adding elective courses and reducing preclinical course hours.[16] Western Sydney University in Australia also reduced required scholastic time. Faculty allowed students to take "well-being days" for self-care and were surveyed on their perceptions of the intervention. Students reported a positive experience: well-being days allowed for decreased contact hours and a greater amount of self-care and peer support, although they expressed concern that the program could also be misused by peers or staff, perhaps subjecting the students to unwanted surveillance.[20]

Support for Self-Care and Personal Development

While participation in self-care can be considered an individual-level driver of well-being, the extent to which a school or organization supports self-care can be thought of as an institutional-level driver. Many medical schools have begun to build self-care directly into their curricula to emphasize the importance of these practices for medical students.

At Northwestern University Feinberg School of Medicine (NUFSM) in 2008–2009, students took a required Healthy Living unit, which included an assignment to develop a Behavior Change Plan.[21] Students were asked to choose a health-related behavior which they wished to improve (e.g., the amount they slept or how much they exercised) and then develop a plan to modify that behavior in service of their goal. While only about 40% of students met their goal and the only category within which there was a statistically significant improvement was sleep, more than 80% of students felt that they became healthier as a result of the intervention.

Vanderbilt University School of Medicine (VMS) set out to employ a uniquely proactive approach, which they defined as "programming that staves off problems before they occur."[22] Their program included three core components. First, they created an "advisory college system" in which faculty volunteers were each paired with two students per class year. Then, all students and participating faculty members were divided into four advisory colleges, with student and faculty leadership structures and friendly competition between the colleges. Second, they created a Student Wellness Committee, with attention to multiple domains of well-being. The committee was tasked with developing programming specific to each domain (e.g., cooking classes to promote physical well-being). Third, and finally, they created "VMS LIVE," to support the personal development of medical students with a specific goal for each year of school (e.g., that third-year students learn conflict resolution). This portion of the initiative included emphases on faculty modeling of self-care, contemplation of one's life as a physician, and fostering dialogue about life-giving relationships. Although the program was not designed with an assessment to measure outcomes, the individual interventions were positively received and superior to previously standard advising with regard to student well-being.[23] Follow-up work during the program's fifth year, however, revealed that, contrary to the authors' hypothesis, recollection of participation in the Vanderbilt Wellness Program was not associated with decreased levels of burnout.[24] Nonetheless, participation in the program was high. Most students reported weekly or monthly contact with their mentors and engaged in wellness-related activities. Interestingly, the overall rate of burnout among Vanderbilt students was somewhat lower than that of students elsewhere, regardless of participation in the program, leading the authors to conclude that the institutional *value* placed on emotional well-being rather than direct *participation* in the Wellness Program may itself have been responsible for the lower rate of burnout among Vanderbilt students.[24]

Support from Peers and Faculty in the Learning Environment

Other studies have explored more complex causes and consequences of burnout in the clinical years. One such study surveyed clinical medical students at five institutions and found a multitude of facets of the learning environment to be associated with burnout, including levels of perceived supervision and support from superiors and administration, levels of support from peers, feeling that their education was a high priority, and having exposure to a wide variety of medical problems.[25]

Another study made use of the COVID-19 pandemic to assess how classroom attendance affects grades and well-being and what changes result when students can no longer attend class. Using mixed methods within an observational cohort design, authors hypothesized that classroom attendance rates would positively correlate with academic performance and well-being and that removing in-person learning would more adversely affect those who attend class regularly than those who do not. Eighty-two of 120 first-year students consented to participate; 44 completed the pre-COVID survey, and 39 completed the post-COVID survey. Ultimately, there was no association between attendance and grades, no change in well-being metrics before and after COVID, and a small association between attendance and protection from stress and loneliness. The authors took care to note that the study group was overall "'well' and resilient," which may limit generalizability of the findings.[26]

Support for Diversity and Inclusion

A 2007 survey of more than 3,000 medical students at five institutions sought to determine if race and ethnicity were associated with differences in burnout, depressive symptoms, and quality of life. The survey had a response rate of 55%, and the researchers found that minority students were more likely to report that their race negatively affected their medical school experience compared with non-minority students; however, there were no differences in rates of depressive symptoms. Perhaps surprisingly, non-minority students had higher overall risk for burnout compared with minority students.[27] The authors took care to note that there were no differences between different minority groups on dimensions of burnout and thus pooled the data for all minority groups. Another prospective survey of medical students at the same five institutions at two different points in time found no single demographic characteristics associated with resiliency; however, in multivariable analysis, being part of a non-White group was associated with higher odds of resilience to or recovery from burnout.[28] A more recent study also found lower burnout among minority racial and ethnic physicians than among non-Hispanic White physicians.[29] Because experiencing racism clearly has negative impacts on well-being, these findings indicate the need for further research in this area to better understand differences in burnout and how to measure and address important other aspects of well-being for students and trainees from underrepresented backgrounds.

To this point, an institution's general diversity climate may provide additional important information about the relationship between background/identity and well-being. The Medical Student Cognitive Habits and Growth Evaluation (CHANGE) Study surveyed students from a representative sample of 49 medical schools about witnessing or experiencing a variety of mistreatment around matters including race, ethnicity, gender, sexual orientation, poverty, obesity, and disability.[30] They found that a negative diversity climate was associated not only with depressive symptoms among minority groups, but also among all students. Additionally, they noted that 64% of students reported at least some exposure to a negative racial climate.

Individual Drivers of Well-Being in Medical Students

Self-Care

No matter how an individual student begins medical school, as a group, medical students appear to have a decline in self-care, measured by a student's satisfaction with life, physical activity, sleep, and alcohol use, that may well begin early in medical training.[9] An Indiana University survey reported that, over the first year of medical school, socialization and exercise decreased while alcohol use increased.[9] These changes were concurrent with a near doubling of reported depression in the student population. Furthermore, others have found that symptoms of burnout, greater student debt, being single, and being younger are associated with greater risk of alcohol abuse and dependence in medical students.[31]

Additional research has sought to explore which specific activities medical students pursue for self-care, taking care to note that many studies focus on predetermined modulators of well-being, such as sleep and socialization, rather than on student-identified behaviors. In one study, authors surveyed a national sample of medical students and found a diverse array of self-care activities that could generally be organized under the categories of nourishment, hygiene, intellectual and creative health, physical activity, spiritual care, balance and relaxation, time for loved ones, picturing goals, outside activities, and hobbies. While types of student self-care were identified as remarkably diverse, the authors highlighted that students most frequently relied on activities to foster social cohesion (e.g., going out to dinner and spending time with friends and family), while most institutionally recommended activities were relatively solitary in nature, such as exercise and engaging in mindfulness training (with the exception of shadowing practicing physicians).[32]

While some have explored the type of self-care in which students engage, others have attempted to measure the impact of the *amount* of self-care in which students engage.[33] One group sought to answer this question with a survey sent to all US allopathic medical schools in 2015–2016, using rating scales to assess stress, self-care, and quality of life, as well as demographics. The response rate was not reported because the number of students who received the survey could not be determined; however, it was presumed to be relatively low, with responses garnered from 871 students at 49 schools. Although there were more women and non-Hispanic White students in the sample, there were still some notable findings. Women engaged in more self-care than men but also reported greater stress than men. Non-Hispanic White students engaged in more self-care and also experienced less stress than other racial or ethnic groups. Similarly, students in the fourth year reported more self-care than most other years and less stress than all other years. Across all groups, there was an inverse relationship between perceived stress and students' quality of life, but engaging in self-care seemed to attenuate the strength of this relationship.

Debt

Student debt correlates positively with anxiety and negatively with psychological comfort.[34] A multi-institutional study of students at seven American medical schools found that those with greater than $100,000 debt were 1.47 times as likely to experience suicidal ideation as those with less than $50,000 debt.[35] Another study at the University of Toronto found that both current debt and anticipated total debt correlated with self-reported financial stress.[36]

Personal Events and Characteristics

Negative personal events, such as divorce and death of a loved one, contribute strongly to burnout despite burnout typically being a measure of professional distress.[37] Specifically, experiencing a major illness and the overall number of negative personal life events within the past year were associated with greater risk of burnout. Some later work, however, found that while a positive personal event protected students from burnout, negative life events were not associated with an increased risk of burnout.[25]

Another important factor that may serve to drive well-being is help-seeking behavior among medical students. Researchers at Yale University surveyed all undergraduate medical students about their help-seeking behavior around medical illness, psychological distress, grades, and other stressors and also administered a modified Maslach Burnout Inventory. The response rate was 35%. Researchers found that students who had previously sought academic help and had supportive relationships with faculty members were more likely to seek mental health care when needed and that students who reported burnout were less likely to seek help when needed.[38]

Drivers of Well-Being in GME Trainees

In graduate medical education (GME), professional demands and obligations often encroach into personal time for family and interests outside medicine. "Residency" is so-named because GME trainees used to live and work inside the hospital. It is perhaps not therefore surprising that our GME trainees and our training system still struggle with what a modern version of GME trainee well-being might look like. Here, we explore potential drivers of well-being and burnout in residents at the institutional and individual levels, recognizing that these levels can sometimes overlap. While the institutional drivers of well-being for medical students come primarily from the medical educational institutions in which they learn, residents' well-being is broadly impacted by the many interwoven entities in which they learn and work: residency programs, academic departments, educational institutions, clinic sites, and hospital systems.

Institutional Drivers of Well-Being in Residents

Residency is a time of immersion in a chosen field, which contrasts with the broader exposure to different topics and fields in medical school. Residency training programs prepare physicians for independent practice through a combination of work and learning. Programs are organized into rotations and clinical experiences that are designed to teach specialty-specific knowledge and skills that prepare residents for independent practice. This training environment, which includes educational pedagogy, experiential learning through interactions with the medical system and patients, and the development of relationships with peers and faculty, can serve as a primary driver of well-being in residents and fellows.

Determining cause-and-effect relationships for well-being in our GME trainees has been a challenge. Many factors within the working and learning environment, rather than individual characteristics, are now seen as the major drivers of burnout in residents.[10,39–41] Both positive and negative elements within the medical system are associated with burnout in residents and fellows. These factors can be categorized according to the demands placed on individuals that drive burnout or the resources within the system that might help to mitigate or prevent burnout. Although studies of physician drivers have made distinctions between unit-level, institutional-level, and national drivers,[42] studies involving residents acknowledge these complex factors, but have generally not determined the relative contribution of each factor separately.

Program- and System-Level Demands That Drive GME Trainee Well-Being

The demands that residents and fellows experience are influenced by their training program, the institutional environment, and the health care system as a whole. Yet, because of their unique role in the physician training hierarchy, residents likely do not experience these demands in the same way as medical students or practicing physicians. Residents and fellows are in a unique position of having two official statuses: employees held accountable for serious work productivity and patient care, and learners responsible for substantial knowledge acquisition. Residents have already had success as learners by nature of having completed medical school, and they must now figure out how to maintain their learning identity while simultaneously succeeding as productive and knowledgeable physicians. The addition of this new responsibility can create vulnerability in a hierarchical environment with heavy work demands.

Workload

The workload of residents is large, and the results of studies of the relationship between workload, burnout, and well-being are mixed. Workload and emotional demands of work both had significant positive associations with emotional exhaustion, yet in one study only emotional demands were significantly correlated with depersonalization.[43] Insufficient time in the day to complete the assigned workload and perceptions of having excessive paperwork were significantly associated with two of three burnout subscales.[44] Extra hours spent in electronic health records outside of work correlated with emotional exhaustion in a study of psychiatry residents.[45] A qualitative study examining well-being trajectories of first-year residents in the context of challenges, supports, and adaptations over time found that well-being decreased with the presence of heavy work demands.[46] In contrast, two longitudinal studies conducted between 2003 and 2008 found no relationship between self-reported workload or call frequency and burnout in residents.[47-49] Although the evidence for a direct association with burnout in residents remains mixed, given the generally heavy workload for most residents, differences attributable purely to workload may also be more difficult to discern among residents than among practicing physicians.

Hours Worked

A specific work demand of residents and fellows that has received much attention is the vast number of hours they regularly work. National work-hour limitations were implemented by the Accreditation Council for Graduate Medical Education (ACGME) in 2003, then revised in 2011 and 2017. The regulations limited total work to 80 hours in a week, specified details of mandatory time free of clinical work and education, and regulated the maximum time for individual shifts. The intention of these work-hour limits was to increase time for resident rest in order to provide safer patient care, but many studies have looked at the relationship between work hours and burnout. Studies exploring the impact of these work-hour limits on burnout and well-being have also found mixed results.

Initial correlations between work hours and emotional exhaustion were found after the implementation of the 2003 work-hour limitations.[50,51] In early 2004, a study of internal medicine residents found that fewer residents met criteria for emotional exhaustion in 2004 than in 2001, and that the average emotional exhaustion subscale scores were also lower in 2004. No significant differences in the depersonalization or personal accomplishment subscales were found.[50] In a study of otolaryngology residents, hours that residents worked in 2005 were predictive of emotional exhaustion even after adjusting for potential confounders.[51]

While these studies showed associations between the onset of work-hour restrictions in 2003 and decreasing burnout, subsequent results have not consistently demonstrated this trend. Several longitudinal studies found no relationship found between self-reported work hours and burnout in residents.[47-49] Similarly, in a large national study of more than 16,000 internal medicine residents in the United States, the prevalence of burnout in 2008 was similar to rates prior to the 2003 ACGME work-hour reforms.[52]

Another national study, the Individualized Comparative Effectiveness of Models Optimizing Patient Safety and Resident Education (iCOMPARE) trial, measured educational experience, in-training exam scores, resident and program director satisfaction, overall resident well-being, and resident burnout.[53] This study randomly divided 63 internal medicine residency programs and compared those governed by standard ACGME 2011 duty-hour policies and those assigned to have more flexible policies without shift length limits or mandatory time off between shifts. Both groups were limited to the same average total number of hours worked per week (80 hours), which was still obviously quite a large number of hours. While first-year residents in programs without mandates on shift length or time off between shifts were more likely to report dissatisfaction with educational quality and overall well-being, there was no difference between groups in rates of burnout, which was high for both groups.

Changes in markers of resident well-being over time were measured between 2001 and 2012. This study found that resident perceptions of the 2011 work-hour limitations were generally negative, even though residents had lower rates of burnout and depression in 2012 than in 2001 and 2004.[54] In 2012, 61% of these internal medicine residents were burned out, compared with 76% in 2001. However, only 23% of the residents at the end of the study thought that the 2011 duty-hour policy had positively impacted their well-being. Senior residents actually perceived that the changed work-hour limits had negative impacts on their well-being, education, and patient care.[54] While it is difficult to determine the exact nature of the relationship between work hours and well-being, it may be that other factors in the health system simultaneously changed other aspects of work that are important to well-being, such as the nature and meaning of work, or that the loss of autonomy and control resulting from work-hour changes had a negative impact on work experience. As further described below, these studies also suggest that resulting work compression negatively contributes to well-being.

Work Compression

A 2012 study found that increased work compression seemed to be contributing greatly to decreases in resident well-being after the implementation of the ACGME work hour limits.[55] Even with work-hour restrictions, resident hours spent working are often still quite extensive. It may be that without a change in the amount of work needed to be done, the limitation on hours worked actually compressed work tasks into a shorter period of time thereby increasing work intensity within the shorter period. Taken in combination with the findings about workload and work hours, it is likely that efforts to address work compression are needed in conjunction with any efforts to reduce hours, in addition to efforts to enhance time spent in meaningful work.

Demands of Providing Clinical Care and Making Errors

Several factors related to the stresses and responsibilities of patient care also contribute to resident well-being. Some of these new challenges include making medical errors, seeing patients receive suboptimal care, having interactions with difficult and complicated patients, and having to make medical decisions in the face of uncertainty. Encountering these scenarios may increase the likelihood of burnout. A longitudinal study of internal medicine residents examined self-reported medical errors and found that self-perceived errors were an independent predictor of subsequent worsening in all domains of burnout.[56] Similarly, residents who self-reported instances of providing what they considered suboptimal patient care were more inclined to be burned out.[57] Self-reported interactions with patients perceived as difficult or complicated were also associated with a higher risk of burnout in residents in a study of 150 residents at two hospitals in 13 specialties.[44]

While the above studies looked at self-reports, other studies examined documented errors and those observed by others in the clinical environment. In a clinical surveillance study with nurse and physician observers, errors by more than 500 pediatric residents on an inpatient rotation were measured and categorized as either harmful or nonharmful. Results found no statistically significant association between burnout and harmful, nonharmful, or total number of errors.[58] Another study of documented medication errors found no correlation between burnout and the number of medication errors seen in collected chart review data.[59] In contrast, another study found a small decrease in medication prescription errors in residents with burnout compared to those without.[60] Although the significance of this one study is unclear, this finding does raise questions about the nature of relationships among medical errors, stress, and burnout and warrants further research. Additionally, the *perception* of one's experience with an error may be as important as the error itself.

One research team explored the stress residents experience when faced with the uncertainty of making some medical decisions and looked at the relationships among stress, uncertainty, burnout, and resilience. Residents who had burnout had higher levels of stress due to uncertainty and lower levels of resilience than their non-burned out peers.[61] This finding suggests that education aimed at increasing residents' tolerance of uncertainty may help improve resiliency and reduce burnout.

Program- and System-Level Resources That Drive Resident Well-Being

Learning Environment and Autonomy-Supervision Balance

When GME trainees perceive that they have adequate support from their program and institution to succeed, they have less burnout, better resilience, better job satisfaction, and less work–life strain.[62] They also perceive a better workplace climate and are more likely to have high performance on their in-service examinations. Specific support resources that have correlated with improved well-being and perceived clinical learning environment include educational stipends, provision of review questions for standardized testing, in-service board preparation, and support for poor performers.[62] A Dutch study that assessed the learning climate by measuring feedback, coaching, assessment, supervision, patient handovers, and professional relationships found that a better learning climate (as measured by these components) was associated with lower emotional exhaustion and depersonalization.[63] A Canadian qualitative study of first-year residents also found that their well-being changed with different rotations. Residents reported greater well-being when they had exposure to more valued learning opportunities compared with fewer and when they felt more competent.[46] Specifically, residents described lower valued learning opportunities as "scut" work on rotations with short staffing and less overall learning on service-heavy rotations.

In contrast, well-being may be hindered when GME trainees feel pressure to project an image of expertise.[64] In a qualitative study of surgical residents, participants described how they can feel pressure to portray an impression of being "all-knowing," "quick," "decisive," and "confident," even when feeling the opposite. They reported that creating this impression of competence was taxing and required a lot of "mental energy." Although residents felt that projecting confidence positively influenced evaluations and learning opportunities, this effort also had unintended negative consequences on learning, well-being, and patient care. One example was that trainees trying to display confidence in their ability to perform a procedure were reluctant to ask questions, admit knowledge gaps, or ask for help when needed.

The ultimate goal of resident learning is independent practice, which is achieved through increased autonomy as training progresses. A study of emergency medicine residents distinguished between two types of autonomy: administrative and clinical.[65] Residents with low levels of both administrative and clinical autonomy were significantly more likely to be burned out. An Argentinean study examined correlations between burnout and the residency educational environment as represented by the three concepts: role autonomy, teaching, and social support. Autonomy and personal accomplishment had a strong positive correlation, while a significant negative correlation was found between autonomy and both exhaustion and depersonalization.[66] Dutch medical residents whose survey responses indicated that they experienced little or no work-related autonomy were more likely to be burned out, with thematic analysis finding that new residents were the most challenged by a lack of control over patient scheduling and a desire to take extra time with patients.[67]

Scheduling Control and Flexibility

In a study of GME trainees from 13 specialties in two hospitals examining a collection of stressors and protective factors identified by GME trainees, a lack of control over office processes and schedules correlated with burnout.[44] Two self-reported factors were associated with the absence of burnout and were therefore perhaps protective: feeling like one "has a say" in the training program and feeling like one has some control over one's schedule. Additional studies have identified that rigid schedules interfered with work–home integration and increased the challenges of completing personal tasks.[68] This encroachment in turn left trainees feeling that their personal needs were inconsequential, a perception that was more common in burned out residents compared with those without burnout.[57] In one qualitative study of GME trainees from seven specialties, schedule flexibility was more important to overall well-being than work-hour limitations.[69]

Expectation Alignment and Well-Being Mindset

Residents generally enter their training program with a set of expectations about how they will develop into independent physicians and how they will maintain their own well-being. First-year residents have reported feeling underprepared for residency, especially in the areas of behavioral adaptability, mindset, emotional health, and financial health.[70] Programs and institutions can help address these areas in formal orientations and continued efforts throughout training.

When program orientations are strong and prepare residents for what lies ahead, they help to align expectations with the reality of training and increase resident well-being. Residents report increased well-being when they considered program and rotation orientations to be strong. Qualities of rotation orientations that were considered strong included not only expectations related to the development of knowledge competency, but also an introduction to the setting and patients, clarification of role expectations, and electronic medical record training.[46]

Resident perspectives on maintaining a well-being mindset during training are quite varied and may not be ideal. Some residents may take a cynical view, stating that the pursuit of personal well-being often seems futile in residency.[71] Others believe they must temporarily compromise their well-being, describing residency as "a time for temporary imbalance" and that during residency they have chosen to invest in professional development instead of other domains.[69]

Residency programs have an opportunity to thoughtfully promote an alternative perspective about an achievable plan for maintaining well-being in residency. These efforts can begin at orientation and should continue throughout training to address the many transitions that occur during a training program. While a temporary shift toward a focus on professional development and away from relationships and physical and mental health may seem to benefit careers in the short term, this focus has the danger of sliding into self-sacrifice, which can be detrimental.[69] Indeed, residents who reported it was critical to have a "survival attitude" to manage stress were significantly more likely to be burned out.[57] The residency community should work with residents to build shared expectations of well-being in residency that are achievable and can be supported by program resources.

Supportive Team and Professional Relationships

Supportive professional relationships are important in shaping resident well-being and when missing, contribute to burnout in residents.[72] Well-being in residency has been described as having a highly fluctuating pattern that coincides with levels of supervisor and colleague support as well as changes in rotations.[46] In a 2006 multi-specialty study of residents at a single institution, having strong and supportive relationships was the only factor significantly associated with levels of emotional exhaustion, depersonalization, and personal accomplishment in a study of perceived well-being factors associated with burnout.[44] First-year family medicine and surgical residents in Canada who felt higher levels of support from their team reported increased overall well-being, and well-being decreased when they felt lower team support.[46] Another study found that support from colleagues was more important to males in protecting against burnout, and support from family or partners was more important to females.[43]

Peer support is very important for resident well-being, and a lack of support is associated with resident burnout. Poor collaboration between peers was the strongest factor found to be associated with high emotional exhaustion and depersonalization in a study of the residency learning climate.[63] A qualitative study of residents from multiple specialties found that residents associated conflict with colleagues with lower states of well-being.[69] Programs can support strong peer relationships by encouraging collaboration and productive methods of conflict resolution.

Support for Diversity and Inclusion

When team members are mistreated, individuals' well-being is negatively impacted. Residents who experienced mistreatment, including discriminating, abusive, or harassing behavior, were more likely than those who did not report mistreatment to have symptoms of burnout.[73,74] Experiencing negative interpersonal interactions or unfair treatment predicted subsequent burnout 1 year later among both men and women in a study of more than 3,500 residents from a multitude of specialties.[11] However, women were found to experience more negative interactions and were more likely to be burned out in their third year of residency than their male colleagues. A study of more than 7,000 surgical residents from across the United States looked at many forms of mistreatment, including gender and racial discrimination, sexual harassment, and abuses that were verbal, emotional, or physical. Although the largest source of reported mistreatment came from patients and families, mistreatment by faculty accounted for nearly 20% of the reports among surgical residents and more than 40% of the reports from pediatric residents, with women residents again experiencing more frequent mistreatment overall.[74] Pediatric residents experiencing mistreatment also reported higher stress levels and a lower quality of life. Exposure to unprofessional conduct by faculty, senior residents, and nurses is associated with higher burnout and cynicism scores among internal medicine residents.[75] Unprofessional conduct included observing medical record falsification, feeling humiliated by a member of the team, observing criticism of services and specialties, and observing others being disrespected. These studies highlight the importance of systems to combat harassment, discrimination, and mistreatment in the learning environment.

Support from Faculty and Mentorship

The educational and emotional support or lack of support residents feel from faculty influences well-being and burnout. Residents who rated their teachers more favorably and experienced explicit teaching from supervisors had lower emotional exhaustion scores,[76] and dissatisfaction with clinical faculty in general was associated with increased likelihood to meet burnout criteria.[77] More specifically, dissatisfaction with emotional support from supervisors was a strong predictor of both emotional exhaustion and depersonalization.[78] Finally, residents who viewed relationships with supervisors as mutually supportive had lower emotional exhaustion and depersonalization scores. In these mutually beneficial relationships, residents described receiving teaching and support for professional development, and supervisors reported feeling supported through work completed by residents.[79]

When faculty–trainee relationships are viewed by residents as unsupportive of their learning and professional development, burnout may be more likely. Stress in resident–faculty relationships in neurosurgery residents was found to be associated with emotional exhaustion.[80] Faculty making high demands and residents having lack of independence correlated with higher emotional exhaustion in pediatric residents in three different hospitals.[51] Likewise, working with faculty members who were considered to be hostile was a predictor of burnout in a national study of surgical residents.[81]

Mentoring programs are one specific way that faculty can provide support to trainees. These programs can vary in content and structure but may include educational, personal, and career guidance and support. In a national survey, residents who indicated that a structured surgical mentoring program was available to them had lower burnout scores,[82] while residents who were not satisfied with mentoring relationships were more likely to be burned out.[83]

Individual Drivers of Well-Being and Burnout in GME Trainees

Individual characteristics and experiences influence how workload and level of support are perceived and may also have significant impact on well-being.[84] It is important to understand and address individual drivers concurrently as programmatic and institutional changes are considered. Early research found associations between burnout and personal health, both mental and physical. While most of this research is cross-sectional and cannot point to causation, these individual differences may account for the differential impact of programmatic changes on some residents and not others. In addition, as discussed in future chapters, attention to the individual drivers of trainee well-being, including mental health, is an important in any comprehensive well-being program.

Self-Care

Self-care habits such as exercise, sleep, healthy eating, and meditation have been frequently studied in the context of well-being and burnout. These habits and resulting health effects are often measured in studies of well-being. So, while it is important to examine what drives self-care in residents and fellows, data show mixed results. Select personal well-being promotion strategies have correlated with higher resident mental well-being, including stressing personal–professional balance, taking a positive outlook, and appreciating personal religious/spiritual practices.[85]

Resident well-being habits also often change during residency. In studies looking at personal patterns before and after starting residency, several studies found significant changes in personal practices. In a 2014 study, 40% of residents reported not achieving physical activity guidelines, and 79% of residents reported that their level of physical activity has decreased since they began medical training.[86] Residents who wished they could exercise more frequently (96.8%) were twice as likely to be emotionally exhausted.[87] Burned out residents were significantly more likely to rate physical exercise as essential or significant to managing stress levels.[57] These studies on changes in exercise frequency and mismatch between current and desired frequency of exercise may help to make sense of earlier studies that looked only at presence and absence of regular exercise in residents, which have shown mixed results. Some studies found an association between frequency of exercise and lower burnout,[86,88–90] while others found no significant relationship between burnout subscales and frequency of exercise.[48,91]

The impact of residency training itself on self-care habits (rather than personal motivation or desire) is supported by studies that examined changes in health behaviors after starting residency. In a small study looking at health behaviors prior to residency and in residency, first-year resident respondents reported that their overall health was worse than the prior year. Residents reported getting an average of 1 hour less sleep per night and exercising on average 1 day fewer per week. The percentage of people who reported not eating breakfast increased by 22% during residency, and residents ate out at lunch at more than double the rate they did prior to residency.[92] A larger study with residents from several specialties, including obstetrics and gynecology, family practice, internal medicine, pediatrics, and surgery, found similar results. Surveys conducted before and after the start of residency found that residents reported a significant reduction in eating low-fat meals, sleep hours, hours spent exercising, and time spent with family.[93] Residents in this study also reported a significant increase in the number of important events they missed since beginning residency training. Although overall well-being and burnout were not measured in these studies, the quality of GME trainees' physical and social health—significant components of well-being—decreased after beginning residency, as measured by self-care related well-being metrics.

These studies suggest that, given the resources and support to make healthy self-care choices, residents would do so but often cannot in their present environments. This reinforces the idea that well-being in residency is a shared responsibility. Self-care deficiencies in residents may not be due to a knowledge deficit but rather to structural barriers such as time and access.

Social Support

It is beneficial to residents' well-being when their relationships with those outside of the working and learning environment are supportive and understanding. In a study of GME trainees from 13 specialties at a single institution, social support was the only demographic variable found to be associated with all three burnout subscales: emotional exhaustion, depersonalization, and personal accomplishment.[44] When residents reported increased perceived social support, emotional exhaustion decreased, depersonalization decreased, and personal accomplishment increased. Residents with higher loneliness scores were more likely to have high emotional exhaustion and depersonalization, although personal accomplishment was not impacted.[94]

Studies have consistently reported an association between work–home conflict and higher burnout among residents.[43,67,80] A Dutch study found that the likelihood of burnout increased when work interfered with home life. Yet social support from family, partners, or colleagues seemed protective against burnout, and this protection was found to be stronger in females. In males, social support from colleagues and participation in decision-making at work was protective.[43] In a study that examined work–life factors in pediatric residents, two factors were found to be associated with burnout: frequent perceived conflicts between personal and professional life, and dissatisfaction with life as a resident.[95] Low satisfaction in an intimate partner relationship was not associated with burnout.

Qualitative studies have explored the pressures of dual-role responsibilities felt by residents and how they contribute to work–life imbalance.[96,97] One study included 13 focus groups and 35 interviews with 96 GME trainees and revealed two themes about what contributes to work–life imbalance.[97] First, GME trainees felt they had to prioritize work over home life, and, when frequent transitions at work and home disrupted personal relationships, resulting stress impacted learning and deprived GME trainees of support to cope with work difficulties. A second study found themes related to gender differences and traditional gender roles in surgical residents. When participants discussed the dual-role responsibilities of being a parent/partner and a surgeon, there was a greater perceived impact on well-being for women GME trainees. Women GME trainees felt the need to more frequently meet demands and pressures outside the hospital, while GME male trainees felt social pressure to work tirelessly for their families and to prioritize job responsibilities over family obligations.[96]

Residents' relationships may also be influenced by evolving professional identity. As professional identities develop and strengthen, residents saw residency as all-consuming (time, emotion, motivation, energy), leaving them less time for family and friends. They reported that being a doctor superseded their personal relationships, and, as such, they created a relationship hierarchy and modified their existing relationships. While family and friends could support residents forgoing personal responsibilities from home, residents expected others in their lives to compromise their expectations. The residents used coping mechanisms (e.g., adjusting social plans and work schedules, compromise, use of technology) to manage the conflict and protect their relationships. Despite using coping strategies, residents articulated a strong identity dissonance—a clash between their professional and personal identities. To resolve, some gravitated toward relationships with others who shared their professional identity or sought social comparison as affirmation.[98]

Coping with Stress and Anxiety

As described above, some of the differing stressors for residents as compared to medical students include work compression, excessive workload and work hours, frequent overnight calls, limited autonomy, lack of timely feedback, stressful relationships with supervisors, and perceptions that their personal needs are not important to their training program. In one study, residents who were burned out were more likely to report common resident stressors, such as insufficient sleep, shifts in excess of 24 hours, and not enough leisure time, as major personal stressors.[57]

Life stressors outside medicine may also be related to resident burnout but likely to a lesser degree. In one study, while recent family stress was associated with increased likelihood of burnout,[77] the impact of other life stressors seemed less conclusive. Although some studies found a relationship between education debt, financial stress, and burnout,[52,80] others have found that education debt was not predictive of burnout.[48,99]

The way residents perceive and cope with stress influences their well-being and burnout. Having good coping skills is one of several self-reported protective factors associated with the absence of burnout.[44] Higher overall stress and a lack of stress coping in residents was found to be associated with burnout.[100] More specifically, residents who utilized strategies of acceptance, active coping, positive reframing, and humility/personal application have been found to have lower scores in the burnout domains of emotional exhaustion and depersonalization. In contrast, coping strategies of denial or disengagement were associated with higher emotional exhaustion and depersonalization scores.[101] Another study found that dispositional (inherent tendency towards) mindfulness in residents was associated with lower risk of burnout.[102] Finally, higher levels of anxiety in the fourth year of medical school were associated with higher instances of burnout as a second-year resident in a large longitudinal study.[103]

Empathy and Emotional Intelligence

Several studies have found associations between empathy, emotional intelligence, and well-being. Emotional intelligence was found to be strongly predictive of general psychological well-being and was negatively correlated with both the emotional exhaustion and depersonalization domains of burnout in a study of surgical residents from a single institution.[104] In another study, higher empathy during the fourth year of medical school was associated with lower reported symptoms of burnout during residency.[103] *Cognitive empathy* refers to an individual's ability to understand another person's perspective regarding their experience, where the emotive subscale measures individual's tendency to respond emotionally to the feelings experienced by others. A 2005 study of internal medicine residents examined cognitive and emotive empathy and found that only cognitive empathy was statistically significantly related to well-being.[85] A qualitative study of French general practice residents further explored the complex relationship between burnout and empathy in GME trainees, finding that while empathy is helpful for both provider satisfaction and good patient relationships, empathy also must be carefully controlled in order to avoid exhaustion or burnout.[105] This work could be expanded to further understand this complex relationship and focus teaching approaches for empathy and emotional intelligence in order to achieve well-being and mitigate burnout.

Personality Styles

Personality styles may influence how residents experience burnout. Correlations between personality and burnout among residents point to some interesting potential drivers of well-being in this population. Two longitudinal studies found relationships between personality measures in an initial survey and burnout at a later time. One study found that residents self-identifying as calm were significantly less likely to have burnout. This study, which examined burnout in residents entering and finishing their first year, also found that having a disorganized personality style at the start of the intern year was associated with an increased likelihood of developing burnout during the year.[48] Interesting correlations between Myers-Briggs and Maslach Burnout Inventory subscales found that Perceiving residents were less emotionally exhausted; Feeling residents were less depersonalized; and

Extroverted, intuitive residents had greater sense of personal accomplishment.[91] Another study looking at the Big Five personality traits found that neuroticism in residency was predictive of emotional exhaustion during residency and 5 years later into clinical practice. Lower levels of agreeableness were related to high levels of depersonalization. Extroverted residents reported lower levels of emotional exhaustion later in practice.[84]

Conclusion

Existing models for understanding well-being, as described in Chapter 1, are helpful in making sense of the voluminous literature about the drivers of medical student and resident well-being and burnout. Many of the findings described in this chapter fall into Maslach's six areas of worklife that may intensify or alleviate burnout: workload, control, rewards, community, fairness, and values.[106] These areas are similar to seven dimensions that Shanafelt and Noseworthy found contribute to burnout and engagement in physicians: workload, efficiency, flexibility/control over work, work–life integration, alignment of individual and organizational values, social support/community at work, and the degree of meaning derived from work.[42] While these models do not specifically include residents or students, taken in combination with the literature reviewed in this chapter, they can help institutions identify overall drivers for burnout and well-being in medical students and residents in order to begin to understand potential interventions.

Table 4.1 outlines these two models and highlights similarities with system-level drivers found in literature about well-being and burnout in medical students and

TABLE 4.1 System drivers of well-being and burnout: A comparison

Leiter and Maslach's six areas of worklife	Shanafelt and Noseworthy's drivers of burnout and engagement	Institutional drivers of well-being and burnout in medical students	Institutional drivers of well-being and burnout in residents
Workload	Workload Resources and efficiency	Support for learning	Workload, hours worked, work compression Demands of clinical care and making errors
Control	Flexibility/control over work Work-life integration	Scheduling control and flexibility	Scheduling control and flexibility
Rewards	Meaning	Personal development and meaning	Focus on learning and meaning
Community	Social support/community at work	Support from peers and faculty	Supportive team Supportive faculty
Fairness		Support for diversity	Support for diversity
Values	Alignment of individual and organizational values	Learning environment	Learning environment Expectation alignment

Leiter MP, Maslach C. Six areas of worklife: A model of the organizational context of burnout. *J Health Hum Serv Adm.* 1999;21(4):472–489; Shanafelt TD, Noseworthy JH. Executive leadership and physician well-being: Nine organizational strategies to promote engagement and reduce burnout. *Mayo Clin Proc.* 2017;92(1):129–146.

residents, aligning these models with material presented in this chapter. It is interesting to note commonalities, differences, and gaps, particularly in the areas of workload, rewards, fairness, and values.

All populations seem to require attention to workload but in slightly different ways. The physician model adds the related concept of efficiency, which is also seen in the resident literature around work hours, time demands, and work compression. Medical student "work" is essentially to learn, so having support for learning to take place is the organizational support needed for their well-being. Residents also have the role of learner, but it is in addition to the role of worker. They require support from organizations to be able to focus on their learning and not solely on completing clinical work. Resident workload also includes adjusting to the many new demands of providing clinical care that they are experiencing for the first time.

The differences in the areas of rewards, fairness, and values are interesting. More research in these areas for residents and medical students could help the medical community understand drivers of well-being and burnout more completely. Of particular note is support for diversity and inclusion. It is encouraging that literature related to well-being and burnout in this area is emerging. Increased investigations should continue, and institutions should consider how their support for diversity impacts the areas of rewards, fairness, and values. Approaches to decreasing burnout and increasing well-being for both medical students and residents need to address these drivers that are present within the medical culture and educational system. Additional drivers such as rewards, fairness, and values should also be explored, particularly in the context of supporting diversity. The aims of such efforts should seek to promote more than the absence of burnout and include an environment in which all GME trainees flourish, achieve high well-being, and acquire the skills necessary to promote resilience. Achieving these aims will help foster the competency, dedication, and professionalism of future doctors, both during the training process and over the course of their careers.

Summary Points

- Medical student stress is influenced by the learning environment; lacking support from faculty, residents, staff, and peers; rotation organization; mistreatment; and grading schema.
- Preclinical pass–fail grading and other curricular reforms such as reductions in course hours, learning communities, and well-being days appear to protect well-being without compromising educational benefits such as USMLE and Step 1 performance, although benefits may not be durable through the clinical years.
- Students' perception that the curriculum prioritizes student well-being and that faculty and school officials care about their well-being may confer protection from burnout.

- Negative racial climates are disappointingly common and are associated not only with depressive symptoms among minority groups, but also among all students. Improving diversity climates will likely benefit all students.
- Despite these interventions, burnout continues to increase among medical students, and further, high-quality research is needed to test the wide-scale applicability and durability of these and other interventions.
- Medical students begin their undergraduate medical education with higher levels of well-being relative to their non-medical peers.
- Medical students who are most likely to maintain their well-being are more likely to socialize, exercise, moderate their alcohol use, sleep adequately, and have relatively less debt. Some students maintain well-being despite academic, social, and financial stressors.
- An inverse relationship is seen between perceived stress and students' quality of life, but engaging in self-care seems to mitigate the strength of this relationship.
- Medical students with a previous willingness to seek help for academic problems and good relationships with faculty members are more likely to seek help when needed and in turn preserve their well-being.
- Demands such as insufficient time to complete work, excessive paperwork, time spent working in electronic health records outside the workday, and the emotional demands of resident work all contribute to burnout in GME trainees.
- While workload and the number of hours worked initially seemed to be drivers of burnout and well-being, it now appears that efforts to reduce work compression may be the important intervention.
- The demands of providing clinical care include the stress of seeing patients receiving suboptimal care, having interactions with difficult and complicated patients, and the stress of making medical decisions in the face of uncertainty. When GME trainees experience these demands, they are more likely to experience burnout. The relationship between medical errors and burnout is less clear and warrants further research.
- GME trainees who perceive that they have adequate support from their program and institution have had less burnout, better resilience, better job satisfaction, and less work–life strain. Support measures that are valued include educational stipends, review questions and board preparation, remediation support, the presence of valued learning opportunities, and opportunities to demonstrate competence and have autonomy.
- Experiences that fail to include a focus on learning negatively impact resident well-being. Examples of these experiences include "scut" work on rotations with short staffing, less learning on service-heavy rotations, and pressure to falsely project an image of expertise.

- Flexibility and control over schedules correlates with increased well-being and decreased burnout in residents. Control related to office processes and feeling like one has a "say" in their training program may also be protective against burnout.

- Strong program orientations can positively impact resident well-being by helping to align resident expectations with the realities of training. Content areas to consider are clarification of knowledge and role expectations, introduction to the clinical setting and patient population, electronic medical record training, well-being mindset, and emotional and financial health.

- Creating an environment free from mistreatment, discrimination, abuse, harassment, negative interpersonal experiences, unfair treatment, and unprofessional conduct is important; residents who experience mistreatment are more likely to have burnout symptoms.

- Strong and supportive relationships with team members is related to overall well-being in residents and decreased burnout. Peer support is important for resident well-being, and a lack of support is associated with resident burnout. Programs can enhance strong and supportive peer relationships by encouraging collaboration and productive methods of conflict resolution.

- Faculty support of GME trainees can result in decreased likelihood of burnout. Practices that have been found to be helpful include providing emotional support, engaging in mutually supportive relationships, encouraging professional development, promoting independence, and providing educational, personal, and career mentoring.

- Certain personal well-being promotion strategies correlated with higher resident mental well-being, including stressing personal–professional balance, taking a positive outlook, and appreciating personal religious/spiritual practices.

- Self-care deficiencies in GME trainees are not likely due to a knowledge deficit but rather to structural barriers such as time and access. Studies suggest that since GME trainees well-being habits often change for the worse during residency, well-being in GME trainees requires both individual commitment and institutional resources.

- Work–home conflict is associated with higher burnout in residents. GME trainee well-being changes as an increasing sense develops of having to prioritize work over home life and seeing residency as all-consuming, which occurs as resident professional identities develop and strengthen. However, social support from family, partners, or colleagues seemed protective against burnout.

- Having good coping skills, a higher tolerance of uncertainty, and using certain stress management strategies seem to help protect residents against burnout.

- Emotional intelligence and empathy are positively related to well-being and negatively related to burnout. However, the relationship between empathy and burnout may be more complex and must be carefully controlled to avoid emotional exhaustion.

- Personality styles may influence how GME trainee experience burnout and well-being.

> **Putting It into Practice**
>
> • Use Table 4.1 to develop a map of the institutional well-being drivers of burnout in residents or medical students at your institution.
> • Reflect on whether drivers of burnout are experienced differently for different groups in your institution.
> • Consider aspects of driver dimensions for which you do not have sufficient information and ways to gather data to learn more about the extent to which each driver is a factor at your institution.

References

1. Sklar DP. Fostering student, resident, and faculty wellness to produce healthy doctors and a healthy population. *Acad Med.* 2016;1(9):1185–1188.
2. Wasson LT, Cusmano A, Meli L, et al. Association between learning environment interventions and medical student well-being: a systematic review. *JAMA.* 2016;316(21):2237–2252.
3. Brazeau CM, Shanafelt T, Durning SJ, et al. Distress among matriculating medical students relative to the general population. *Acad Med.* 2014;89(11):1520–1525.
4. Sciolla AF, Wilkes MS, Griffin EJ. Adverse childhood experiences in medical students: implications for wellness. *Acad Psychiatry.* 2019;43(4):369–374.
5. Thompson D, Goebert D, Takeshita J. A program for reducing depressive symptoms and suicidal ideation in medical students. *Acad Med.* 2010;85(10):1635–1639.
6. Felitti VJ, Anda RF, Nordenberg D, et al. Relationship of childhood abuse and household dysfunction to many of the leading causes of death in adults: the Adverse Childhood Experiences (ACE) study. *Am J Prev Med.* 1998;14(4):245–258.
7. Campbell JA, Walker RJ, Egede LE. Associations between adverse childhood experiences, high-risk behaviors, and morbidity in adulthood. *Am J Prev Med.* 2016;50(3):344–352.
8. Dyrbye LN, West CP, Satele D, et al. Burnout among U.S. medical students, residents, and early career physicians relative to the general U.S. population. *Acad Med.* 2014;89(3):443–451.
9. Ball S, Bax A. Self-care in medical education: effectiveness of health-habits interventions for first-year medical students. *Acad Med.* 2002;77(9):911–917.
10. Dyrbye L, Shanafelt T. A narrative review on burnout experienced by medical students and residents. *Med Educ.* 2016;1(1):132–149.
11. Dyrbye LN, West CP, Herrin J, et al. A longitudinal study exploring learning environment culture and subsequent risk of burnout among resident physicians overall and by gender. *Mayo Clin Proc.* 2021; 96(8): 2168–2183.
12. Santen SA, Holt DB, Kemp JD, Hemphill RR. Burnout in medical students: examining the prevalence and associated factors. *South Med J.* 2010;103(8):758–763.
13. Rohe DE, Barrier PA, Clark MM, Cook DA, Vickers KS, Decker PA. The benefits of pass-fail grading on stress, mood, and group cohesion in medical students. *Mayo Clin Proc.* 2006;81(11):1443–1448.
14. Reed DA, Shanafelt TD, Satele DW, et al. Relationship of pass/fail grading and curriculum structure with well-being among preclinical medical students: a multi-institutional study. *Acad Med.* 2011;86(11):1367–1373.
15. Bloodgood RA, Short JG, Jackson JM, Martindale JR. A change to pass/fail grading in the first two years at one medical school results in improved psychological well-being. *Acad Med.* 2009;84(5):655–662.
16. Slavin SJ, Schindler DL, Chibnall JT. Medical student mental health 3.0: improving student wellness through curricular changes. *Acad Med.* 2014;89(4):573–577.

17. Chin WW, Salisbury WD, Pearson AW, Stollak MJ. Perceived cohesion in small groups: adapting and testing the Perceived Cohesion Scale in a small-group setting. *Small Group Res.* 1999;30(6):751–766.

18. Slavin S. Reflections on a decade leading a medical student well-being initiative. *Acad Med.* 2019;94(6):771–774.

19. Mazurkiewicz R, Korenstein D, Fallar R, Ripp J. The prevalence and correlations of medical student burnout in the pre-clinical years: a cross-sectional study. *Psychol Health Med.* 2012;17(2):188–195.

20. Byrnes C, Ganapathy VA, Lam M, Mogensen L, Hu W. Medical student perceptions of curricular influences on their wellbeing: a qualitative study. *BMC Med Educ.* 2020;20(1):288.

21. Kushner RF, Kessler S, WC. M. Using behavior change plans to improve medical student self-care. *Acad Med.* 2011;86(7):901–906.

22. Drolet BC, Rodgers S. A comprehensive medical student wellness program—design and implementation at Vanderbilt School of Medicine. *Acad Med.* 2010;85(1):103–110.

23. Sastre EA, Burke EE, Silverstein E, et al. Improvements in medical school wellness and career counseling: a comparison of one-on-one advising to an Advisory College Program. *Med Teach.* 2010;32(10):e429–e435.

24. Real FJ, Zackoff MW, Davidson MA, Yakes EA. Medical student distress and the impact of a school-sponsored wellness initiative. *Med Sci Educ.* 2015;25(4):397–406.

25. Dyrbye LN, Thomas MR, Harper W, et al. The learning environment and medical student burnout: a multicentre study. *Med Educ.* 2009;43(3):274–282.

26. Salzman J, Williamson M, Epsina-Rey A, Kibble J, Kauffman C. Effects of voluntary attendance patterns on first-year medical students' wellness and academic performance during COVID-19. *Adv Physiol Educ.* 2021;45(3):634–643.

27. Dyrbye L, Thomas M, Eacker A, et al. Race, ethnicity, and medical student well-being in the United States. *Arch Intern Med.* 2007;167:2103–2109.

28. Dyrbye LN, Power DV, Massie FS, et al. Factors associated with resilience to and recovery from burnout: a prospective, multi-institutional study of US medical students. *Med Educ.* 2010;44(10):1016–1026.

29. Garcia LC, Shanafelt TD, West CP, et al. Burnout, depression, career satisfaction, and work-life integration by physician race/ethnicity. *JAMA Netw Open.* 2020;3(8):e2012762.

30. Hardeman RR, Przedworski JM, Burke S, et al. Association between perceived medical school diversity climate and change in depressive symptoms among medical students: a report from the Medical Student CHANGE Study. *J Natl Med Assoc.* 2016;108(4):225–235.

31. Jackson ER, Shanafelt TD, Hasan O, Satele DV, Dyrbye LN. Burnout and alcohol abuse/dependence among U.S. medical students. *Acad Med.* 2016;91(9):1251–1256.

32. Ayala EE, Omorodion AM, Nmecha D, Winseman JS, Mason HRC. What do medical students do for self-care? A student-centered approach to well-being. *Teach Learn Med.* 2017;29(3):237–246.

33. Ayala EE, Winseman JS, Johnsen RD, Mason HRC. U.S. medical students who engage in self-care report less stress and higher quality of life. *BMC Med Educ.* 2018;18(1):189.

34. Marci CD, Roberts TG. The increasing debt of medical students: how much is too much? *JAMA.* 1998;280(21):1879–1880.

35. Dyrbye LN, Thomas MR, Massie FS, et al. Burnout and suicidal ideation among U.S. medical students. *Annals of Internal Medicine.* 2008;149:334–341.

36. Morra DJ, Regehr G, Ginsburg S. Anticipated debt and financial stress in medical students. *Med Teach.* 2008;30(3):313–315.

37. Dyrbye LN, Thomas MR, Huntington JL, et al. Personal life events and medical student burnout: a multicenter study. *Acad Med.* 2006;81(4):374–384.

38. Gold JA, Johnson B, Leydon G, Rohrbaugh RM, Wilkins KM. Mental health self-care in medical students: a comprehensive look at help-seeking. *Acad Psychiatry.* 2015;39(1):37–46.

39. National Academies of Sciences, Engineering, and Medicine. *Taking Action Against Clinician Burnout: A Systems Approach to Professional Well-Being.* The National Academies Press; 2019. Accessed August 29, 2021. https://www.nap.edu/catalog/25521/taking-action-against-clinician-burnout-a-systems-appro ach-to-professional.

40. Prins JT, Gazendam-Donofrio SM, Tubben BJ, van der Heijden FM, van de Wiel HB, Hoekstra-Weebers JE. Burnout in medical residents: a review. *Med Educ.* 2007;41(8):788–800.

41. Ripp JA, Privitera MR, West CP, et al. Well-being in graduate medical education: a call for action. *Acad Med.* 2017;1(7):914–917.

42. Shanafelt TD, Noseworthy JH. Executive leadership and physician well-being: nine organizational strategies to promote engagement and reduce burnout. *Mayo Clin Proc.* 2017;92(1):129–146.

43. Verweij H, van der Heijden F, van Hooff MLM, et al. The contribution of work characteristics, home characteristics and gender to burnout in medical residents. *Adv Health Sci Educ Theory Pract.* 2017;22(4):803–818.

44. Eckleberry-Hunt J, Lick D, Boura J, et al. An exploratory study of resident burnout and wellness. *Acad Med.* 2009;1(2):269–277.

45. Domaney NM, Torous J, Greenberg WE. Exploring the association between electronic health record use and burnout among psychiatry residents and faculty: a pilot survey study. *Acad Psychiatry.* 2018;42(5):648–652.

46. Hurst C, Kahan D, Ruetalo M, Edwards S. A year in transition: a qualitative study examining the trajectory of first year residents' well-being. *BMC Med Educ.* 2013;1:96.

47. Campbell J, Prochazka AV, Yamashita T, Gopal R. Predictors of persistent burnout in internal medicine residents: a prospective cohort study. *Acad Med.* 2010;85(10):1630–1634.

48. Ripp J, Babyatsky M, Fallar R, et al. The incidence and predictors of job burnout in first-year internal medicine residents: a five-institution study. *Acad Med.* 2011;86(10):1304–1310.

49. Ripp JA, Bellini L, Fallar R, Bazari H, Katz JT, Korenstein D. The impact of duty hours restrictions on job burnout in internal medicine residents: a three-institution comparison study. *Acad Med.* 2015;90(4):494–499.

50. Goitein L, Shanafelt TD, Wipf JE, Slatore CG, Back AL. The effects of work-hour limitations on resident well-being, patient care, and education in an internal medicine residency program. *Arch Intern Med.* 2005;165(22):2601–2606.

51. Golub JS, Weiss PS, Ramesh AK, Ossoff RH, Johns MM, 3rd. Burnout in residents of otolaryngology-head and neck surgery: a national inquiry into the health of residency training. *Acad Med.* 2007;82(6):596–601.

52. West CP, Shanafelt TD, Kolars JC. Quality of life, burnout, educational debt, and medical knowledge among internal medicine residents. *JAMA.* 2011;306(9):952–960.

53. Desai SV, Asch DA, Bellini LM, et al. Education outcomes in a duty-hour flexibility trial in internal medicine. *N Engl J Med.* 2018;378(16):1494–1508.

54. Krug MF, Golob AL, Wander PL, Wipf JE. Changes in resident well-being at one institution across a decade of progressive work hours limitations. *Acad Med.* 2017;92(10):1480–1484.

55. Auger KA, Landrigan CP, del Rey JAG, Sieplinga KR, Sucharew HJ, Simmons JM. Better rested, but more stressed? Evidence of the effects of resident work hour restrictions. *Acad Pediatr.* 2012;12(4):335–343.

56. West CP, Huschka MM, Novotny PJ, et al. Association of perceived medical errors with resident distress and empathy: a prospective longitudinal study. *JAMA.* 2006;296(9):1071–1078.

57. Shanafelt TD, Bradley KA, Wipf JE, Back AL. Burnout and self-reported patient care in an internal medicine residency program. *Annals of Internal Medicine.* 2002;136(5):358–367.

58. Brunsberg KA, Landrigan CP, Garcia BM, et al. Association of pediatric resident physician depression and burnout with harmful medical errors on inpatient services. Article. *Acad Med.* 2019;94(8):1150–1156.

59. Fahrenkopf AM, Sectish TC, Barger LK, et al. Rates of medication errors among depressed and burnt-out residents: prospective cohort study. *BMJ.* 2008;336(7642):488–491.

60. Kwah J, Weintraub J, Fallar R, Ripp J. The effect of burnout on medical errors and professionalism in first-year internal medicine residents. *J Grad Med Educ.* 2016;8(4):597–600.

61. Simpkin AL, Khan A, West DC, et al. Stress from uncertainty and resilience among depressed and burned-out residents: a cross-sectional study. *Acad Pediatr.* 2018;18(6):698–704.

62. Lee N, Appelbaum N, Amendola M, Dodson K, Kaplan B. Improving resident well-being and clinical learning environment through academic initiatives. *J Surg Res.* 2017;215:6–11.

63. Vendeloo SN, Brand P, Verheyen C. Burnout and quality of life among orthopaedic trainees in a modern educational programme. *The Bone & Joint Journal.* 2014;96-B(8):1133–1138.

64. Patel P, Martimianakis MA, Zilbert NR, et al. Fake it 'til you make it: pressures to measure up in surgical training. *Acad Med*. 2018;1(5):769–774.

65. Kimo Takayesu J, Ramoska EA, Clark TR, et al. Factors associated with burnout during emergency medicine residency. *Acad Emerg Med*. 2014;21(9):1031–5.

66. Llera J, Durante E. Correlation between the educational environment and burn-out syndrome in residency programs at a university hospital. *Archivos Argentinos de Pediatria*. 2014;112(1):6–11.

67. Ringrose R, Houterman S, Koops W, Oei G. Burnout in medical residents: a questionnaire and interview study. *Psychol Health Med*. 2009;14(4):476–486.

68. Geurts S, Rutte C, Peeters M. Antecedents and consequences of work-home interference among medical residents. *Soc Sci Med*. 1999;48(9):1135–1148.

69. Ratanawongsa N, Wright SM, Carrese JA. Well-being in residency: a time for temporary imbalance? *Med Educ*. 2007;41(3):273–280.

70. Diller D, Osterman J, Tabatabai R. Qualitative analysis of well-being preparedness at an emergency medicine residency program. *West J Emerg Med*. 2019;1(1):122–126.

71. Edmondson EK, Kumar AA, Smith SM. Creating a culture of wellness in residency. *Acad Med*. 2018;1(7):966–968.

72. IsHak WW, Lederer S, Mandili C, et al. Burnout during residency training: a literature review. *J Grad Med Educ*. 2009;1(2):236–242.

73. Hu YY, Ellis RJ, Hewitt DB, et al. Discrimination, abuse, harassment, and burnout in surgical residency training. *N Engl J Med*. 2019;381(18):1741–1752.

74. Kemper KJ, Schwartz A. Bullying, discrimination, sexual harassment, and physical violence: common and associated with burnout in pediatric residents. *Acad Pediatr*. 2020;20(7):991–997.

75. Billings ME, Lazarus ME, Wenrich M, Curtis JR, Engelberg RA. The effect of the hidden curriculum on resident burnout and cynicism. *J Grad Med Educ*. 2011;3(4):503–510.

76. Mougalian S, Lessen D, Levine R, et al. Palliative care training and associations with burnout in oncology fellows. *J Support Oncol*. 2013;11(2):95–102.

77. Martini S, Arfken CL, Churchill A, Balon R. Burnout comparison among residents in different medical specialties. *Acad Psychiatry*. 2004;28(3):240–242.

78. Prins JT, Hoekstra-Weebers JE, van de Wiel HB, et al. Burnout among Dutch medical residents. *Int J Behav Med*. 2007;14(3):119–125.

79. Prins J, Gazendam-Donofrio S, Dillingh G, Wiel H, Heijden F, Hoekstra-Weebers J. The relationship between reciprocity and burnout in Dutch medical residents. *Med Educ*. 2008;42:721–728.

80. Sargent MC, Sotile W, Sotile MO, Rubash H, Barrack RL. Stress and coping among orthopaedic surgery residents and faculty. *J Bone Joint Surg Am*. 2004;86-A(7):1579–1586.

81. Attenello FJ, Buchanan IA, Wen T, et al. Factors associated with burnout among US neurosurgery residents: a nationwide survey. *J Neurosurg*. 2018;1(5):1349–1363.

82. Elmore LC, Jeffe DB, Jin L, Awad MM, Turnbull IR. National survey of burnout among US general surgery residents. *J Am Coll Surg*. 2016;223(3):440–451.

83. Oladeji LO, Ponce BA, Worley JR, Keeney JA. Mentorship in orthopedics: a national survey of orthopedic surgery residents. *J Surg Educ*. 2018;75(6):1606–1614.

84. McManus IC, Keeling A, Paice E. Stress, burnout and doctors' attitudes to work are determined by personality and learning style: A twelve-year longitudinal study of UK medical graduates. *BMC Med*. 2004;2:29.

85. Shanafelt TD, West C, Zhao X, et al. Relationship between increased personal well-being and enhanced empathy among internal medicine residents. *J Gen Intern Med*. 2005;1(7):559–564.

86. Olson SM, Odo NU, Duran AM, Pereira AG, Mandel JH. Burnout and physical activity in Minnesota internal medicine resident physicians. *J Grad Med Educ*. 2014;6(4):669–674.

87. Becker JL, Milad MP, Klock SC. Burnout, depression, and career satisfaction: cross-sectional study of obstetrics and gynecology residents. *Am J Obstet Gynecol*. 2006;195(5):1444–1449.

88. Lebensohn P, Dodds S, Benn R, et al. Resident wellness behaviors: relationship to stress, depression, and burnout. *Fam Med*. 2013;45(8):541–549.

89. Sargent MC, Sotile W, Sotile MO, Rubash H, Barrack RL. Quality of life during orthopaedic training and academic practice: part 1: orthopaedic surgery residents and faculty. *J Bone Joint Surg.* 2009;91(10):2395–2405.

90. Weight CJ, Sellon JL, Lessard-Anderson CR, Shanafelt TD, Olsen KD, Laskowski ER. Physical activity, quality of life, and burnout among physician trainees: the effect of a team-based, incentivized exercise program. *Mayo Clin Proc.* 2013;88(12):1435–1442.

91. Lemkau JP, Purdy RR, Rafferty JP, Rudisill JR. Correlates of burnout among family practice residents. *J Med Educ.* 1988;63(9):682–691.

92. Wee CE, Petrosky J, Mientkiewicz L, Liu X, Patel KK, Rothberg MB. Changes in health and well-being during residents' training. *South Med J.* 2020;1(2):70–73.

93. Perry MY, Osborne WE. Health and wellness in residents who matriculate into physician training programs. *Am J Obstet Gynecol.* 2003;1(3):679–683.

94. Shapiro J, Zhang B, Warm EJ. Residency as a social network: burnout, loneliness, and social network centrality. *J Grad Med Educ.* 2015;7(4):617–623.

95. Sagalowsky ST, Feraco AM, Baer TE, Litman HJ, Williams DN, Vinci RJ. Intimate partner relationships, work-life factors, and their associations with burnout among partnered pediatric residents. *Acad Pediatr.* 2019;1(3):263–268.

96. Dahlke AR, Johnson JK, Greenberg CC, et al. Gender differences in utilization of duty-hour regulations, aspects of burnout, and psychological well-being among general surgery residents in the United States. *Ann Surg.* 2018;268(2):204–211.

97. Rich A, Viney R, Needleman S, Griffin A, Woolf K. 'You can't be a person and a doctor': the work-life balance of doctors in training-a qualitative study. *BMJ Open.* 2016;6(12):e013897.

98. Law M, Lam M, Wu D, Veinot P, Mylopoulos M. Changes in personal relationships during residency and their effects on resident wellness: a qualitative study. *Acad Med.* 2017;1(11):1601–1606.

99. Dyrbye LN, West CP. Enhancing resident well-being: illuminating the path forward. *J Gen Intern Med.* 2018;33(4):400–402.

100. Hillhouse JJ, Adler CM, Walters DN. A simple model of stress, burnout and symptomatology in medical residents: a longitudinal study. *Psychol Health Med.* 2000;5(1):63–73.

101. Doolittle BR, Windish DM, Seelig CB. Burnout, coping, and spirituality among internal medicine resident physicians. *J Grad Med Educ.* 2013;5(2):257–261.

102. Lebares CC, Guvva EV, Ascher NL, O'Sullivan PS, Harris HW, Epel ES. Burnout and stress among US surgery residents: psychological distress and resilience. *J Am Coll Surg.* 2018;226(1):80–90.

103. Dyrbye LN, Burke SE, Hardeman RR, et al. Association of clinical specialty with symptoms of burnout and career choice regret among US resident physicians. *JAMA.* 2018;320(11):1114–1130.

104. Lin DT, Liebert CA, Tran J, Lau JN, Salles A. Emotional intelligence as a predictor of resident well-being. *J Am Coll Surg.* 2016;1(2):352–358. doi:10.1016/j.jamcollsurg.2016.04.044

105. Picard J, Catu-Pinault A, Boujut E, Botella M, Jaury P, Zenasni F. Burnout, empathy and their relationships: a qualitative study with residents in general medicine. *Psychol Health Med.* 2016;21(3):354–361. doi:10.1080/13548506.2015.1054407

106. Leiter MP, Maslach C. Six areas of worklife: a model of the organizational context of burnout. *J Health Hum Serv Adm.* Spring 1999;21(4):472–489.

5

What's at Stake?

Consequences of Burnout

Ingrid Philibert and Lyuba Konopasek

Overview: What's at Stake

Physician burnout affects medical students, graduate medical education (GME) trainees, individual physicians in practice, their patients, their teams and colleagues, their institutions, and the health care system and society. Physicians experiencing burnout are less engaged with their patients and other professional responsibilities. In the professional role of the physician, the impact of burnout can manifest in a variety of ways, including decreased empathy, increased cynicism, and reduced work effort. Consequences include increased sick days (absenteeism), lower professional effectiveness in the workplace (presenteeism), reduced participation in team-based models of care, lower quality of care, and higher rates of errors.[1] Burnout also is associated with an increased likelihood of job turnover and plans to leave the profession as a whole or enter into nonclinical work.[1] Physicians experiencing burnout are less likely to be effective teachers and role models for medical students, GME trainees, and other health professions students,[2] leading to an overall negative impact on the clinical learning environment. The financial cost of physician burnout in the United States due to turnover, attrition from clinical work, and reduced productivity has been estimated to be up to $4.6 billion annually.[3] This chapter aggregates information on the consequences of burnout in physicians across the continuum of education and practice; includes estimates of the impact of burnout on patients, institutions, and the US health care system; and highlights areas in need of further study. Each section begins with data on consequences for physicians in practice, the group for which the most information is available, followed by data for medical students and resident physicians. The negative impact of burnout in those supervising educators themselves on the medical student and GME trainee learning environment is also considered. One limitation in much of the data is that most studies on burnout are cross-sectional, and therefore directionality can often not be determined: in some cases burnout may result from some of these factors, rather than causing these consequences, or the relationship may be bidirectional. The chapter therefore concludes with a discussion of new areas for study, such as the consequences of burnout in women and minority physicians, the impact of COVID-19 on physician burnout, and the need to collect data on the impact of interventions to reduce burnout, its consequences, and associated costs.

What Is Known: Research on the Consequences of Burnout in Physicians

The past two decades have seen an enhanced focus on physician well-being, including attention to the impact of job burnout and its consequences. This emphasis has emerged in the context of an added understanding of the stresses faced by physicians, including clinical demands and productivity pressures, documentation expectations that lessen physician face-to-face contact with patients, and challenges to professional and personal life integration. Burnout among US physicians is reported to be higher than in any other occupational sector,[1] with studies showing that up to 50% or more of physicians-in-training,[4] and a slightly lower percentage of physicians in practice experience burnout. Between 2011 and 2017, there was an observed decline in the prevalence of burnout among practicing physicians[5]; no comparable data are available for medical learners.

The consequences of burnout have been studied over the past 50 years and include low morale, reduced work engagement, negative consequences for personal relationships, job turnover, physical exhaustion, depression, and suicide.[6–9] One limitation of the research, noted in the National Academy of Medicine's 2019 report "Taking Action Against Clinician Burnout,"[1] is the challenge of quantifying the magnitude of these consequences of burnout and their associated costs. To date, formal estimates of the financial consequences of burnout focus exclusively on the cost due to reduced clinical work or turnover and exit from the profession. Some have argued that, in addition to moral and ethical arguments for organizations to address physician burnout, the economic consequences alone provide a sufficient rationale for organizations to invest in interventions to reduce physician burnout. This business case is strengthened by the relationship between burnout and lower quality and safety of care and patient satisfaction, which pose additional threats to success and sustainability of organizations when physician burnout is not addressed.[10] The business case for investing in physician well-being is further discussed in Chapter 12.

An article in the occupational literature[11] posits the existence of a "burnout cascade," and a systematic review of 43 articles used this model to assign the consequences of burnout to three categories: reduced activity, distress, and despair.[12] This phenomenon suggests that burnout is a complex, dynamic phenomenon.[11] The cascade can begin with an individual who faces excessive job demands and in turn devotes additional time, effort, and creativity to meet potentially unrealistic and unattainable goals,[11] putting the most dedicated individuals potentially at higher risk.[13] If the effort to meet the demands is unsustainable, the burnout cascade may follow.[11,12] The burnout cascade manifests in stages.[11]

1. *Exhaustion*: Loss of energy, chronic fatigue, fewer extra-role behaviors, and negative effects on interpersonal interactions
2. *Reduced activity*: Resignation, avoidance, less communication, less initiative, less interest in connecting with patients
3. *Distress*: Negativity, cynicism, aggression
4. *Breakdown*: Persistent distress/depression/anxiety, reduced motivation and engagement/participation in practice, medical errors and unprofessional behaviors, turnover intentions
5. *Psychosomatic reactions*: Sleep disturbance, gastrointestinal and cardiovascular disorders, susceptibility to infection, sexual disorders, intake of drugs and alcohol
6. *Degradation*: Severe emotional distress, loss of social contacts, absenteeism, tardiness, loss of productivity, turnover, leaving clinical medicine or the profession
7. *Despair*: Persistent health problems and professional problems, suicidal ideation/suicide

Many of the consequences of burnout in this list are described in the literature and their level of impact ranges from the individual to society at large as shown in Table 5.1.

Consequences of Burnout for Physicians' Mental and Physical Health

Burnout in physicians has been shown to have negative effects on mental and physical health, as well as on physician self-care practices and occupational safety.

General Mental and Physical Health

Few studies to date focus on the impact of burnout on physicians' physical health. However, studies of burnout in the general population show associations with health consequences, including hypercholesterolemia, type 2 diabetes, coronary heart disease, cardiovascular disorders, musculoskeletal pain, fatigue, headaches, gastrointestinal issues, respiratory problems, injuries, and early mortality.[14] In the domain of mental health, a number of studies suggest that burnout is associated with depression in physicians, although the relationship is complex: while some individuals with burnout screen positive for depression symptoms, many do not. Furthermore, not all individuals with depression

TABLE 5.1 Manifestations and consequences of burnout in physicians in training and in practice

Individual physician	Patient	Health care team	Institution	Society
1. CONSEQUENCES OF BURNOUT ON INDIVIDUAL PHYSICIANS' MENTAL AND PHYSICAL HEALTH				
Depression and other mental health problems Self-medication, including alcohol and substance use Physical health conditions Suicidal ideation/suicide	Negative impact on therapeutic relationship with patients	Impact on health care teams Ineffectual role modeling (trainees, junior colleagues, other team members)	Cost of lost professional contribution Cost of providing care to the physician in distress	Cost of lost professional contribution
2. IMPACT OF BURNOUT ON PROFESSIONAL BEHAVIORS, EMPATHY, AND COMMUNICATION				
Declining empathy Reduced patient communication skills Loss of professional agency and caring Cynicism Microaggressions and perceptions of microaggressions in others	Lower patient satisfaction, reduced patient engagement Lower likelihood of providing value-conscious care	Less prosocial behavior Impact on peers and junior learners Ineffective role modelling	Costs associated with low patient satisfaction and engagement and reduced patient activation Costs associated with higher use of health care resources	Lower patient engagement and activation Lower health care quality Higher health care costs
3. IMPACT OF BURNOUT ON PROFESSIONAL EFFICACY AND CONSEQUENCES FOR QUALITY AND SAFETY OF CARE				
Absenteeism, presenteeism Reduced work engagement Lower professional efficacy Lower cognitive and learning efficacy	Lower patient satisfaction, reduced patient activation Reduced quality and safety of care	Reduced team efficacy Reduced quality and safety of care Ineffective role modeling	Cost of reduced productivity Costs associated with quality and safety problems	Reduced access to care Lower health care quality Lower patient safety Higher health care costs
4. CONSEQUENCES FOR CAREER SATISFACTION, TURNOVER, AND ATTRITION FROM THE PROFESSION				
Reduced clinical work effort/hours, including decisions to select part-time clinical work Turnover Attrition from clinical medicine or from the profession	Reduced access and continuity of care	Loss of individual expertise Reduced team continuity Reduced interest in a career in clinical medicine Thoughts of dropping out of medical school or discontinuing residency	Cost of turnover and professional attrition	Lost professional contribution Reduced access to care

symptoms meet criteria for burnout.[15] A survey from 2019 found 15% of physicians reporting burnout also indicated suffering from self-reported or clinically diagnosed depression.[16] One challenge in measuring the mental health consequences of burnout is the overlap in symptoms between burnout and depressive disorder, particularly exhaustion, which may result in depression being misclassified as burnout and left untreated.[17] For example, in a large study of physicians, burnout was associated with suicidal ideation but that association dropped away after adjusting for depression. Therefore, it is important to consider burnout and depression as related, although distinct outcomes, particularly when considering approaches to mitigate and treat.

Alcohol and Substance Use

Physicians experiencing burnout also reported using potentially maladaptive coping strategies such as alcohol and drug use. Approximately 10–12% of physicians in general develop at least one substance abuse disorder during their lifetime, a rate similar to that of the general US population.[18] Data from a survey of more than 7,200 US physicians suggest that 12.9% of male physicians and 21.4% of female physicians meet criteria for alcohol abuse or dependence.[19] The same study found alcohol abuse or dependence was associated with burnout ($p < .0001$), depression ($p < .0001$), suicidal ideation ($p = .0004$), lower quality of life ($p < .0001$), lower career satisfaction ($p = .0036$), and recent medical errors ($p = .0011$).[19] One study of the association of burnout and alcohol use in more than 7,000 US surgeons found that individuals meeting criteria for burnout were more likely to have alcohol abuse or dependence than individuals who did not report burnout, with emotional exhaustion and depersonalization Maslach Burnout Inventory (MBI) subdomains strongly associated with alcohol abuse or dependence.[20]

Suicidal Ideation/Suicide

By some estimates, as many as 400 physicians in the United States die by suicide each year,[21] and suicide is the second leading cause of death among US resident physicians (4.1 per 100,000, or approximately five residents per year).[22] Burnout may contribute to increased risk for suicide. In a cross-sectional survey study of 1,354 physicians across all specialties using several burnout measures, each standard deviation increase in burnout was associated with an 85% increased odds of suicidal ideation; yet, after adjusting for depression, this association disappeared.[23] In the adjusted model, each standard deviation increase in depression was associated with a 202% increased odds of suicidal ideation.[23] A study of 81 surgery residents using a burnout metric adapted from existing validated instruments found that community teaching hospital setting and increased number of weekly work hours were both associated with higher rates of burnout and suicidal ideation. Residents in community-affiliated programs were at higher risk.[24] In summary, there is a suggestion that burnout may be associated with suicidality, but it is unclear whether this association persists when controlled for other factors such as depression.

Occupational Health and Safety Risks

Research in resident physicians suggests that there may be an increased risk of occupational injury due to burnout. A 4-year longitudinal study at one institution showed internal medicine residents who reported burnout were at higher risk for blood and body fluid exposures as well as motor vehicle accidents.[25] The MBI burnout subdomain that appeared to place residents at risk for blood or body fluid exposure in the subsequent 3 months was reduced personal accomplishment, while overall burnout and a positive depression screen were individually associated with higher odds of reporting a motor vehicle incident in the subsequent 3 months.[25]

The Impact of Burnout on Professional Behaviors

Reduced Empathy and Patient-Centered Communication

Reduced empathy is mentioned in the early conceptual work on burnout, yet few studies have measured declines in empathy among physicians in practice. Reduced empathy as a consequence of burnout has been found in studies of medical students and residents. The likely reason is that learners undergo regular assessments on empathy, patient communication, and interpersonal skills. In a study of 93 GME trainees, participants completed self-reported measures of stress and burnout using measures of burnout, empathy and patient-centered communication skills collected at the start and end of a 24-hour call shift.[26] The study found a decrease in empathy and patient-centered communications by the end of the call shift. Higher burnout scores were a predictor for larger declines in empathy and patient-centered communication during the latter half of the shift.[26]

A prospective study of 44 internal medicine residents and their patients from one institution found associations between higher MBI depersonalization scores and lower patient ratings of resident empathy.[27] Another study explored the relationship between burnout and empathy in 353 medical students over a 3-year period by measuring two dimensions of empathy: empathic concern and personal distress.[28] It found that students with high levels of *empathic concern* (showing empathy) reported lower burnout, while those with higher reported *personal distress* (feeling empathy) showed significantly higher scores of burnout over 3 years in medical school.[28] Physicians' empathic behaviors are a form of "emotional labor," and physicians in practice and in training who experience burnout may be less able or willing to engage in this form of work to be empathic or demonstrate empathic communications.[29] Another study of 127 fourth-year medical students found higher burnout scores associated with lower scores on the Jefferson Scale of Physician Empathy.[30]

Professional Behaviors

Burnout also may affect physicians' professional behaviors. A survey study of 800 practicing physicians found that, after adjusting for personal and professional characteristics, physicians who reported burnout were also more likely to report engaging in unprofessional behaviors such as documenting tasks they did not perform in the health record or claiming unearned continuing medical education credit.[31] On multivariable analysis, burnout was independently associated with reporting one or more unprofessional behaviors.[31] In a study of 349 palliative care clinicians, perceptions of providing futile and potentially ineffective care were associated with burnout, measured by a validated single item adapted from the MBI, and with avoidant behaviors with patients, families, and colleagues.[32] In a study of more than 1,100 physicians at a large institution, higher scores on the MBI depersonalization domain were associated with a greater odds of complaints about that individual to the institutional ombudsperson (odds ratio [OR] 1.72) [33] Adding to the literature on the association between burnout and professional behavior, research on mandated well-being visits with a teaching institution's Faculty and Staff Assistance Program for 62 internal medicine residents found that burnout scores declined following the intervention, and professionalism concerns for internal medicine decreased significantly, from 17 of 62 (31%) pre-intervention to 1 of 62 (1.6%) following the intervention.[34]

In a study of 82 US psychiatry residents, lower burnout scores were associated with plans to accept Medicaid patients after completion of training; however, residents who experienced assault in the emergency department were less likely to indicate that they would treat publicly insured patients after training.[35]

In a cross-sectional study of 2,566 students in all years at seven US medical schools, students with burnout were more likely to report engaging in unprofessional behaviors (such as reporting patient care tasks that they had not completed or dishonest academic behaviors) than those without burnout (OR, 1.89). Students with burnout were also less likely to report altruistic views regarding physicians' responsibility to society, such as providing care for medically underserved populations (OR, 0.68).[36] In multivariable analysis to adjust for personal and professional characteristics and depression, burnout was the only factor independently associated with reporting unprofessional behaviors (OR, 1.76) or having less altruistic views regarding physicians' responsibility to society (OR, 1.65).[36]

The Impact of Burnout on Professional Efficacy

Reduced Personal Achievement

In a study of 1,272 US emergency medicine physicians using the MBI and a 79-item questionnaire of job- and performance-related attributes, two highly ranked self-reported correlates of burnout were lack of job involvement and negative self-assessment of productivity.[37] In a study of 82 US psychiatry residents, higher burnout scores on a two-item instrument adapted from the MBI were associated with lower self-reported quality of care delivered.[35]

A study of 126 primary care physicians in a health maintenance organization in Israel showed that burnout was associated with higher referrals for tests and specialist care.[38] Another study with a sample of 188 Israeli primary care physicians showed that burnout measured by the MBI negatively affected mood, which in turn resulted in less communication with patients, more prescribing, and higher rates of referrals.[39]

A study of videotaped consultations from a national sample of 126 general practice physicians in the Netherlands showed that physicians with lower personal accomplishment MBI subdomain scores communicated less effectively, were less patient-centered, and had less eye contact with their patients compared to respondents with more positive personal accomplishment scores.[40]

In a study of 82 US medical students at the start of their third year, higher burnout scores were associated with lower self-reported efficacy, expressed as disagreement with the statements "I have control over my daily schedule" (p = 0.0286) and "I am confident that I will have the knowledge and skills necessary to become an intern when I graduate."[41]

Educational Attainment and Engagement in Professional Development

In a study of 458 general practitioners in Denmark, physicians who reported burnout were less likely to be members of a continuing medical education (CME) group or to take part in improvement outreach visits with other general practices.[42]

In a study of more than 16,000 US residents using two items adapted from the MBI, respondents who reported daily emotional exhaustion symptoms had mean in-training examination (ITE) scores that were lower than the comparison, and residents who reported a quality of life that was "as bad as it can be" had (ITE) scores that were 4.2 points lower (P < .001) than those who reported their quality of life was "as good as it can be."[43] A study of more than 2,500 recently graduated family medicine residents registering for the American Board of Family Medicine showed a relationship between burnout and lower scores on professional conduct and accountability milestones (OR, 1.41). However, in that study, no statistically significant association was found between burnout and lower ITE scores.[44]

Suboptimal Role Modeling and Impact on the Learning Environment

Burnout affects physician colleagues, other team members, and learners within the clinical environment. Physicians experiencing burnout are suboptimal role models for learners and peers, may contribute to a negative work environment, and can in turn put others at risk for burnout.[2] One study of 127 medical students at the beginning of their fourth year found that higher scores on the MBI were associated with lower student ratings of the professional climate created by faculty, residents, and other medical students.[30]

Consequences of Burnout on Satisfaction with Clinical Medicine as a Career Choice

Job Turnover

The relationship between burnout and job turnover has been examined in several studies. A longitudinal study of 472 primary care clinicians found a high prevalence of burnout (52%), low engagement (only 32% with high engagement), and high potential turnover (30% indicating plans to change the institution at which they practice in the next 2–3 years).[45] Burnout and low work engagement were both shown to be predictors of potential clinician turnover.[45] In a longitudinal study of 688 physicians at two university-affiliated hospitals between 2013 and 2015, 26% reported burnout on the MBI and 28% indicated an intention to leave.[46] By 2015, 13% of the physicians in the original sample had actually left.[46] After adjusting for specialty, work hours, sleep loss, anxiety, and depression in a logistic regression model, physicians who experienced burnout had 168% higher odds of leaving the institution compared to those who did not report burnout, and the cost of recruitment incurred due to departure attributable to burnout was estimated to be between $15.5 million and $55.5 million.[46] A study of more than 1,100 US physicians found that emotional exhaustion was associated with a greater odds of leaving the organization, while depersonalization and overall burnout score were not.[33]

Reducing Clinical Hours or Leaving Clinical Practice

In a study of more than 1,300 emergency physicians from the 1990s that used a single-item burnout measure, 25% of respondents reported burnout and 23% indicated plans to leave emergency medicine within 5 years.[47] A longitudinal study of more than 2,500 physicians showed that higher burnout scores on the MBI correlated with actual reductions in percentage of full-time equivalent (FTE) work over the following 24 months, measured by administrative and payroll records.[48] Controlling for age, sex, and specialty in longitudinal analysis, each 1-point increase in the 7-point emotional exhaustion domain on the MBI was associated with a greater likelihood of reducing FTE commitments over the following 24 months (OR, 1.43).[47] In a cross-specialty study of 6,680 physicians, burnout and dissatisfaction with work–life integration as related to the electronic health record were each independent predictors of physicians' stated intent to reduce clinical hours, leave clinical practice, or leave the profession.[49] Another large multispecialty study of 2,000 US physicians found that individuals experiencing burnout were less likely to report a commitment to direct patient care and clinical practice.[50]

Leaving the Medical Field or Regretting Specialty Choice

Burnout is associated with thoughts of leaving the medical field across the continuum of training and practice, including among medical students. In one study, 11% of 2,222 medical students at five schools reported serious thoughts of dropping out within the previous year.[50] In a prospective sample of 858 students in the same cohort, burnout, lower mental or physical quality of life, and depressive symptoms at baseline predicted thoughts of dropping out during the following year. For burnout, each 1-point increase in the emotional exhaustion and/or depersonalization score and each 1-point decrease in personal accomplishment score was associated with a 7% increase in the odds of serious thoughts of dropping out.[51] While no studies to date have directly examined the impact of burnout on GME trainee decisions to drop out of training, a study of Canadian medical students and GME trainees found that higher levels of psychological distress were associated with a 6.04 greater likelihood of thoughts of dropping out of medical training in the past year for both medical students and residents.[52] A study of 415 urology residents found that 47% of all respondents and 65% of second-year residents met criteria for burnout and that 1 in 6 respondents reported they regretted their career choice.[53] Similarly, in a study of 408 vascular surgery trainees, 45% reported symptoms of burnout, 10% reported thoughts of attrition, and 8% reported thoughts of changing specialty.[54]

Societal Consequences of Burnout: Quality and Safety, Patient Satisfaction, and Cost of Care

Given the multitude of effects of burnout on the individual and on the health care team, it is not surprising that burnout is associated with a number of consequences for society and the health care system as a whole. These consequences to society are summarized in Box 5.1.

BOX 5.1 Potential Societal Consequences and Costs of Physician Burnout

Physicians and medical learners who experience burnout may be more likely to:

- Reduce their participation and engagement in patient care, with the potential for reduced patient trust in physicians and the health care system.
- Limit their efforts to improve care, resulting in lower quality and increased cost.
- Lessen their focus on patient safety, resulting in higher medical errors and potentially malpractice exposure. Studies show a potentially bidirectional relationship between burnout and errors, with medical errors increasing burnout, which in turn may contribute to future medical errors.
- Have increased thoughts of dropping out of medical school or residency, regret their career or specialty choice, reduce their clinical practice hours, leave their current institution, and/or exit from clinical medicine.
- Provide suboptimal role modeling for students, residents, and junior colleagues.
- Advocate against clinical medicine as a desirable career choice for students and GME trainees.

Quality and Safety of Care

A meta-analysis encompassing 82 studies and 210,669 clinicians found statistically significant negative relationships between burnout and quality of care and burnout and patient safety.[55] Moderators of the relationship between burnout and quality of care included the burnout dimension (emotional exhaustion, depersonalization), unit of analysis (individual vs. hospital unit), and metric type of quality of care (provider metric vs. patient satisfaction).[55] Studies that assessed patient satisfaction as the outcome showed lower associations with burnout.[55] Moderators of the relationship between burnout and patient safety included safety indicator type, study population (physicians vs. interprofessional teams), country of study, and the metric used to assess safety (safety perceptions vs. safety events).[55] A systematic review of 12 articles also found moderate evidence for an association between burnout and reduced quality and safety of care. In this study, the variability in the way quality and safety of care was measured and how burnout was assessed likely attenuated the relationship between burnout and quality and safety of care.[56]

A longitudinal study of 184 internal medicine residents found that higher scores on the MBI were associated with an increased odds of self-reporting a major medical error in the subsequent 3 months.[57] Self-reports of medical errors were also associated with worsening burnout, depressive symptoms, and decreased quality of life, suggesting a possible bidirectional relationship between errors and clinician distress.[57] In another study of 115 internal medicine residents, respondents with higher MBI scores were more likely to self-report providing at least one type of suboptimal patient care (53% vs. 21%).[58] When domains of burnout were evaluated separately, only the depersonalization dimension was associated with suboptimal patient care.[58] An additional longitudinal study of 32 US first-year internal medicine residents found a slightly lower rate of medication prescription errors in residents with higher burnout scores at the end of their first year.[59]

In a study of more than 6,500 physicians in practice, respondents who self-reported medical errors were more likely to report symptoms of burnout (77.6% vs 51.5%), fatigue (46.6% vs 31.2%), and recent suicidal ideation (12.7% vs 5.8%).[60] In multivariate analysis, self-reports of errors were independently associated with burnout (OR, 2.22), fatigue (OR, 1.38), and lower work unit safety grades measured by the Agency for Healthcare Research and Quality Survey on Patient Safety (OR, 1.70), after adjusting for demographic and clinical characteristics.[60] Added evidence for a complex relationship between depression, burnout, and medical errors comes from a meta-analysis of 11 studies involving 21,517 physicians, showing a higher relative risk for errors by physicians reporting depression.[61] An analysis of the four longitudinal studies in the sample (4,462 physicians) showed a bidirectional relationship between physician depressive symptoms and medical errors.[62]

Medico-Legal Risk

Several cross-sectional studies suggest an association between malpractice suits and burnout. A 2010 study of more than 7,900 US surgeons found an association between burnout (measured with a two-item instrument adapted from the MBI), an increased rate of medical errors, and greater medico-legal risk.[62] A second study in more than 7,000 surgeons showed an association between recent malpractice claims, depression (OR, 1.27), and burnout (measured by a two-item instrument adapted from the MBI (OR, 1.17) after controlling for personal and professional characteristics.[63]

A factor in the increased risk for malpractice claims could be suboptimal communication and lower expressed empathy by individuals experiencing burnout. In a study of 1,354 practicing physicians, each standard deviation increase in burnout was associated with an increase in self-reported medical errors (OR, 1.48); in contrast, depression was not associated with self-reported medical errors (OR, 1.01).[23]

Patient Satisfaction

A few studies have assessed the relationship between expressed empathy and patient satisfaction, suggesting that higher scores on the depersonalization component of burnout may contribute to lower patient satisfaction. The relationship is complex and influenced by many factors. One study of 28 emergency medicine physicians and 423 patients found that burnout (as measured by the Copenhagen Burnout Inventory [CBI]) had no association with patient satisfaction.[64] However, when empathy (measured with the Jefferson Scale of Empathy [JSE]) and CBI scores were analyzed collectively, the adjusted OR increased, and the highest adjusted OR (8.37) was found for a model that combined high patient-assessed physician empathy, a low CBI score, and high physician scores on the JSE.[64] A prospective study using 178 matched pairs of physicians and hospitalized patients found that depersonalization (assessed by the MBI) was associated with lower patient satisfaction and a longer post-discharge recovery period after controlling for severity of illness and demographic factors.[65]

Cost of Care

Cost-conscious approaches to care are important to health care systems that already assume a sizable and rising share of annual spending. The data for the impact of burnout on the cost of care are limited. A multivariable analysis of data from a survey study of 800 practicing physicians showed that burnout (using the MBI) was independently associated with respondents reporting a less favorable attitude toward cost-conscious approaches to care.[31] In two studies of Israeli primary care physicians, burnout (measured by the MBI) was associated with increased test ordering, higher prescribing rates, and more referral rates for specialty care, all of which likely contributed to increased health care costs.[38,39]

Societal Costs of Turnover and Reduced Clinical Hours

At the level of the health care system, the costs associated with burnout have been quantified for two potential consequences: reduced participation in work by physicians experiencing burnout and turnover or exit from the clinical workforce due to burnout. Within the United States, the cost of these consequences has been estimated at $4.6 billion annually, with multivariate probabilistic sensitivity analyses ranging from $2.6 billion to

$6.3 billion. This estimate suggests a combined economic cost of burnout resulting from reduced clinical hours, turnover, and exit from clinical work of approximately $7,600 per US physician each year.[3] Beyond the financial consequences, turnover due to burnout may reduce expertise in the workforce and limit access to care. While not quantifiable, reduced physician engagement and participation and physician turnover have the potential to also decrease patients' trust in the health care system.

Consequences of Burnout for the Medical Education Continuum

Much of the above literature has focused on consequences of burnout for physicians in general. In this section, we discuss specific implications for those in medical training. Academic institutions create the environment where physicians learn the art and science of medicine and form their professional identities across the education continuum from medical school to residency and into clinical practice. Burnout is higher in medical students, residents, and early-career physicians than in general population controls[66] and may already be present in students entering medical school. A longitudinal study of freshman and sophomore premedical students at one university showed that students with higher levels of burnout reported a significant decrease in interest in a medical career over the study period, and this relationship persisted after controlling for sociodemographic factors and educational achievement.[67]

Because studies of burnout rely predominantly on self-report, many of the manifestations and consequences of burnout, including impact on the learning and clinical environment, have not been extensively characterized. Much of the consideration of these issues in the medical education community is described in editorials which focus on the need to address burnout in physicians and medical learners and the academic or professional challenges faced by learners across the medical education continuum. Opinion pieces suggests that students and GME trainees who are burned out may have more difficulty with critical elements of medical education such as learning clinical medicine, task completion, team and mentor relationships, and career progression. While much of the evidence to support these specific consequences is still emerging, this conversation in the literature suggests that unaddressed burnout in medical students may persist into residency and practice beyond, with potentially cumulative and increasingly severe consequences for clinicians, patients, and the health care system as a whole. Additionally, the effects of burnout in faculty and residents may be propagated across the continuum when students or GME trainees have negative experiences in the clinical learning environment, potentially leading to a cycle in which burnout in supervisors begets burnout for those in training. This theory requires further study, but some relevant cross-sectional data in support of consequences in the learning environment are presented below.

Consequences in the Learning Environment
for Medical Students

There is evidence of a relationship between the medical student learning environment and the clinical environment for residents, although most of these studies are cross-sectional and therefore causality cannot be inferred. Nevertheless, they are described here to provide a comprehensive view of our current understanding on the interplay between burnout and other important elements of the learning environment. Studies have linked learner intimidation, harassment, and mistreatment events in the learning environment to learner reports of burnout. A multispecialty study of Canadian resident physicians found that those who reported experiencing intimidation or harassment also reported higher burnout and reduced satisfaction with both their residency training program and their choice of medicine as a career.[68] A study of more than 600 third-year medical students from 24 different schools found that students who reported mistreatment by faculty or residents had higher burnout scores (as measured by the two-item modified MBI), compared with students who indicated that mistreatment was nonexistent or infrequent.[69] Another study of 1,701 medical students measuring burnout with the MBI found that characteristics of the learning environment associated with burnout differed between the pre-clerkship and clerkship years and may suggest an impact of faculty or supervising resident well-being and burnout on student burnout.[70] In pre-clerkship students, dissatisfaction with school infrastructure and lower perceived levels of faculty support were associated with burnout. In the clerkship phase of medical student learning, each 1-point increase in agreement with a statement regarding the student's current supervising resident or intern level of cynicism was associated with a 1.35 higher odds of reporting burnout.[70] Conversely, a prospective cohort analysis of 792 medical students at five schools that assessed resilience and recovery from burnout (using the MBI) reported that faculty and staff support and other attributes of the learning environment were associated with student resilience or recovery from burnout.[71] For students who recovered from burnout (meeting burnout criteria in year 1 but not in year 2), satisfaction with support provided by faculty, satisfaction with the learning environment, and student perception of faculty interest in student education increased the odds for recovery by 38%, 29%, and 29%, respectively.[1] In addition, positive perception of faculty interest in student education was also associated with a 59% increase in the odds of recovery.[71]

For residents, a less positive perception of the learning environment also was associated with higher reports of burnout after adjusting for age, gender, training year, and specialty.[72] In one study of 762 resident physicians at a single US institution, higher burnout scores (on a two-item modified MBI burnout instrument) were associated with fewer resident reports of observed faculty professional behavior.[72] A longitudinal study of 2,888 US second- and third-year resident physicians from a national sample (on a two-item modified MBI burnout instrument) showed that burnout was associated with higher reports of negative interpersonal experiences in the learning environment.

Residents who reported negative experiences in year 2 were more likely to have burnout at year 3 (OR, 1.32).[73] Burnout experienced by faculty may also have a negative impact on faculty teaching skill. One study of faculty and residents in a single US urology residency training program found that higher faculty burnout (on the MBI) was associated with lower faculty self-assessed teaching ability and, to a lesser degree, resident ratings of faculty teaching ability.[74] While additional studies are needed, evidence and anecdote to date suggest that when physician leaders experience burnout, the resultant impact on the working and learning environment may discourage junior colleagues from fully engaging in the profession and propagate early cynicism in learners. Taken together, these studies highlight the overall consequence of burnout for the entire health care workforce; burnout that affects one member of the health care team is likely to also affect other members of the team, with learners uniquely vulnerable to these impacts.

Consequences of Burnout in Minority and Female Physicians and Medical Students

Burnout in Underrepresented in Medicine Minority Physicians and Medical Students

Until the most recent decade, burnout was studied predominantly in majority populations. While some more recent studies have explored the contribution of minority status to burnout and aspects of the working and learning experience of minority medical students, residents, and practicing physicians, there likely is underreporting of burnout and its consequences specifically in these groups.[75] Attributes of the learning environment that disproportionately affect minority medical students and resident physicians include the conscripted curriculum,[76] microaggressions, microinsults, and microinvalidations.[77] A conscripted curriculum occurs when teachers ask students of color to publicly discuss their social experiences with race, especially when not paired with objective representation of these matters in didactic materials.[76] This experience may result in a more emotionally exhausting and unrewarded student experience compared with that of nonminority peers[76] that in turn may contribute to burnout.

While a number of studies have explored the prevalence of burnout and related measures of well-being in Asian, Black, and Hispanic/Latinx physicians, limited research has focused on the consequences of burnout in these groups. A systematic review of 15 studies of racial/ethnic differences in burnout for physicians and medical students found no significant differences in burnout among underrepresented in medicine students (URiM) and non-URiM groups across medical students, residents, academic faculty, and physicians in practice, yet it did note some nuanced findings.[75] Studies that used less well-defined metrics for burnout were less likely to show differences among racial/ethnic groups.[75] A study of 1,701 students at five medical schools that used the MBI found higher burnout in minority medical students associated with experiences of discrimination, prejudice, and isolation, which may have contributed to meeting established cutoff scores for overall burnout and emotional exhaustion and depersonalization.[78] Another study reported similar rates of burnout for minority and nonminority students, yet found that a larger percentage of minority students met criteria for low personal accomplishment, and the mean personal accomplishment score was lower for minority students.[79] A prospective study of 792 medical students that used the MBI showed minority medical students had higher odds of successfully recovering from burnout and higher odds of resiliency compared to White students.[71]

Consequences of Burnout in Women Physicians

A secondary analysis of data from a longitudinal study of midcareer emergency medicine physicians showed that more women reported that burnout (measured by a single item) was a significant problem. When men and women respondents were stratified by years in practice, women had a 707% higher odds of reporting plans to leave the profession.[80] In contrast, a study of 456 radiology faculty physicians at 11 academic institutions using the Professional Fulfillment Index (PFI) found higher rates of burnout and lower professional fulfillment in women faculty, yet this finding was accompanied by lower reports of intention to leave by female faculty.[81]

In a study of 282 internal medicine program directors, female program directors reported that work–home conflict was associated with burnout (as measured by two-item modified MBI) and distress.[82] Female program directors also were more likely to report recent work–home conflicts and resolving these conflicts more commonly in favor of work and less often in a way that balances their work and home responsibilities.[83] Due to the cross-sectional nature of this study, determining causality is not possible: it may be that female physicians with burnout are more likely to consequently have work–home conflict or that those who have work conflict are more likely to develop burnout. Overall, while there may be a suggestion that burnout may contribute to attrition of female physicians, the literature is not clear yet on this point, and more research is needed to better understand potential differential consequences of burnout for female physicians.

Consequences of Burnout in LGBTQ+ Physicians

The single study to date that has explored the consequences of burnout in LGBTQ+ residents showed that LGBTQ+ surgery residents reported similar perceptions of the learning environment, career satisfaction, and burnout as other residents, but were more likely to report plans to leave their program or consider suicide. Increased risk for suicide was reduced after adjusting for mistreatment, which was commonly experienced by this group.[84] Again, while this study suggests that those who identify as LGBTQ+ may have important differences in drivers or consequences of well-being at work, further research is needed to better understand potential differential consequences of burnout for those who identify as LGBTQ+.

Areas for Future Research on Consequences of Burnout

The COVID-19 Pandemic, Physician Burnout, and Its Consequences

The coronavirus (COVID-19) pandemic has placed added strain on a US health care system already stretched tight to meet the needs of patients.[85] The long-lasting nature of the COVID-19 pandemic poses particular risks for physician burnout as a result of ongoing high work demands. To date, few studies have analyzed the consequences of burnout resulting from or exacerbated by the experience of physicians during the pandemic. One study that highlighted the complex relationship between existing physician burnout and the impact of the pandemic found that prior-year burnout was associated with the highest risk of developing symptoms for COVID-19–related posttraumatic stress disorder, major depressive disorder, and general anxiety disorder, while higher perceived support from hospital leadership was associated with a lower risk for negative outcomes.[86] Another study of 225 residents and faculty at a single New York institution during the peak of the pandemic also showed that burnout, depression, and suicidal ideation were associated with a history of prior depression/anxiety but also with the frequency of in-house call.[87] Again, institutional support during the pandemic was thought to have reduced burnout and the negative impacts for physicians at the front line.[87] Ongoing research on the consequences of burnout in physicians from the burden of working during the pandemic is needed. Some of the emerging literature on this topic is further described in Chapters 9 and 18.

A Need to Consider Different Dimensions of Burnout

Research on its consequences suggests that burnout may manifest differently for different groups and that it is not a static construct, as described in Chapter 2. The potential for different patterns across the three subconstructs of the MBI suggests there may be different "latent" burnout profiles: (1) burnout (high on all MBI dimensions), (2) overextended (high on emotional exhaustion), (3) disengaged (high on depersonalization), and (4) ineffective (low on personal achievement).[88] Each profile may have a particular set of relationships with the consequences of burnout. These latent profiles and the dynamic burnout cascade described at the beginning of the chapter may help explain some of the mixed associations between burnout and its consequences. Further study also is needed to examine the complex relationship and potential overlap between burnout and mental health outcomes, such as depression and suicidality, with a focus on antecedents and consequences.

Summary Points

- Physician burnout is present across the medical education continuum and has consequences for individuals and institutions.
- Unaddressed burnout in medical students may persist into the graduate medical education phase and into practice.

- Attributes of the learning environment may have a significant effect on burnout, resilience and recovery, and may mitigate or perpetuate burnout among other members of the health care team.
- Consequences of burnout place a burden on physicians and their families, patients and the health care system and society.
- Further research to better understand the consequences of burnout among specific groups may help to target interventions to mitigate these impacts.

Putting It into Practice

- Academic and career mentoring are critical in ensuring that students adapt well to the medical curriculum and explore specialty choice with confidence and thought to their future well-being and work–life balance.
- Interventions to evaluate and improve the learning environment should be followed by periodic evaluation of the impact on learner perceptions and burnout prevalence.
- Addressing burnout in leadership, faculty, and residents is critical due to their role modeling and the negative impact of supervisor burnout and cynicism on the learning environment.
- Medical schools and teaching institutions should strive to create a culture that "normalizes" help-seeking for performance, mental health, and social isolation.

References

1. National Academies of Sciences, Engineering, and Medicine. *Taking Action Against Clinician Burnout: A Systems Approach to Professional Well-Being.* National Academies Press; 2019. Accessed February 23, 2021. https://doi.org/10.17226/25521.
2. Christakis NA, Fowler JH. Social contagion theory: examining dynamic social networks and human behavior. *Stat Med.* 2013;32(4):556–577.
3. Han S, Shanafelt TD, Sinsky CA, et al. Estimating the attributable cost of physician burnout in the United States. *Ann Intern Med.* 2019. 170(11):784–790.
4. Dyrbye L, Shanafelt T. A narrative review on burnout experienced by medical students and residents. *Med Educ.* 2016;50(1):132–149.
5. Shanafelt TD, West CP, Sinsky C, et al. Changes in burnout and satisfaction with work-life integration in physicians and the general US Working population between 2011 and 2017. *Mayo Clin Proc.* 2019;94(9):1681–1694.
6. Freudenberger HJ. Staff burn-out. *J Soc Issues.* 1974;30(1):159–165.
7. Maslach C. Burn-out. *Human Behavior.* 1976;5:16–22.
8. Maslach C, Jackson SE, Leiter MP. *Maslach Burnout Inventory Manual* (4th ed.). Mind Garden, Inc.; 2017.
9. Maslach, C. The client role in staff burn-out. *J Soc Issues.* 1978;34-111-124.
10. Shanafelt T, Goh J, Sinsky C. The business case for investing in physician well-being. *JAMA Intern Med.* 2017 Dec 1;177(12):1826–1832.
11. Weber A, Jaekel-Reinhard A. Burnout syndrome: a disease of modern societies? *Occup Med (Lond).* 2000 Sep;50(7):512–517.

12. Williams ES, Rathert C, Buttigieg SC. The personal and professional consequences of physician burnout: a systematic review of the literature. *Med Care Res Rev.* 2020;77(5):371–386.

13. Maslach C, Schaufeli W, Leiter M. Job burnout. *Ann Rev Psych.* 2001;52:397–422.

14. Salvagioni DAJ, Melanda FN, Mesas AE, González AD, Gabani FL, Andrade SM. Physical, psychological and occupational consequences of job burnout: a systematic review of prospective studies. *PloS ONE.* 2017;12(10):e0185781.

15. Maslach C, Leiter MP. Understanding the burnout experience: recent research and its implications for psychiatry. *World Psychiatry.* 2016;15(2):103–111.

16. Peckham C. Medscape national physician burnout & depression report 2019. *Medscape.* 2019. Accessed February 23, 2021. https://www.medscape. Com/slideshow/ 2019-lifestyle-burnout-depression-6011056#2.

17. Oquendo MA, Bernstein CA, Mayer LES. A key differential diagnosis for physicians-major depression or burnout? *JAMA Psychiatry.* 2019;76(11):1111–1112.

18. Hughes PH, Brandenburg N, Baldwin DC, Jr. Prevalence of substance use among US physicians. *JAMA.* 1992;267(17):2333–2339.

19. Oreskovich MR, Shanafelt T, Dyrbye LN, et al. The prevalence of substance use disorders in American physicians. *Am J Addict.* 2015;24(1):30–38.

20. Oreskovich MR, Kaups KL, Balch CM, et al. Prevalence of alcohol use disorders among American surgeons. *Arch Surg.* 2012;147(2):168–174.

21. Kishore S, Dandurand DE, Mathew A, Rothenberger D. *Breaking the Culture of Silence on Physician Suicide.* National Academy of Medicine; 2016.

22. Yaghmour NA, Brigham TP, Richter T, et al. Causes of death of residents in ACGME-accredited programs 2000 through 2014: implications for the learning environment. *Acad Med.* 2017;92(7):976–983.

23. Menon NK, Shanafelt TD, Sinsky CA, et al. Association of physician burnout with suicidal Ideation and Medical Errors. *JAMA Netw Open.* 2020;3(12):e2028780.

24. Kinslow K, Sutherland M, McKenney M, Elkbuli A. Reported burnout among U.S. general surgery residents: a survey of the association of program directors in surgery members. *Ann Med Surg (Lond).* 2020;60:14–19.

25. West CP, Tan AD, Shanafelt TD. Association of resident fatigue and distress with occupational blood and body fluid exposures and motor vehicle incidents. *Mayo Clin Proc.* 2012;87(12):1138–1144.

26. Passalacqua SA, Segrin C. The effect of resident physician stress, burnout, and empathy on patient-centered communication during the long-call shift. *Health Commun.* 2012;27(5):449–456.

27. Lafreniere JP, Rios R, Packer H, Ghazarian S, Wright SM, Levine RB. Burned out at the bedside: patient perceptions of physician burnout in an internal medicine resident continuity clinic. *J Gen Intern Med.* 2016;31(2):203–208.

28. von Harscher H, Desmarais N, Dollinger R, Grossman S, Aldana S. The impact of empathy on burnout in medical students: new findings. *Psychol Health Med.* 2018;23(3):295–303. Erratum in: *Psychol Health Med.* 2018;23(10):1282.

29. Larson EB, Yao X. Clinical empathy as emotional labor in the patient physician relationship. *JAMA.* 2005;293:1100–1106.

30. Brazeau CM, Schroeder R, Rovi S, Boyd L. Relationships between medical student burnout, empathy, and professionalism climate. *Acad Med.* 2010;85(10 Suppl):S33–36.

31. Dyrbye LN, West CP, Hunderfund AL, et al. Relationship between burnout, professional behaviors, and cost-conscious attitudes among US physicians. *J Gen Intern Med.* 2020;35(5):1465–1476.

32. Chamberlin P, Lambden J, Kozlov E, et al. Clinicians' perceptions of futile or potentially inappropriate care and associations with avoidant behaviors and burnout. *J Palliat Med.* 2019;22(9):1039–1045.

33. Windover AK, Martinez K, Mercer MB, Neuendorf K, Boissy A, Rothberg MB. Correlates and outcomes of physician burnout within a large academic medical center. *JAMA Intern Med.* 2018;178(6):856–858.

34. Sofka S, Lerfald N, Reece J, Davisson L, Howsare J, Thompson J. Universal well-being assessment associated with increased resident utilization of mental health resources and decrease in professionalism breaches. *J Grad Med Educ.* 2021;13(1):83–88.

35. Dennis NM, Swartz MS. Emergency psychiatry experience, resident burnout, and future plans to treat publicly funded patients. *Psychiatr Serv.* 2015;66(8):892–895.

36. Dyrbye LN, Massie FS Jr, Eacker A, et al. Relationship between burnout and professional conduct and attitudes among US medical students. *JAMA*. 2010;304(11):1173–1180.

37. Goldberg R, Boss RW, Chan L, et al. Burnout and its correlates in emergency physicians: four years' experience in a wellness booth. *Acad Emerg Med*. 1996;3:1156–1164.

38. Kushnir T, Greenberg D, Madjar N, Hadari I, Yermiahu Y, Bachner YG. Is burnout associated with referral rates among primary care physicians in community clinics? *Fam Pract*. 2014;31:44–50.

39. Kushnir T, Kushnir J, Sarel A, Cohen AH. Exploring physician perceptions of the impact of emotions on behaviour during interactions with patients. *Fam Pract*. 2011;28:75–81.

40. Zantinge EM, Verhaak PF, de Bakker DH, van der Meer K, Bensing JM. Does burnout among doctors affect their involvement in patients' mental health problems? A study of videotaped consultations. *BMC Fam Pract*. 2009;10:60.

41. Mazurkiewicz R, Korenstein D, Fallar R, Ripp J. The prevalence and correlations of medical student burnout in the pre-clinical years: a cross-sectional study. *Psychol Health Med*. 2012;17(2):188–195.

42. Brøndt A, Sokolowski I, Olesen F, Vedsted P. Continuing medical education and burnout among Danish GPs. *Br J Gen Pract*. 2008;58(546):15–19.

43. West CP, Shanafelt TD, Kolars JC. Quality of life, burnout, educational debt, and medical knowledge among internal medicine residents. *JAMA*. 2011;306(9):952–960.

44. Davis C, Krishnasamy M, Morgan ZJ, Bazemore AW, Peterson LE. Academic achievement, professionalism, and burnout in family medicine residents. *Fam Med*. 2021;53(6):423–432.

45. Willard-Grace R, Knox M, Huang B, Hammer H, Kivlahan C, Grumbach K. Burnout and health care workforce turnover. *Ann Fam Med*. 2019;17(1):36–41.

46. Hamidi MS, Bohman B, Sandborg C, et al. Estimating institutional physician turnover attributable to self-reported burnout and associated financial burden: a case study. *BMC Health Serv Res*. 2018;18(1):851.

47. Doan-Wiggins L, Zun L, Cooper MA, Meyers DL, Chen EH. Practice satisfaction, occupational stress, and attrition of emergency physicians. Wellness Task Force, Illinois College of Emergency Physicians. *Acad Emerg Med*. 1995;2(6):556–563.

48. Shanafelt TD, Mungo M, Schmitgen J, et al. Longitudinal study evaluating the association between physician burnout and changes in professional work effort. *Mayo Clin Proc*. 2016;91(4):422–31.

49. Sinsky CA, Dyrbye LN, West CP, Satele D, Tutty M, Shanafelt TD. Professional satisfaction and the career plans of US physicians. *Mayo Clin Proc*. 2017;92(11):1625–1635.

50. Tak HJ, Curlin FA, Yoon JD. Association of intrinsic motivating factors and markers of physician well-being: a national physician survey. *J Gen Intern Med*. 2017;32(7):739–746.

51. Dyrbye LN, Thomas MR, Power DV, et al. Burnout and serious thoughts of dropping out of medical school: a multi-institutional study. *Acad Med*. 2010;85(1):94–102.

52. McLuckie A, Matheson KM, Landers AL, et al. The relationship between psychological distress and perception of emotional support in medical students and residents and implications for educational institutions. *Acad Psychiatry*. 2018;42(1):41–47.

53. Koo K, Javier-DesLoges JF, Fang R, North AC, Cone EB. Professional burnout, career choice regret, and unmet needs for well-being among urology residents. *Urology*. 2021;157:57–63.

54. Chia MC, Hu YY, Li RD, et al. Prevalence and risk factors for burnout in U.S. vascular surgery trainees. *J Vasc Surg*. 2021;75(1):308–315.

55. Salyers MP, Bonfils KA, Luther L, et al. The relationship between professional burnout and quality and safety in healthcare: a meta-analysis. *J Gen Intern Med*. 2017;32(4):475–482.

56. Dewa CS, Loong D, Bonato S, Trojanowski L. The relationship between physician burnout and quality of healthcare in terms of safety and acceptability: a systematic review. *BMJ Open*. 2017;7(6):e015141.

57. West CP, Huschka MM, Novotny PJ, et al. Association of perceived medical errors with resident distress and empathy: a prospective longitudinal study. *JAMA*. 2006;296(9):1071–8.

58. Shanafelt TD, Bradley KA, Wipf JE, Back AL. Burnout and self-reported patient care in an internal medicine residency program. *Ann Intern Med*. 2002;136(5):358–67.

59. Kwah J, Weintraub J, Fallar R, Ripp J. The effect of burnout on medical errors and professionalism in first-year internal medicine residents. *J Grad Med Educ*. 2016;8(4):597–600.

60. Tawfik DS, Profit J, Morgenthaler TI, et al. Physician burnout, well-being, and work unit safety grades in relationship to reported medical errors. *Mayo Clin Proc.* 2018;93(11):1571–1580.

61. Pereira-Lima K, Mata DA, Loureiro SR, Crippa JA, Bolsoni LM, Sen S. Association between physician depressive symptoms and medical errors: a systematic review and meta-analysis. *JAMA Netw Open.* 2019;2(11):e1916097.

62. Shanafelt TD, Balch CM, Bechamps G, et al. Burnout and medical errors among American surgeons. *Ann Surg.* 2010;251(6):995–1000.

63. Balch CM, Oreskovich MR, Dyrbye LN, et al. Personal consequences of malpractice lawsuits on American surgeons. *J Am Coll Surg.* 2011;213(5):657–667.

64. Byrd J, Knowles H, Moore S, et al. Synergistic effects of emergency physician empathy and burnout on patient satisfaction: a prospective observational study. *Emerg Med J.* 2021;38(4):290–296.

65. Halbesleben JR, Rathert C. Linking physician burnout and patient outcomes: exploring the dyadic relationship between physicians and patients. *Health Care Manage Rev.* 2008;33(1):29–39.

66. Dyrbye LN, West CP, Satele D, et al. Burnout among U.S. medical students, residents, and early career physicians relative to the general U.S. population. *Acad Med.* 2014;89(3):443–51.

67. Grace MK. Depressive symptoms, burnout, and declining medical career interest among undergraduate pre-medical students. *Int J Med Educ.* 2018;9:302–308.

68. Ferguson C, Low G, Shiau G. Resident physician burnout: insights from a Canadian multispecialty survey. *Postgrad Med J.* 2020;96(1136):331–338.

69. Cook AF, Arora VM, Rasinski KA, Curlin FA, Yoon JD. The prevalence of medical student mistreatment and its association with burnout. *Acad Med.* 2014;89(5):749–754.

70. Dyrbye LN, Thomas MR, Harper W, et al. The learning environment and medical student burnout: a multicentre study. *Med Educ.* 2009;43(3):274–282.

71. Dyrbye LN, Power DV, Massie FS, et al. Factors associated with resilience to and recovery from burnout: a prospective, multi-institutional study of US medical students. *Med Educ.* 2010;44(10):1016–1026.

72. Dyrbye LN, Leep Hunderfund AN, Moeschler S, et al. Residents' perceptions of faculty behaviors and resident burnout: a cross-sectional survey study across a large health care organization. *J Gen Intern Med.* 2021 Jul;36(7):1906–1913. Epub. 2021 Jan 22.

73. Dyrbye LN, West CP, Herrin J, et al. A longitudinal study exploring learning environment culture and subsequent risk of burnout among resident physicians overall and by gender. *Mayo Clin Proc.* 2021;96(8):2168–2183.

74. Lewis JM, Yared K, Heidel RE, et al. Emotional intelligence and burnout related to resident-assessed faculty teaching scores. *J Surg Educ.* 2021;78(6):e100–e111.

75. Lawrence JA, Davis BA, Corbette T, Hill EV, Williams DR, Reede JY. Racial/ethnic differences in burnout: a systematic review. *J Racial Ethn Health Disparities.* 2021;11:1–13.

76. Olsen LD. The conscripted curriculum and the reproduction of racial inequalities in contemporary U.S. Medical Education. *J Health Soc Behav.* 2019;60(1):55–68.

77. Sue DW, Capodilupo CM, Torino GC, et al. Racial microaggressions in everyday life: implications for clinical practice. *Am Psychol.* 2007;62(4):271–286.

78. Dyrbye LN, Thomas MR, Eacker A, et al. Race, ethnicity, and medical student well-being in the United States. *Arch Intern Med.* 2007;167(19):2103–2109.

79. Dyrbye LN, Thomas MR, Huschka MM, et al. A multicenter study of burnout, depression, and quality of life in minority and nonminority US medical students. *Mayo Clin Proc.* 2006;81(11):1435–1442.

80. Lall MD, Perman SM, Garg N, et al. Intention to leave emergency medicine: mid-career women are at increased risk. *West J Emerg Med.* 2020;21(5):1131–1139.

81. Higgins MCSS, Nguyen MT, Kosowsky T, Unan L, Mete M, Rowe S, Marchalik D. Burnout, professional fulfillment, intention to leave, and sleep-related impairment among faculty radiologists in the United States: an epidemiologic study. *J Am Coll Radiol.* 2021;5:S1546–1440(21)00315-X.

82. Shanafelt TD, Raymond M, Kosty M, et al. Satisfaction with work-life balance and the career and retirement plans of US oncologists. *J Clin Oncol.* 2014;32(11):1127–1135.

83. West CP, Halvorsen AJ, Swenson SL, McDonald FS. Burnout and distress among internal medicine program directors: results of a national survey. *J Gen Intern Med.* 2013;28(8):1056–1063.

84. Heiderscheit EA, Schlick CJR, Ellis RJ, et al. Experiences of LGBTQ+ residents in US general surgery training programs. *JAMA Surg.* 2021:e215246.

85. Blumenthal D, Fowler EJ, Abrams M, Collins SR. Covid-19: implications for the health care system. *N Engl J Med.* 2020;383(15):1483–1488. Epub 2020 Jul 22.

86. Feingold JH, Peccoralo L, Chan CC, et al. Psychological impact of the COVID-19 pandemic on frontline health care workers during the pandemic surge in New York City. *Chronic Stress (Thousand Oaks).* 2021 Feb 1;5:2470547020977891. doi:10.1177/2470547020977891

87. Al-Humadi S, Bronson B, Muhlrad S, Paulus M, Hong H, Cáceda R. Depression, suicidal thoughts, and burnout among physicians during the COVID-19 pandemic: a survey-based cross-sectional study. *Acad Psychiatry.* 2021;45(5):557–565.

88. Leiter MP, Maslach C. Latent burnout profiles: a new approach to understanding the burnout experience. *Burnout Res.* 2016; 3(4): 89–100.

Design Considerations for a Comprehensive Well-Being Program

Components of a Comprehensive Well-Being Program

Jennifer G. Duncan, Michael Maguire, and Stuart J. Slavin

Introduction

Well-being is a multidimensional concept that often includes facets of physical, emotional, and mental health, as well as positive feelings associated with being challenged and achieving success in various aspects of personal and professional life.[1,2] As such, the learning environment and its impact on sense of accomplishment can have a major influence on well-being. While there are multiple drivers of medical student and graduate medical education (GME) trainee distress and burnout,[3] it is of key importance to recognize that each individual is impacted differently by these drivers. Therefore, well-being programs should not offer a "one-size-fits-all" approach. A successful program should include a variety of resources and initiatives within the larger domains that we address, including efforts aimed at supporting personal/individual health, improving the learning environment for all students and residents/fellows, and increasing access to mental health services. This chapter provides an introduction to these elements as components of a well-being program (Box 6.1). It also serves as an overview of content that is discussed in further depth in Chapters 7 (individual-level interventions), 8 (system-level interventions), and 9 (mental health resources).

BOX 6.1 Components of a Comprehensive Well-being Program

Individual Factors and Health
  Physical health
  Individual skill-building
  Support programming
  Peer support, discussion groups, coaching
  Well-being assessments

Efficiency and Function of the Learning Environment
  Curriculum design and assessments
  Clinical learning environment structure
  Educational needs of different team members

Culture and Climate of the Learning Environment
  Educational structure
  Team culture and community
  Balance of supervision and autonomy
  Environment of inclusion
  Meaning and purpose in work

Mental Health Support
  Building awareness
  Mental health screening
  Counseling and psychiatric services
  Clinician peer support programs
  Crisis planning

Individual Factors and Health

A wide range of individual strategies and tools can be used to manage stress and distress associated with work and with life overall. This topic will be explored in more detail in Chapter 7. In this chapter, we provide an overview of some common self-care activities, skill-building to promote resilience, and peer support programming.

Physical Health

Promotion of self-care activities has been a centerpiece of many well-being programs for medical learners. Common strategies include meditation/ mindfulness, yoga, exercise and physical activity, nutrition, and sleep regulation/fatigue mitigation.[4] Self-care promotion should also include attention to physical and mental health needs. Chapter 7 will describe additional individually - focused interventions in further detail.

Nutrition

Nutrition is a pillar of good health and well-being and promotion of healthy and nutritious eating is a mainstay of many well-being programs. Medical students and GME trainees may have had variable nutrition education; thus, attention to increasing knowledge related to healthy eating is important.[5,6] However, other barriers exist that also need to be addressed. For example, students and GME trainees may feel that they do not have the time and energy to prepare and eat healthy meals. Additionally, recent data indicate that food insecurity is an important problem to assess and address, at least in medical students, with difficulty accessing food and lack of financial means to purchase food being major causes of insecurity.[7,8] Increasing access to healthy, nutritious food at school and work is essential if we are to be successful in promoting healthy eating. One of the more promising approaches to promotion of healthy eating is the use of teaching kitchens.[9,10] This approach moves beyond the typical knowledge-based approach to the promotion of culinary skill-building and may be more effective in long-lasting behavior change.

Exercise

Physical activity has been shown to have a positive association with medical student and GME trainee well-being.[11,12] A number of interventions can be instituted to promote physical activity, including lectures and workshops focusing on the value of physical activity (not just for well-being but also for cognitive functioning), discounted or free gym membership, and creation of gyms that are conveniently located and have hours that health care students can utilize. Other barriers to exercise should also be considered since it can become difficult for those without a preexisting routine to initiate exercise habits amid a busy medical school schedule. Attention could therefore be paid to finding ways to encourage those who do not exercise regularly to adopt a regular exercise regimen rather than using a one-size-fits-all approach to the issue.

Sleep

Sleep is foundational for good mental health. Medical students, and particularly GME trainees, are at risk for getting inadequate sleep. Inadequate sleep has been associated with burnout in an array of workers.[13] Medical schools and residency programs commonly provide lectures to encourage good sleep practices that focus on topics such as the negative impact of inadequate sleep on cognition, mental health, and physical health; recognizing signs of fatigue; sleep hygiene; and approaches to fatigue mitigation. However, fatigue must not be viewed as solely a self-care concern, given the largely environmental nature of the problem resulting from the structure of medical training. In the pre-clerkship period, initiatives to reduce the content overload that characterizes this phase of education are needed. In the clerkship phase, careful assessment of the utility of various activities could improve the time crunch students feel on many clerkships. Efforts must continue to be made to implement programs that reduce the temporal demands on students and GME trainees in order to improve sleep opportunities.

Promotion of self-care activities is critically important, but not sufficient to address the mental health needs of health professions students. However, systems can deploy strategies that support trainees in developing self-care skills and overcoming barriers to healthy living as one component of a comprehensive approach to well-being.

Skill-Building to Promote Well-Being

A number of techniques or approaches show promise in helping students and GME trainees manage the stresses inherent in their educational paths. These strategies include skills in cognitive restructuring, positive psychology, narrative medicine, and contemplative practice.

Mindfulness

Mindfulness and meditation have been widely used to help manage stress and promote calm and well-being for individuals in the broader society for many years. Mindfulness training has become mainstream at many medical schools and academic medical centers over the past decade. The typical approach to promotion of mindfulness is encouragement of formal meditation practice. Mindful meditation practices have been shown in a number of studies to be effective in reducing stress and adverse mental health outcomes in medical students.[14,15] A potential problem with formal practice, however, is that given the busy schedules and demands placed on medical students and residents, many may not desire or be able to maintain a regular meditation practice (e.g., 15 minutes or more per day). One author of this chapter (SJS) routinely asks medical audience members to raise their hands if they have a regular meditation practice of more than 15 minutes per day, and never have more than 3% raised their hands. Encouraging this type of practice, particularly if less time-consuming alternatives are not offered, may therefore have limited population-based efficacy at best and potentially engender resentment at worst for being seen as unaware of these time-based limitations. Informal mindfulness practices, therefore, can and should be offered as an alternative if students are not interested in developing a formal mindfulness practice. Informal strategies take no extra time in the day and can be built into regular daily activities. Such informal practice typically involves focusing on one of the senses for brief (e.g., 30- to 60-second) intervals and, as thoughts appear, noticing them, letting them go, and then returning attention to one of the senses. An example would be to walk down a hallway or path and focus just on hearing sounds. Another would be to focus simply on the movement of the hands and the sensations during a 20-second hand wash. While these practices may not result in the highest attainment of mindfulness, their efficacy has been demonstrated in some studies, and their relative accessibility and ease of use make them an attractive alternative for busy people.[16,17]

Cognitive Restructuring

Medical students and GME trainees have been found to commonly possess potentially detrimental mindsets, such as impostor phenomenon and maladaptive perfectionism.[18-22] These mindsets may be coupled with cognitive distortions; that is, unconscious processes that can lead to heightened anxiety during challenging situations or events and can contribute to personal distress and adverse mental health outcomes. Cognitive restructuring is a technique for addressing and managing these cognitive distortions. This strategy forms the basis of cognitive behavioral therapy, which remains the gold standard treatment for anxiety, is helpful in depression, and can be effective in managing some of the mindsets and thought processes mentioned above. Rather than only using these techniques once a mental illness develops, evidence suggests that students and GME trainees can be taught these strategies to help *prevent* adverse mental health outcomes.[23,24]

Positive Psychology

The positive psychology movement, promoted by Martin Seligman at the University of Pennsylvania, utilizes a model called Positive Emotions, Engagement, Relationships, Meaning and Purpose, and Accomplishment (PERMA) to cultivate positive mental health outcomes and promote happiness. Attention to each of these areas is postulated to have the potential to enhance well-being and happiness. A range of strategies and tools, both individual and environmental, can be used to promote strength in each of these areas.[25] For example, cultivating positive emotions can be enhanced by using a simple strategy called "three good things."[26] In this practice, individuals can be encouraged to have a journal next to their bed and, before going to sleep, write down three good things that they experienced that day. Creating small interventions to promote connection with others through social events and brief additions to rounds to encourage a deeper knowledge of colleagues' backgrounds and interests can also be utilized.

Arts, Humanities, and Self-Reflection

Many health professions schools have expanded their arts and humanities programs and/or encouraged students and trainees to engage in an array of self-reflection activities to help cultivate a number of skills, including observation, empathy, and critical thinking.[4,27,28] Many of these modalities can be used to promote well-being, particularly those that focus on narrative medicine and reflective writing. As with all individually focused well-being interventions (discussed further in Chapter 7), one question that needs to be considered is whether to make these required or elective offerings. If required, some students or trainees may find them uncomfortable to participate in and may see the interventions and assignments as extra burdens in an already overscheduled life. However, elective activities may convey an implicit message that these exercises are less important, and fewer individuals will have the potential to benefit from the activities.

Individual and Group Support Programming

Medical schools and training programs have instituted a range of programs to help support students, including peer support, facilitated reflection, big sibling programs, Balint-type support groups, and coaching programs. These strategies focus on normalizing and processing the challenges of patient care and being a physician.

Peer Support

Peer-based support programming can take different forms and utilize several different models. Some schools and programs have developed big sibling programs that pair more senior students or trainees with those who are more junior. Others have provided select students and GME trainees with training in active listening and psychological first aid and have made them accessible as resources for students in distress (formal peer support programs are discussed further in the section "Clinician Peer-Support Programs" below). Peer supporters are generally not mental health providers, but they can act as mental health first responders, providing support, care, and referral to formal mental health support when needed, thereby facilitating the linkage to mental health care that some students or GME trainees might not otherwise access.[29–31]

Discussion Groups

Facilitated discussion or Balint-type groups have been used fairly widely, most commonly in residency training programs and particularly, but not exclusively, in family medicine and psychiatry programs. In Balint groups, facilitated discussions allow participants to bring forward emotionally challenging or distressing situations from the clinical setting to process together under the leadership of a trained facilitator. Some programs have expanded the scope of these discussions to address challenges residents face outside of work.[32]

Coaching

Coaching programs have proliferated in recent years in the physician world and are beginning to be developed at the medical school and GME trainee levels. A coaching program developed in partnership between certified physician coaches and senior medical students at one medical school has been very well received by students. Coaching in a residency programs has also been associated with improved coping skills and lower levels of emotional exhaustion.[25–27]

Well-Being Assessments

In addition to providing programming to build skills and support personal development, regularly providing access to screening tools for students and GME trainees to self-assess their current state of well-being may be beneficial. Physicians often lack awareness about their personal levels of distress and how their distress compares to others. Providing screening tools may help students and physicians-in-training gain a better understanding of their personal levels of distress and potentially prompt them to either seek help sooner than they would have otherwise or to at least consider adaptations to their individual strategies for stress and health management. As described in detail in Chapter 2, there are a variety of tools available, ranging from free to cost-associated, including the Mini-Z, Mayo Well-Being Index, various burnout inventories (e.g. Maslach, Oldenburg), the Stanford Professional Fulfillment Index,[33] and short screening tools for depression and anxiety. Coupling these screening tools with information about available resources in the various dimensions of well-being can be a useful mechanism for enhancing the support provided to trainees.

Efficiency and Function of the Learning Environment

While the aforementioned tools directed at the individual can be of considerable support, the impact of the learning environment itself is crucial to the well-being of students, trainees, and faculty alike. Chapter 8 explores system-level interventions in detail, but in this chapter we provide an overview of some of the key considerations in the efficiency and function of the learning environment. The learning environment is a critical intersection between system and personal drivers that can have significant impact on joy in work (and learning), emotional well-being, burnout, and fatigue. Medical education inherently is challenging because its learning environment spans multiple settings with different climates and stressors as well as transient stakeholders. With respect to the learning environment throughout the continuum of medical education, education leaders must address drivers of burnout and fatigue with careful consideration of educational structure design, assessment, and promotion of meaningful experiences that reduce non-educational activities and administrative tasks. Figure 6.1 depicts a model of this balance of factors that contributes to efficiency and function within the learning environment.

In both undergraduate and graduate medical education, a delicate tension exists between workload and education. Within the clinical and nonclinical environments, leaders must constantly strive toward high-value educational and meaningful experiences while reducing irrelevant or non-educational activities. Additionally, assessment and promotion at each step of training should be intentional, transparent, and competency-based.

Curriculum Design and Assessments

In undergraduate medical education, regardless of the timing within a medical school's curriculum or class format, fundamental components of basic science medical education must be mastered in a nonclinical setting. It is crucial for medical schools to routinely

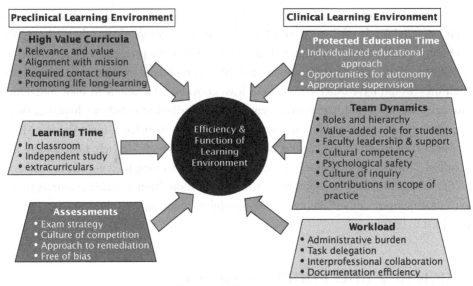

FIGURE 6.1 Factors contributing to efficiency and functioning of the learning environment.

review each component of a curriculum's nonclinical material for relevance and value. While institutions may have unique curricula based on overarching goals aligned with a school's educational mission, it is important that no curriculum is overly influenced by an individual professor's interest, bias, or strengths as a researcher. Schools should continually evaluate the efficacy of curriculum delivery in order to offer the highest yield for students to achieve competency.[24,34] Such approaches could possibly further well-being by enhancing a sense of effectiveness and values alignment.

Furthermore, a school's curriculum often continually expands with the rapid growth of information in the hard sciences and social sciences as exemplified by the recent pandemic. Often, topics are added to a curriculum because of perceived gaps, evolving science, or because of social change, without the removal of any existing content. These ad hoc additions not only require more contact hours for the learner but also may not give the topic the proper attention it requires. The end result is additional stress, cognitive load, and potential burnout.[34,35] Curricula should be frequently and intentionally reviewed to remove excess but also have space intentionally designed to allow for just-in-time learning about emerging topics.

As part of efforts to support well-being through curricular content and structure, assessment strategies should also be considered. Often, a student's preclinical education is modular, with a set period of time spent on a topic, culminating with a final examination. Different schools may employ different methods of testing and grading; however, structures that promote competition among learners could be reconsidered to promote collaboration and teamwork, competency development, and lifelong learning. Traditional final exams or a few large-scale examinations over a prolonged course unit can create periods of stress and cramming interspersed with prolonged periods of laxity. Perhaps a more ideal structure might include regular, low-stress assessments with the ability to provide individualized feedback on competency development, which can allow remediation when a learner is identified as struggling with a particular competency. (See the section "Building Awareness" for further discussion on the contribution of curricular design to a culture of well-being.[36])

The curricular load for medical students and GME programs is also important. For medical schools, attention to the specific structure of the curriculum in terms of time spent in the clinical versus the nonclinical environment and the number of tests taken can be beneficial in improving well-being.[37] Time spent learning should also be evaluated to achieve appropriate balance. Learning time should not just be based on "in-person, in-class" hours but also include reasonable expectations for independent study and extracurricular activity. Extracurriculars, in particular, are an important part of the preclinical period in UME and often allow students to personalize and enrich their education, potentially gain clinical exposure through observerships or preceptorships, and begin to develop and define career aspirations. However, it is again crucial that students are not overextended and that extracurricular activity does not add unmanageable obligations. While the Accreditation Council for Graduate Medical Education (ACGME) sets work hours for required activities, programs should seek to account for time required for conferences, mandated onboarding modules, and other human resources requirements in addition to clinical workload.

Clinical Learning Environment Structure

In the clinical learning environment, the tension between workload and education is even more prevalent than in the preclinical learning environment. First, clinical and administrative demands present a crunch on available time for educational activity and can reduce opportunities for work–life integration, which in turn may threaten well-being (see further discussion in Chapter 8). Additionally, regardless of an institution's preclinical curricular design, the clinical learning environment incorporates many unique aspects that have a potential impact on the learner's educational experience and well-being. These new elements include team formation, interprofessional collaboration, and a frequent emphasis on communication, which are, at best, simulated or performative in the preclinical learning environment but frequently not encountered at all until clinical training. These new scenarios can present challenges for learners and may require the utilization of additional skills, such as emotional intelligence and communication tools often emphasized in the preclinical years but with few opportunities to put into practice or develop.

Meeting Educational Needs of Team Members

After a lengthy nonclinical period, new clinical medical students are often excited to experience patient care and be part of the medical team. As with any team formation, roles need to be delineated. Medical students must be helped to find ways to contribute to the team's work demands while being challenged by a lack of familiarity and ability within a new clinical space. They can often feel lost, forgotten, or even unwanted in these situations. Because of the demands placed on the faculty and GME trainee members of the team, the education of the most junior learner—the medical student—may not be prioritized. Medical student education is often centered at the bedside, whereas for GME trainees, bedside teaching may feel burdensome as it has the potential to interfere with the completion of work demands. Faculty should be intentional in providing high-value and appropriate educational experiences to all learners, both as a group and, when warranted, individually. It is crucial to develop teams that are high functioning and have enough bandwidth to nurture the individual needs of their members.[38,39] Ideally, by improving efficiency and intentionality of design, the team should be able to prioritize education to enhance meaning and sense of value among all members of the team. Chapter 8 further describes cultural and organization efforts that can optimize team functionality and improve team dynamics.

Workload

Attention to the overall workload for students and GME trainees is important; however, defining workload is not entirely straightforward. For learners in particular, work is associated with ongoing learning (cognitive), emotional experiences, and physical tasks. The Physician Task Load index is one means of conceptualizing this workload and is described in more detail in Chapter 8.[40] Strategies for improving the clinical learning environment for medical students and GME trainees as well as faculty include reduction of administrative burden, standardization of task delegation, and intentional design for each member of the interprofessional team to do the work for which they are uniquely trained.[41] Work-sharing within a team includes delegation within the nucleus of the medical team, which might include multiple undergraduate learners, GME trainees, and a faculty member, but also efficient delegation and collaboration among additional interprofessional team members, such as nurses, social workers, pharmacists, and physical and occupational therapists.[42] As workload is distributed across a team, not only will patient care likely be improved, but also stress, time, and individual energy expenditure will be spared, leaving more time to be allotted for education. Additionally, efficiency of the documentation process can be enhanced and workload for GME trainees and faculty can be decreased in multiple ways to reduce clerical burden and enhance education time, such as by improving the usability of the electronic health record (EHR), reducing overall administrative tasks and documentation time, and by having medical students contribute to note-writing in a meaningful, nonredundant manner. Overall, attention to the interplay between work demands and resources available to support task completion, cognitive load, and emotional stressors is critical. Strategies to improve optimize workload to support well-being and the concept of the Job Demand-Resources model will be explored further in Chapter 8.[43]

Balance of Workload and Education for GME Trainees

The tension between workload demands and educational time is often greatest in the GME trainee and should be carefully considered, with educational time protected regularly, because, in addition to being essential to competency development, it contributes to meaning in work and increased self-efficacy. A priority must be placed on GME trainee education, and it should be individualized so that trainees can achieve proficiency in areas of need while streamlining areas in which they are competent. Furthermore, once a trainee achieves a level of competency to ensure efficiency and function, they must actually be allowed to practice autonomously. Supervision must still happen, but not at the expense of the trainee's time, which could otherwise be spent on educational or workload activities. A common pitfall in the tension between workload, education, well-being, and time away from the clinical space is related to the amount of redundancy in practice. Faculty are crucial change agents in enabling high-functioning, highly efficient teams. The faculty team leader has the ability to assist, when needed, to reduce workload, maximize efficiency, and promote educational opportunities. Additionally, faculty can enhance team function by understanding the individual and group needs of the various team learners. When designing an ideal learning environment, one consideration should be ensuring faculty development in areas of leadership, emotional intelligence, and competency with regards to teaching. This emphasis, in turn, requires ensuring that faculty are also well supported with protected time for their own development.

Culture and Climate of the Learning Environment

The overall climate (structure, experiences, and perceptions) and culture (shared values) within the learning environment play a major role in the well-being of students and GME trainees. Numerous factors in the learning environment contribute to stress, including the design of curricula, the system or process for grading and evaluation, the culture within teams, opportunities for mentorship and advising, the level of supervision versus autonomy, and the atmosphere of inclusion. As medical schools and training programs design well-being programs, specific attention must be paid to each of these factors in the learning environment.

Educational Structure

Feedback and Grades

The educational structure within schools and programs can play a significant role in the stress experienced by GME trainees. This includes the process for grades or evaluations, approach to feedback or remediation, and curricular design. In medical school, specifically, pass–fail grading systems have been associated with improved stress and overall well-being without an adverse impact on academic performance.[37,44-46] While GME trainees do not receive grades, evaluation of performance is often a similar stressor for residents and fellows.[47] Many residents and fellows have concerns about their performance, and lack of regular and clear feedback, often coupled with the presence of impostor syndrome, can contribute to significant distress.[18,22] Provision of consistent, specific, and actionable feedback is one mechanism for combating this phenomenon.[22,48] In a similar manner, a compassionate approach to remediation of students and GME trainees and a climate in which mistakes are not punished can be effective means of reducing distress among learners. In an ideal setting, timely, specific, and honest feedback will provide learners with a clear sense of areas in need of improvement, such that they are not surprised by the need for formal remediation. Structured remediation plans that have clear objective goals and are focused on competencies are important. It can also be helpful to couple remediation with additional resources for mental health or coaching support because the need for remediation is often a major stressor for any learner. Additionally, a mental health or psychosocial concern could be driving the need for remediation. Cultures that promote question-asking and that recognize mistakes as part of the learning process are beneficial in supporting the overall well-being of learners.

Formal Well-Being Curricula and Advising Systems

Medical schools and GME programs often provide specific curricula focused on well-being. These sessions can include education about self-care, physician distress, and help-seeking as well as provide opportunities for building some of the skills discussed earlier in the chapter and in further detail in Chapter 7. Some medical schools have restructured their curricula to create learning communities that offer an opportunity for longitudinal peer and faculty mentor interactions.[49] Students in one school indicated that they felt that faculty in these learning communities were very attentive to wellness, mentoring, and career advice.[50] Formal faculty advising and coaching programs for both medical students and GME trainees have also been shown to be beneficial in fostering personal and professional development and improving well-being.[51-57]

Team Culture and Community

The culture within teams in the learning environment is also a critical component of overall well-being. Interpersonal relationships in the workplace can serve as both a source of conflict and a source of support, thus impacting overall well-being.[58,59] Cultural competency and psychological safety are key components of a healthy learning environment. Attention to a collaborative team approach to supporting patient care has been shown to reduce distress in GME trainees by impacting the overall workflow and workload in a clinical area.[42] Conversely, interpersonal conflicts between team members and an overall sense of not being valued are major contributors to distress among learners.[59-63] Providing opportunities for recognition of work and expression of gratitude can have an important impact.[64,65] One center created a mechanism for genuine and humorous expression of gratitude that was uncoupled from performance awards and noted an overall improve-ment in civility within the workplace.[66]

Creating opportunities for social connection and community-building is another key well-being program component. Community-building can take on many forms, in-cluding structured interactions, such as in learning communities or from support groups, and more informal opportunities for connection through social gatherings or group physical activity. Programs can also consider creating opportunities for sharing experi-ences in groups, such as narrative medicine groups or storytelling events, which can en-hance connection with others through recognition of shared vulnerabilities.[27,67,68] These types of events have the additional benefit of helping learners who may feel alone in their struggle with a particular issue to see that many others have similar experiences.

Balance of Supervision and Autonomy

There is an important link between autonomy and well-being. For years, social science researchers have documented a relationship between choice in how one approaches work and life and overall satisfaction, happiness, and mood symptoms.[1,69,70] It is important to note that autonomy is not equivalent to independence, and therefore supervision and autonomy are not mutually exclusive. Daniel Pink, in his book *Drive*,[71] highlights that autonomy is about choice and can come in four forms: task, time, technique, and team. In the context of medical training, while clinical supervision is essential, autonomy can include choice regarding which research topic one pursues (task), choice in vacation time (schedule), or choice in which antibiotic one uses to treat an infection (technique). While choosing team members is more of a challenge in the health care setting, there may be opportunities to allow some choice for students in group learning settings and for GME trainees in settings where they might be able to choose a clinical mentor. These choices do have to be balanced with adequate supervision of learners in a manner commensurate with their level of training. Medical students could be provided opportunities to choose which patients they follow and be allowed to make suggestions for care while still being provided with direct supervision, teaching, and feedback. For residents and fellows, the supervision should be modified as they progress through training. This concept is em-phasized by the ACGME, which requires that faculty should provide enough supervision and oversight to ensure safe, effective patient care while allowing residents increasing independence and authority.[72]

Providing physicians-in-training the opportunity to choose treatment approaches, as long as there is no harm to the patient, is imperative for professional identity for-mation, emerging independence, and developing confidence in their abilities. Studies of residents demonstrate a direct link between a sense of control or autonomy and increased confidence, sense of mastery, and well-being.[73] The important balance between autonomy and supervision was highlighted in a recent qualitative study where GME trainees ver-balized the sense of meaning and learning that they experienced when enabled to make decisions for patients while also noting that difficult decisions, such as those involving dying patients, can be burdensome and the availability of faculty support and supervision is beneficial.[74]

Environment for Diversity, Equity, and Inclusion

The stressful demands of medical school and GME training may predispose students and trainees to burnout and poor life satisfaction at baseline. For individuals who belong to marginalized groups, the experience can be even more challenging. These individuals often face added obstacles, including subconscious bias, microaggressions, offensive interactions, overt discrimination or harassment, and systems that have historically not rewarded their race or gender.[75,76] Individuals who report mistreatment or experience offensive behavior in the workplace have higher rates of burnout and depressive symptoms.[77-79] Attention to ensuring an inclusive environment is an important factor in any comprehensive well-being program. All efforts should involve cooperation between hospitals and associated schools of medicine so that the entire clinical environment is aligned in terms of values related to diversity. Diversity, equity, and inclusion initiatives need to occur at multiple levels (see Chapter 8), including attention to larger institutional initiatives aimed at recruiting and supporting underrepresented minorities in medicine; development of curriculum and training related to health disparities, equity, bias, "isms," and allyship; and provision of support in various forms such as affinity groups, support groups, and other community-building efforts at both the local level (in divisions, departments, or individual medical student classes) and across medical centers. Concerted efforts to address mistreatment events in a systematic way are important; these must include attention to protecting those who report these incidents and confidentiality for the offending individual while also working to close the loop with mistreatment reporters after an event so that learners feel that leadership takes all events seriously.

Meaning and Purpose in Work

Having a purpose is a key factor for an individual to find meaning in one's work; this can provide direction for goal-setting and drive both engagement and innovation in the workplace. Purpose serves as a foundation for the development of professional identity.[80,81] Studies demonstrate an association between burnout, life satisfaction, and a commitment to patient care.[81] Others have found that finding meaning in work is protective from burnout.[82,83] The learning climate needs to attend to and leverage the underlying calling students and GME trainees have to the medical profession. When there is misalignment between this calling and the work that individuals are asked to complete, it can fuel distress. Physicians who spend less time doing the activities they find meaningful have higher rates of burnout.[84] Institutions should attend to these issues as they relate to professional identity formation and the educational and clinical work that is being required by asking critical questions about the purpose and meaning of the work being performed by students and trainees.

Mental Health Support

As institutions consider the components of a comprehensive well-being program, support for mental health must be included. We know that medical students, residents, and fellows have higher levels of burnout, but they also have higher risk for mental health diagnoses compared to other professions.[23,85–87] As described in previous chapters and further detailed in Chapter 9, burnout and mental illness are distinct, though likely related, entities. Labeling changes in a student or GME trainee's demeanor as burnout, without consideration for other causes could have serious consequences by not matching interventions with the underlying problem at hand. Addressing burnout and more serious mental illness with a proactive approach may be beneficial in reducing overall distress and potentially preventing more severe mental illness for some people. Unfortunately, there remains significant stigma associated with mental illness and help-seeking behavior.[24,88,89]

Building Awareness

Systems that openly discuss student and physician distress and mental health needs may help to reduce fears related to help-seeking.[90] Educational efforts, promotion of regular well-being and mental health assessments, and the establishment of mechanisms for support by supervisors and peers, as well as awareness and access to individual counseling can all send important messages to students and GME trainees about institutional support for help-seeking.

Significant importance should be placed on the education of all students, GME trainees, faculty, and staff about the emotional stressors and risk for mental health disorders among medical students and physicians-in-training. The importance of this education is underscored by the specific requirement by the ACGME to address well-being topics as part of the common program requirements (see the Introduction).[59] Public health awareness campaigns related to mental health have also been beneficial in increasing knowledge and reducing stigma.[91–93] Educational efforts in medical schools and training programs can serve a similar purpose. This type of awareness-building may help to identify struggling students and GME trainees early, potentially reducing risks for more serious mental health crises.

Beyond just education aimed at helping to identify students or GME trainees who are experiencing distress, educational curricula can also ensure trained individuals are armed with appropriate resources for referring any student or GME trainee who might be identified as needing help. Each institution needs to clearly delineate the resources available for students and trainees. Given the need to reach large populations of individuals who interact with medical students and physicians-in-training, multiple modalities for delivering education may need to be considered. In some cases, education around mental health needs can be left up to individual GME training programs and the school of medicine separately. In other cases, institutions may choose to provide centralized resources for broad education across the continuum of learning. Medical schools and GME programs generally also partner with clinical leaders at affiliated sites or institutions to ensure the essential education of clinic and hospital staff as well, as these individuals typically work closely with students and GME trainees.

An added structural approach to raising awareness can be through psychological first-aid training.[94,95] Psychological first-aid training offers peer-level education on how to best check in with a colleague who might be struggling or who is known to have a recent stressor. While there are formal psychological first-aid training courses, many institutions have modified this approach to offer shorter workshops or sessions that serve to provide basic information and tips on how to listen actively and offer empathetic support. This type of education could be provided broadly to faculty, staff, and learners as a means of enhancing support within the environment. A necessary component of psychological first aid is helping people recognize when colleagues need a referral to a higher level of support.

Mental Health Screening

In addition to anonymous screening tools focused on overall well-being, platforms have been developed that provide more direct connection between at-risk learners and mental health professionals. The American Foundation for Suicide Prevention's Interactive Screening Platform (ISP) is one example of a population-level suicide prevention program. The ISP allows individuals to anonymously submit a stress and depression questionnaire and receive a response from a licensed mental health provider via an anonymous portal. The response time is coupled to the degree of distress displayed in the assessment, with the most distressed individuals receiving a response within 24 hours. This platform aims to identify at-risk individuals and get them mental health support quickly; it also allows for a personal connection between a counselor and the individual submitting the assessment. In one study, among more than 2,800 faculty, residents, and students, 13% completed an online questionnaire and, among those, 27% were noted to have significant risk for depression and/or suicide.[96] Among those noted to be at-risk, only 15% were already engaged in counseling. Thus, the ISP platform was able to identify a population of high-risk individuals, and nearly 50% of those accepted referrals for mental health care. Because the ISP platform does need to be linked to established counseling resources or employee assistance programs (EAPs) within the institution, it does require a significant investment of institutional financial and personnel resources.

If a population-level screening tool is not feasible for an institution due to lack of sufficient institutional resources, there are a variety of targeted screening tools for mental health conditions that can be utilized in assessing the mental health status of students and GME trainees. Most often these instruments are used as point-of-care assessments by primary care or mental health providers in their assessment and tracking of outcomes for their patients, but they can also be used in larger-scale data collection and have been used in many studies focused on well-being. It is important for institutions to align their screening approach with the available resources they have in place to respond to positive screens, in order to maintain trust in the institutional approach to responding to mental health needs.

Counseling and Psychiatric Services

Beyond education and assessment, medical schools and training programs should provide resources for learners to access mental health services for both counseling and psychiatric care. Data demonstrate a high incidence of stress and burnout, as well as mental health disorders such as depression and anxiety, among medical students and GME trainees, and high rates of suicidal ideation.[23,85–88,97] Additionally, physicians and medical students often do not seek care for themselves.[98] Multiple barriers exist to care-seeking, including concerns about stigma associated with mental health diagnoses, perceived weakness associated with the need for support, and concerns about implications for future residency applications, licensure, and credentialing.[11,88,99] It is important to consider mechanisms of support that protect confidentiality while also attending to awareness campaigns that help to reduce stigma and address concerns about the impact on licensure. Regardless of the approach taken, it is important for a mental health program to track satisfaction, utilization, ease of access, and barriers to seeking help in order to assess whether the needs of learners and GME trainees are being met.

As is further discussed in Chapter 9, there are a variety of potential approaches to providing counseling and psychiatric resources and the specific approach chosen should depend on feasibility and infrastructure within individual institutions. In many cases, the approach taken by medical schools is different from the approach taken by GME programs, but in some institutions the resources provided are shared. Some medical schools offer internal counseling and psychiatric services through student counseling or mental health centers that are either coupled with the larger counseling program at a university or function as a separate program within the school of medicine.[100] The specific scope of practice may vary among institutions in terms of services provided (short- vs. long-term) and specific conditions treated. Establishing resources for referral outside of the institution is also important, both for conditions not within scope of practice and for those who prefer to be seen in a different setting. The counselors in these programs often are also involved in building awareness and education across the learning environment.

For GME programs, a similar approach to providing internal services has also been found to be quite effective, especially when coupled with campaigns aimed at reducing stigma and promoting help-seeking.[101,102] Institutions which choose to have an internal resource model need to consider funding for clinical full-time equivalent (FTE), space, and administrative support. Dr. Sydney Ey and colleagues estimated that the cost for a midsize academic center might start at $200,000 and increase as a program grows.[101] When these services are offered internally, attention needs to be paid to documentation, in terms of using the institutional medical record system, a separate system, or paper charts. For many GME programs, the resources for counseling and psychiatric services are provided through EAPs. There are various structures within EAPs, and the access and usability should be assessed at each institution.

An additional approach used at several centers or individual programs has been to establish required, or "opt-out," counseling appointments for all new trainees and in some cases trainees across multiple years.[103–105] This approach aims to reduce the stigma associated with help-seeking by normalizing it for all. Recent data indicate that the use of an opt-out mental health service model can also be associated with fewer observed professionalism breaches, presumably the consequence of untreated mental health conditions.[91]

Clinician Peer Support Programs

Separate from formal mental health services, many institutions have found value in offering peer support services. These types of programs acknowledge the stress placed on physicians during their daily work, including the stress of poor outcomes, adverse events, mistakes, and even interprofessional conflict. In many instances, these individual events may not prompt an individual to seek out mental health support, but such individuals may find value in speaking to another physician or peer.[29] Peer support programs provide an opportunity for physicians/students to process these challenging events with another colleague, often from a different specialty, and to receive support.[30,31] Peer supporters are trained to provide support for a variety of concerns and to refer to a higher level of support if needed. While many peer support programs have involved faculty-level supporters, the COVID-19 pandemic led many programs to broaden their peer support programs to include residents and fellows. Others added programming that include peer supporters assigned as longitudinal "buddies" to discuss ongoing challenges and stressors in the workplace.[106]

Crisis Planning

Regardless of the number of services offered at an institution, all schools and GME programs need to ensure that they have plans in place for responding to crises.[107] These crises can come in the form of a trainee death or a learner in acute crisis needing emergent care. Established processes for who to call in a crisis and the sequence of events of where students and GME trainees in crisis will receive support and by whom can ensure that learners and GME trainees get care expediently and with appropriate confidentiality. Clear messaging to all learners and program leaders about crisis phone numbers and resources should be part of a comprehensive well-being program.

Conclusion

Given the multidimensional nature of well-being, it is important for institutions to adopt a broad approach in designing well-being programs. Medical student and GME trainee well-being are impacted by both personal factors and institutional or systems factors; thus it is critical for schools and programs to address both. Addressing personal factors without addressing factors related to the learning climate and culture risks creating more frustration and stress among learners who might feel that the institution is ignoring factors outside of their control which contribute to their sense of well-being. Having an array of choices within the broad areas of well-being that we outline in this chapter offers the best opportunity to reach as many students and GME trainees as possible. What is clear is that not all learners need the same thing; therefore offering options for an array of resources is critical. A comprehensive well-being program should offer support for personal growth and development as well as individual mental health. This support should include educational opportunities as well as resources for individualized counseling. Additionally, the institution should address as many factors as possible related to the learning climate and culture in order to create an environment that is inclusive, meaningful, and efficient. This chapter serves as a prelude to Chapters 7, 8, and 9, which will further explore how to incorporate individual interventions, systems interventions, and mental health interventions into medical school and residency and fellowship training.

Summary Points

- Well-being is multidimensional and should be addressed with an array of options that span both personal factors and institutional/systems factors.
- Attention to personal health and cognitive/emotional skill-building is useful for preparing students and GME trainees to manage the training environment and for ongoing professional development.
- Providing opportunities for connection and community offers students and GME trainees support throughout training.
- Design of curricula, attention to educational needs, assessments, remediation, and the balance of supervision and autonomy are all important areas to address in order to support student and GME trainee well-being
- Careful attention to the intersection between education and workload is critical to ensure students and GME trainees have meaningful experiences and develop a sense of purpose and accomplishment, which are key contributors to overall well-being.
- Attention to the culture within teams and diversity and inclusion are critical systems-related initiatives that can have a large impact on student and GME trainee well-being.

Putting It into Practice

- Review the components of a comprehensive well-being program shown in Box 6.1 and consider which elements currently exist at your institution and which areas present opportunities for expansion.
- Further explore individual interventions in Chapter 7, system-level interventions in Chapter 8, and mental health access and interventions in Chapter 9.

References

1. Deci EL, Ryan RM. *Intrinsic Motivation and Self-Determination in Human Behavior*. Plenum Press; 1985.
2. Wallace JE, Lemaire JB, Ghali WA. Physician wellness: a missing quality indicator. *Lancet*. Nov 14 2009;374(9702):1714–1721. doi:10.1016/S0140-6736(09)61424-0
3. Shanafelt TD, Noseworthy JH. Executive leadership and physician well-being: nine organizational strategies to promote engagement and reduce burnout. *Mayo Clin Proc*. Jan 2017;92(1):129–146. doi:10.1016/j.mayocp.2016.10.004
4. Quinn MA, Grant LM, Sampene E. A curriculum to increase empathy and reduce burnout. *Wis Med J*. 2020;2020(4):258–262.
5. Daley BJ, Cherry-Bukowiec J, Van Way CW, 3rd, et al. Current status of nutrition training in graduate medical education from a survey of residency program directors: a formal nutrition education course is necessary. *JPEN J Parenter Enteral Nutr*. Jan 2016;40(1):95–99. doi:10.1177/0148607115571155
6. Van Horn L, Lenders CM, Pratt CA, et al. Advancing nutrition education, training, and research for medical students, residents, fellows, attending physicians, and other clinicians: building competencies and interdisciplinary coordination. *Adv Nutr*. Nov 1 2019;10(6):1181–1200. doi:10.1093/advances/nmz083
7. Flynn MM, Monteiro K, George P, Tunkel AR. Assessing food insecurity in medical students. *Fam Med*. Jun 2020;52(7):512–513. doi:10.22454/FamMed.2020.722238
8. Zhou AG, Mercier MR, Chan C, Criscione J, Angoff N, Ment LR. Food insecurity in medical students: preliminary data from Yale School of Medicine. *Acad Med*. Jun 1 2021;96(6):774–776. doi:10.1097/ACM.0000000000004048
9. Eisenberg DM, Imamura A. Teaching kitchens in the learning and work environments: the future is now. *Glob Adv Health Med*. 2020;9:2164956120962442. doi:10.1177/2164956120962442
10. Hauser ME, Nordgren JR, Adam M, et al. The first, comprehensive, open-source culinary medicine curriculum for health professional training programs: a global reach. *Am J Lifestyle Med*. 2020;14(4):369–373. doi:10.1177/1559827620916699
11. Dyrbye LN, West CP, Sinsky CA, Goeders LE, Satele DV, Shanafelt TD. Medical licensure questions and physician reluctance to seek care for mental health conditions. *Mayo Clin Proc*. 2017;92(10):1486–1493. doi:10.1016/j.mayocp.2017.06.020
12. Lebensohn P, Dodds S, Benn R, et al. Resident wellness behaviors: relationship to stress, depression, and burnout. *Fam Med*. 2013;45(8):541–549.
13. Stewart NH, Arora VM. The impact of sleep and circadian disorders on physician burnout. *Chest*. 11 2019;156(5):1022–1030. doi:10.1016/j.chest.2019.07.008
14. Daya Z, Hearn JH. Mindfulness interventions in medical education: a systematic review of their impact on medical student stress, depression, fatigue and burnout. *Med Teach*. 2018;40(2):146–153. doi:10.1080/0142159X.2017.1394999
15. Polle E, Gair J. Mindfulness-based stress reduction for medical students: a narrative review. *Can Med Educ J*. 2021;12(2):e74–e80. doi:10.36834/cmej.68406
16. Gilmartin H, Goyal A, Hamati MC, Mann J, Saint S, Chopra V. Brief mindfulness practices for healthcare providers - a systematic literature review. *Am J Med*. 10 2017;130(10):1219.e1–1219.e17. doi:10.1016/j.amjmed.2017.05.041
17. Shankland R, Tessier D, Strub L, Gauchet A, Baeyens C. Improving mental health and well-being through informal mindfulness practices: an intervention study. *Appl Psychol Health Well Being*. 02 2021;13(1):63–83. doi:10.1111/aphw.12216
18. Gottlieb M, Chung A, Battaglioli N, Sebok-Syer SS, Kalantari A. Impostor syndrome among physicians and physicians in training: a scoping review. *Med Educ*. 02 2020;54(2):116–124. doi:10.1111/medu.13956
19. Henning K, Ey S, Shaw D. Perfectionism, the imposter phenomenon and psychological adjustment in medical, dental, nursing and pharmacy students. *Med Educ*. 1998;32(5):456–464. doi:10.1046/j.1365-2923.1998.00234.x
20. Hu KS, Chibnall JT, Slavin SJ. Maladaptive perfectionism, impostorism, and cognitive distortions: threats to the mental health of pre-clinical medical students. *Acad Psychiatry*. Aug 2019;43(4):381–385. doi:10.1007/s40596-019-01031-z

21. Leach PK, Nygaard RM, Chipman JG, Brunsvold ME, Marek AP. Impostor phenomenon and burnout in general surgeons and general surgery residents. *J Surg Educ.* 2019;76(1):99–106. doi:10.1016/j.jsurg.2018.06.025

22. Seritan AL, Mehta MM. Thorny laurels: the impostor phenomenon in academic psychiatry. *Acad Psychiatry.* 2016;40(3):418–421. doi:10.1007/s40596-015-0392-z

23. Guille C, Zhao Z, Krystal J, Nichols B, Brady K, Sen S. Web-based cognitive behavioral therapy intervention for the prevention of suicidal ideation in medical interns: a randomized clinical trial. *JAMA Psychiatry.* 2015;72(12):1192–1198. doi:10.1001/jamapsychiatry.2015.1880

24. Slavin SJ, Schindler DL, Chibnall JT. Medical student mental health 3.0: improving student wellness through curricular changes. *Acad Med.* 2014;89(4):573–577. doi:10.1097/ACM.0000000000000166

25. Positive Psychology Center. Accessed June 2, 2021. https://ppc.sas.upenn.edu/.

26. Sexton JB, Adair KC. Forty-five good things: a prospective pilot study of the Three Good Things well-being intervention in the USA for healthcare worker emotional exhaustion, depression, work-life balance and happiness. *BMJ Open.* 2019;9(3):e022695. doi:10.1136/bmjopen-2018-022695

27. Klugman CM. Medical humanities teaching in North American allopathic and osteopathic medical schools. *J Med Humanit.* 2018;39(4):473–481. doi:10.1007/s10912-017-9491-z

28. Winkel AF, Feldman N, Moss H, Jakalow H, Simon J, Blank S. Narrative medicine workshops for obstetrics and gynecology residents and association with burnout measures. *Obstet Gynecol.* 2016;128 Suppl 1:27S–33S. doi:10.1097/AOG.0000000000001619

29. Hu YY, Fix ML, Hevelone ND, et al. Physicians' needs in coping with emotional stressors: the case for peer support. *Arch Surg.* 2012;147(3):212–217. doi:10.1001/archsurg.2011.312

30. Lane MA, Newman BM, Taylor MZ, et al. Supporting clinicians after adverse events: development of a clinician peer support program. *J Patient Saf.* 2018;14(3):e56–e60. doi:10.1097/PTS.0000000000000508

31. Shapiro J, Galowitz P. Peer support for clinicians: a programmatic approach. *Acad Med.* 2016;91(9):1200–1204. doi:10.1097/ACM.0000000000001297

32. Slavin S, Shoss M, Broom MA. A program to prevent burnout, depression, and anxiety in first-year pediatric residents. *Acad Pediatr.* 2017;17(4):456–458. doi:10.1016/j.acap.2016.12.016

33. Trockel M, Bohman B, Lesure E, et al. A brief instrument to assess both burnout and professional fulfillment in physicians: reliability and validity, including correlation with self-reported medical errors, in a sample of resident and practicing physicians. *Acad Psychiatry.* 2018;42(1):11–24. doi:10.1007/s40596-017-0849-3

34. Zgheib NK, Dimassi Z, Arawi T, Badr KF, Sabra R. Effect of targeted curricular reform on the learning environment, student empathy, and hidden curriculum in a medical school: a 7-year longitudinal study. *J Med Educ Curric Dev.* 2020;7:2382120520953106. doi:10.1177/2382120520953106

35. Irby DM, Cooke M, O'Brien BC. Calls for reform of medical education by the Carnegie Foundation for the Advancement of Teaching: 1910 and 2010. *Acad Med.* 2010;85(2):220–227. doi:10.1097/ACM.0b013e3181c88449

36. Yielder J, Wearn A, Chen Y, et al. A qualitative exploration of student perceptions of the impact of progress tests on learning and emotional wellbeing. *BMC Med Educ.* 2017;17(1):148. doi:10.1186/s12909-017-0984-2

37. Reed DA, Shanafelt TD, Satele DW, et al. Relationship of pass/fail grading and curriculum structure with well-being among preclinical medical students: a multi-institutional study. *Acad Med.* 2011;86(11):1367–1373. doi:10.1097/ACM.0b013e3182305d81

38. Cruess RL, Cruess SR, Boudreau JD, Snell L, Steinert Y. A schematic representation of the professional identity formation and socialization of medical students and residents: a guide for medical educators. *Acad Med.* 2015;90(6):718–725. doi:10.1097/ACM.0000000000000700

39. Teheux L, Coolen E, Draaisma JMT, et al. Intraprofessional workplace learning in postgraduate medical education: a scoping review. *BMC Med Educ.* 2021;21(1):479. doi:10.1186/s12909-021-02910-6

40. Harry E, Sinsky C, Dyrbye LN, et al. Physician task load and the risk of burnout among US physicians in a national survey. *Jt Comm J Qual Patient Saf.* 2021;47(2):76–85. doi:https://doi.org/10.1016/j.jcjq.2020.09.011

41. West CP, Dyrbye LN, Shanafelt TD. Physician burnout: contributors, consequences and solutions. *J Intern Med.* 2018;283(6):516–529. doi:10.1111/joim.12752

42. Smith CD, C. Balatbat S, Corbridge AL, et al. Implementing optimal team-based care to reduce clinician burnout. *NAM Perspectives*. Discussion paper, National Academy of Medicine; 2018. Accessed June 2, 2021. Implementing Optimal Team-Based Care to Reduce Clinician Burnout - National Academy of Medicine (nam.edu)

43. Demerouti E, Bakker AB. The job demands–resources model: challenges for future research. *SA Journal of Industrial Psychology*. 2011;37(2):a#974, 9 pages. doi:10.4102/sajip.v37i2.974

44. Bloodgood RA, Short JG, Jackson JM, Martindale JR. A change to pass/fail grading in the first two years at one medical school results in improved psychological well-being. *Acad Med*. 2009;84(5):655–662. doi:10.1097/ACM.0b013e31819f6d78

45. Dyrbye L, Shanafelt T. A narrative review on burnout experienced by medical students and residents. *Med Educ*. 2016;50(1):132–149. doi:10.1111/medu.12927

46. Spring L, Robillard D, Gehlbach L, Simas TA. Impact of pass/fail grading on medical students' well-being and academic outcomes. *Med Educ*. 2011;45(9):867–877. doi:10.1111/j.1365-2923.2011.03989.x

47. Pereira-Lima K, Mata DA, Loureiro SR, Crippa JA, Bolsoni LM, Sen S. Association between physician depressive symptoms and medical errors: a systematic review and meta-analysis. *JAMA Netw Open*. 11 2019;2(11):e1916097. doi:10.1001/jamanetworkopen.2019.16097

48. Chandra S, Huebert CA, Crowley E, Das AM. Impostor syndrome: could it be holding you or your mentees back? *Chest*. 07 2019;156(1):26–32. doi:10.1016/j.chest.2019.02.325

49. Drolet BC, Rodgers S. A comprehensive medical student wellness program--design and implementation at Vanderbilt School of Medicine. *Acad Med*. Jan 2010;85(1):103–110. doi:10.1097/ACM.0b013e3181c46963

50. Real FJ, Zackoff MW, Davidson MA, Yakes EA. Medical student distress and the impact of a school-sponsored wellness initiative. *Medical Science Educator*. 2015;25(4):397–406. doi:10.1007/s40670-015-0156-0

51. Cameron D, Dromerick LJ, Ahn J, Dromerick AW. Executive/life coaching for first year medical students: a prospective study. *BMC Med Educ*. 2019;19(1):163. doi:10.1186/s12909-019-1564-4

52. Mikhaiel JP, Pollack J, Buck E, et al. Graduating with honors in resilience: creating a whole new doctor. *Glob Adv Health Med*. 2020;9:2164956120976356. doi:10.1177/2164956120976356

53. Palamara K, Kauffman C, Chang Y, et al. Professional development coaching for residents: results of a 3-year positive psychology coaching intervention. *J Gen Intern Med*. 2018;33(11):1842–1844. doi:10.1007/s11606-018-4589-1

54. Deiorio NM, Carney PA, Kahl LE, Bonura EM, Juve AM. Coaching: a new model for academic and career achievement. *Med Educ Online*. 2016;21:33480. doi:10.3402/meo.v21.33480

55. Dyrbye LN, Shanafelt TD, Gill PR, Satele DV, West CP. Effect of a professional coaching intervention on the well-being and distress of physicians: a pilot randomized clinical trial. *JAMA Intern Med*. 2019;179(10):1406–1414. doi:10.1001/jamainternmed.2019.2425

56. Palamara K, Kauffman C, Stone VE, Bazari H, Donelan K. Promoting success: a professional development coaching program for interns in medicine. *J Grad Med Educ*. 2015;7(4):630–637. doi:10.4300/JGME-D-14-00791.1

57. Wolff M, Hammoud M, Santen S, Deiorio N, Fix M. Coaching in undergraduate medical education: a national survey. *Med Educ Online*. 2020;25(1):1699765. doi:10.1080/10872981.2019.1699765

58. Borteyrou X, Truchot D, Rascle N. Development and validation of the Work Stressor Inventory for Nurses in oncology: preliminary findings. *J Adv Nurs*. 2014;70(2):443–453. doi:10.1111/jan.12231

59. Leiter M, Maslach C. The impact of interpersonal environment on burnout and organizational commitment. *J Organ Behav*. 1988;9:297–308.

60. Embriaco N, Azoulay E, Barrau K, et al. High level of burnout in intensivists: prevalence and associated factors. *Am J Respir Crit Care Med*. 2007;175(7):686–692. doi:10.1164/rccm.200608-1184OC

61. Hill MR, Goicochea S, Merlo LJ. In their own words: stressors facing medical students in the millennial generation. *Med Educ Online*. 2018;23(1):1530558. doi:10.1080/10872981.2018.1530558

62. Oskrochi Y, Maruthappu M, Henriksson M, Davies AH, Shalhoub J. Beyond the body: A systematic review of the nonphysical effects of a surgical career. *Surgery*. 2016;159(2):650–664. doi:10.1016/j.surg.2015.08.017

63. Petitta L, Jiang L, Hartel CEJ. Emotional contagion and burnout among nurses and doctors: do joy and anger from different sources of stakeholders matter? *Stress Health.* 2017;33(4):358–369. doi:10.1002/smi.2724

64. Stegen A, Wankier J. Generating gratitude in the workplace to improve faculty job satisfaction. *J Nurs Educ.* 2018;57(6):375–378. doi:10.3928/01484834-20180522-10

65. Waters L. Predicting job satisfaction: contributions of individual gratitude and institutionalized gratitude. *Psychology.* 2012;3:1174–1176.

66. Lee KC, Oppenheim IM, Do D, Lin TC, Rosin R, Merchant RM. Making workplace civility go viral. *NEJM Catalyst.* 2020;1(1). doi:doi:10.1056/CAT.19.1088

67. Olson ME, Walsh MM, Goepferd AK, Trappey B. Sharing stories to build resilience: articulating the common threads that connect us. *J Grad Med Educ.* 2019;11(3):340–341. doi:10.4300/JGME-D-18-00896.1

68. Wesley T, Hamer D, Karam G. Implementing a narrative medicine curriculum during the internship year: an internal medicine residency program experience. *Perm J.* 2018;22. doi:10.7812/TPP/17-187

69. Conzo P, Aassve A, Fuochi G, Mencarini L. The cultural foundations of happiness. *J Econ Psychol.* 2017;62:268–283. https://doi.org/10.1016/j.joep.2017.08.001

70. Diener E. Subjective well-being. *Psychol Bull.* 1984;95(3):542–575.

71. Pink D. *Drive.* Canongate Books; 2011.

72. ACGME. Common Program Requirements (Residency). Updated July 1, 2022. Accessed December 18, 2022. https://www.acgme.org/globalassets/pfassets/programrequirements/cprresidency_2022v3.pdf

73. Raj KS. Well-being in residency: a systematic review. *J Grad Med Educ.* 2016;8(5):674–684. doi:10.4300/JGME-D-15-00764.1

74. Lases SS, Slootweg IA, Pierik EGJM, Heineman E, Lombarts MJMH. Efforts, rewards and professional autonomy determine residents' experienced well-being. *Adv Health Sci Educ Theory Pract.* 2018;23(5):977–993. doi:10.1007/s10459-018-9843-0

75. Nunez-Smith M, Pilgrim N, Wynia M, et al. Race/ethnicity and workplace discrimination: results of a national survey of physicians. *J Gen Intern Med.* 2009;24(11):1198. doi:10.1007/s11606-009-1103-9

76. Osseo-Asare A, Balasuriya L, Huot SJ, et al. Minority resident physicians' views on the role of race/ethnicity in their training experiences in the workplace. *JAMA Network Open.* 2018;1(5):e182723–e182723. doi:10.1001/jamanetworkopen.2018.2723

77. Anderson N, Lett E, Asabor EN, et al. The association of microaggressions with depressive symptoms and institutional satisfaction among a national cohort of medical students. *J Gen Intern Med.* 2021. doi:10.1007/s11606-021-06786-6

78. Hu YY, Ellis RJ, Hewitt DB, et al. Discrimination, abuse, harassment, and burnout in surgical residency training. *N Engl J Med.* 2019;381(18):1741–1752. doi:10.1056/NEJMsa1903759

79. Kemper KJ, Schwartz A, Pediatric resident burnout-resilience study c. bullying, discrimination, sexual harassment, and physical violence: common and associated with burnout in pediatric residents. *Acad Pediatr.* 2020;20(7):991–997. doi:10.1016/j.acap.2020.02.023

80. Steger MF, Kashdan TB. Depression and everyday social activity, belonging, and well-being. *J Couns Psychol.* 2009;56(2):289–300. doi:10.1037/a0015416

81. Tak HJ, Curlin FA, Yoon JD. Association of intrinsic motivating factors and markers of physician well-being: a national physician survey. *J Gen Intern Med.* 2017;32(7):739–746. doi:10.1007/s11606-017-3997-y

82. Ben-Itzhak S, Dvash J, Maor M, Rosenberg N, Halpern P. Sense of meaning as a predictor of burnout in emergency physicians in Israel: a national survey. *Clin Exp Emerg Med.* 2015;2(4):217–225. doi:10.15441/ceem.15.074

83. Rasmussen V, Turnell A, Butow P, et al. Burnout among psychosocial oncologists: an application and extension of the effort-reward imbalance model. *Psychooncology.* 2016;25(2):194–202. doi:10.1002/pon.3902

84. Shanafelt TD, West CP, Sloan JA, et al. Career fit and burnout among academic faculty. *Archives of Internal Medicine.* 2009;169(10):990–995. doi:10.1001/archinternmed.2009.70

85. Dyrbye LN, West CP, Satele D, et al. Burnout among U.S. medical students, residents, and early career physicians relative to the general U.S. population. *Acad Med*. 2014;89(3):443–451. doi:10.1097/ACM.0000000000000134

86. Mata DA, Ramos MA, Bansal N, et al. Prevalence of depression and depressive symptoms among resident physicians: a systematic review and meta-analysis. *JAMA*. 2015;314(22):2373–83. doi:10.1001/jama.2015.15845

87. Mousa OY, Dhamoon MS, Lander S, Dhamoon AS. The MD blues: under-recognized depression and anxiety in medical trainees. *PLoS One*. 2016;11(6):e0156554. doi:10.1371/journal.pone.0156554

88. Gold KJ, Andrew LB, Goldman EB, Schwenk TL. "I would never want to have a mental health diagnosis on my record": a survey of female physicians on mental health diagnosis, treatment, and reporting. *Gen Hosp Psychiatry*. 2016;43:51–57. doi:10.1016/j.genhosppsych.2016.09.004

89. Swapnil S, Mehta BA, Edwards ML, M.D. Suffering in silence: mental health stigma and physicians' licensing fears. *Am J Psychiatry Resid J*. 2018;13(11):2–4. doi:10.1176/appi.ajp-rj.2018.131101

90. Weiner S. Doctors forgo mental health care during pandemic over concerns about licensing, stigma. 2020. Accessed June 2, 2021. https://www.aamc.org/news-insights/doctors-forgo-mental-health-care-during-pandemic-over-concerns-about-licensing-stigma.

91. Collins RL, Wong EC, Breslau J, Burnam MA, Cefalu M, Roth E. Social marketing of mental health treatment: California's mental illness stigma reduction campaign. *Am J Public Health*. 2019;109(S3):S228–S235. doi:10.2105/ajph.2019.305129

92. Evans-Lacko S, London J, Little K, Henderson C, Thornicroft G. Evaluation of a brief anti-stigma campaign in Cambridge: do short-term campaigns work? *BMC Public Health*. 2010;10(1):339. doi:10.1186/1471-2458-10-339

93. Dumesnil H, Verger P. Public awareness campaigns about depression and suicide: a review. *Psychiatr Serv*. 2009;60(9):1203–1213. doi:10.1176/ps.2009.60.9.1203

94. Everly GS. Psychological first aid to support healthcare professionals. *J Patient Saf Risk Manag*. 2020;25(4):159–162. doi:10.1177/2516043520944637

95. Gispen F, Wu AW. Psychological first aid: CPR for mental health crises in healthcare. *J Patient Saf Risk Manag*. 2018;23(2):51–53. doi:10.1177/2516043518762826

96. Moutier C, Norcross W, Jong P, et al. The suicide prevention and depression awareness program at the University of California, San Diego School of Medicine. *Acad Med*. 2012;87(3):320–326. doi:10.1097/ACM.0b013e31824451ad

97. Schernhammer ES, Colditz GA. Suicide rates among physicians: a quantitative and gender assessment (meta-analysis). *Am J Psychiatry*. 2004;161(12):2295–2302. doi:10.1176/appi.ajp.161.12.2295

98. Aaronson AL, Backes K, Agarwal G, Goldstein JL, Anzia J. Mental health during residency training: assessing the barriers to seeking care. *Acad Psychiatry*. 2018;42(4):469–472. doi:10.1007/s40596-017-0881-3

99. Pheister M, Peters RM, Wrzosek MI. The impact of mental illness disclosure in applying for residency. *Acad Psychiatry*. 2020;44(5):554–561. doi:10.1007/s40596-020-01227-8

100. Karp JF, Levine AS. Mental health services for medical students — time to act. *N Engl J Med*. 2018;379(13):1196–1198. doi:10.1056/NEJMp1803970

101. Ey S, Moffit M, Kinzie JM, Brunett PH. Feasibility of a comprehensive wellness and suicide prevention program: a decade of caring for physicians in training and practice. *J Grad Med Educ*. 2016;8(5):747–753. doi:10.4300/JGME-D-16-00034.1

102. Ey S, Moffit M, Kinzie JM, Choi D, Girard DE. "If you build it, they will come": attitudes of medical residents and fellows about seeking services in a resident wellness program. *J Grad Med Educ*. 2013;5(3):486–492. doi:10.4300/JGME-D-12-00048.1

103. Major A, Williams JG, McGuire WC, Floyd E, Chacko K. Removing barriers: a confidential opt-out mental health pilot program for internal medicine interns. *Acad Med*. 2021;96(5):686–689. doi:10.1097/ACM.0000000000003965

104. Sofka S, Grey C, Lerfald N, Davisson L, Howsare J. Implementing a universal well-being assessment to mitigate barriers to resident utilization of mental health resources. *J Grad Med Educ*. 2018;10(1):63–66. doi:10.4300/JGME-D-17-00405.1

105. Sofka S, Lerfald N, Reece J, Davisson L, Howsare J, Thompson J. Universal well-being assessment associated with increased resident utilization of mental health resources and decrease in professionalism breaches. *J Grad Med Educ.* 2021;13(1):83–88. doi:10.4300/JGME-D-20-00352.1

106. Albott CS, Wozniak JR, McGlinch BP, Wall MH, Gold BS, Vinogradov S. Battle buddies: rapid deployment of a psychological resilience intervention for health care workers during the COVID-19 pandemic. *Anesth Analg.* 2020;131(1):43–54. doi:10.1213/ANE.0000000000004912

107. ACGME. After a suicide: a toolkit for physician residency/fellowship programs. Accessed June 2, 2021. https://www.acgme.org/globalassets/PDFs/13287_AFSP_After_Suicide_Clinician_Tool kit_Final_2.pdf

7

Individually Focused Well-Being Interventions

Farah N. Hussain, Mary Elizabeth Yaden, and Oana Tomescu

Introduction

The health and well-being of medical students and GME trainees is central to their development as humanistic providers and compassionate leaders. As we have stressed throughout this book, to make any significant impact on burnout and poor health during medical training and beyond, medical organizations, not just individual trainees, are accountable for interventions that positively impact personal health and well-being. Organizations have a vested interest in the health of individual members: the World Health Organization has emphasized the intrinsic link between an organization's "health" (i.e., productivity, outcomes, status, and optimal functioning), and the health of its individual members.[1] Therefore, medical systems, schools, and training programs have a responsibility to build ecosystems that foster well-being among medical students and GME trainees by nurturing individual growth, engagement, and health. When medical students and GME trainees feel valued, appreciated, and acknowledged, they develop to their fullest potential, exceed the high expectations of our profession, and help their organizations function optimally.

A successful and comprehensive well-being program must address the multifactorial drivers of burnout at all levels. Our Shared Responsibility Framework (Figure 7.1), which is adapted from several frameworks for addressing well-being described in Chapter 1, embraces this philosophy and organizes well-being interventions into four domains: (1) system-level factors that target workplace efficiency, organizational values, and learning environment factors; (2) organizational culture of well-being that fosters diversity, equity,

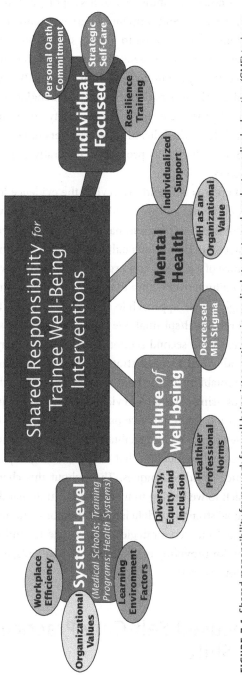

FIGURE 7.1 Shared responsibility framework for well-being interventions in medical students and graduate medical education (GME) trainees.

and inclusion, and propagates healthier professional norms; (3) mental health interventions that champion psychological safety, decrease stigma associated with mental health care, and provide broad access for individualized support; and (4) individual-focused interventions that optimize one's commitment to personal self-care and resilience strategies. While organizations are best suited to impact system-level changes and promote cultural shifts, individuals must also embrace their own responsibility to be as intentional in their self-care practice as they are in their medical training. Because chronic exposure to human suffering makes this profession inherently challenging, individual buy-in and regular engagement in self-care are essential for longevity and well-being. This chapter advocates for a cultural shift in which health care providers not only prioritize their own self-care, but also embrace self-care as protective, restorative, and essential to lifelong learning and serving others.

The goal of this chapter is two-fold: we review the evidence for self-care strategies that promote learner well-being, and we highlight how these individual-focused interventions can be incorporated into programmatic structures and wellness curricula and used to positively impact an organization's culture of well-being. In the first section, we emphasize the importance of a societal and organizational shift toward prioritizing physician well-being and a cultural shift within the profession toward proactive self-care and healthy altruism. We highlight an approach to strategic self-care in three domains: physical, psychological, and relational/spiritual. We then discuss how to strategically optimize the practice of self-care. In the second section, we summarize ways to creatively integrate evidence-based individual-focused strategies into programmatic structures, thus optimizing shared accountability. In the final section, we describe how well-being skills can be taught to trainees using a variety of evidence-based techniques such as mindfulness, compassion, self-compassion, positive psychology, resilience training, creative expression, reflection-based practices, and facilitated discussions. In addition, we provide a framework for a longitudinal curriculum that utilizes small group sessions as a delivery model for these evidence-based techniques. Throughout this chapter, we champion a strengths-based approach to well-being in medical education that does not oversimplify well-being as an individual strength or deficiency. We advocate for reframing the learning and practice of individual-focused strategies as a vehicle for individual longevity and health in the profession, for providing better care to our patients, and for optimizing the health of the organizations we serve.

Individual-Focused Self-Care Practices: A Necessary Shift

The well-being of health care providers is central to their ability to deliver humanistic and compassionate care to their patients. However, this ideal has only recently been championed within the medical profession. Building on the World Health Organization's framework that links organizational "health" to the well-being of its individual members, the "quadruple aim" introduced in Chapter 1 advocates for the addition and inclusion of health care team well-being into health systems improvement efforts.[2] There is growing support for health care organizations' accountability for the well-being of its individual members,[3,4] and this chapter similarly promotes this shared responsibility philosophy.

The initial trend in company-sponsored well-being interventions is exemplified by the "5 PM mindfulness (or yoga, or resilience) class" offered to students/physicians by their organizations. This approach is often met with cynicism and backfires by not only oversimplifying well-being as purely an individual deficiency, but also by failing to acknowledge the complex system-level drivers of burnout. Placing the responsibility solely on individuals breeds resentment and resistance toward individual-focused interventions: the words *wellness*, *resilience*, and *self-care* currently carry a negative connotation for many physicians.[5] In addition, the timing of offered wellness interventions matters: forcing individuals to choose between an enrichment class or going home to attend to their needs and interests outside of work places the burden on the individual. Finally, and most importantly, individually-focused wellness training is insufficient as an isolated intervention. The benefit of organization-directed interventions is clear: system-level interventions seem to have a more significant impact on overall well-being than do individual-focused interventions.[6,7] System-level interventions are described in further detail in Chapter 8. As we describe in the rest of the chapter, individual self-care still has importance for sustaining a lifetime of practice in an inherently challenging profession; thus, messaging the importance of a shared responsibility between the organization and the individual is essential to supporting individuals to adopt self-care strategies that work for them.

A Cultural Shift Toward Healthy Altruism

Pathologic altruism has been defined as "a need to sacrifice oneself for the benefit of others"[8] and as "the willingness of a person to irrationally place another's perceived needs above his or her own in a way that causes self-harm."[9] While this term was not coined specifically about the medical profession, it accurately describes an unhealthy cultural norm that frequently plagues both learners and practicing physicians and manifests as self-care neglect. A cultural shift is needed toward *healthy* altruism. The World Medical Association amended the Declaration of Geneva in 2017 to include a statement charging physicians to care for their own health with the same commitment and intensity they apply to caring for their patients.[10] Two other recent publications, the Charter on Physician Well-Being[11] and Oath to Self-Care and Well-Being,[12] have also stressed that making a personal commitment to one's health is critical for career longevity, professionalism, and personal well-being. Younger generations have entered the profession seeking more integration of work and well-being needs.[13,14] However, for a cultural shift to occur, program-level modifications to the typically inflexible and time-intensive schedules of medical school and clinical training are required in addition to individual buy-in. Schools and training programs can advocate for healthier cultural/professional norms by emphasizing the importance of a personal commitment to self-care at every opportunity: orientation, email communications, recruitment sessions, and wellness curricula, etc. Concurrently, programs must also implement organization-level changes to facilitate the practice of individual-focused strategies by medical students and GME trainees. Every member of the medical profession has an individual responsibility for embracing and propagating healthier norms; in addition, this cultural shift must also be encouraged and facilitated at the organizational level. Culture change is also a shared responsibility opportunity and happens most effectively when embraced by both individuals and organizations.

Strategic Self-Care

Lack of time due to long work hours and high educational and professional demands is a leading driver of poor self-care practices by physicians and learners. Given this limited time, we propose a more proactive and strategic approach to individual health practices. Foremost, a common definition of self-care greatly limits potential benefits by primarily focusing on physical and quality-of-life needs: sleep, healthy nutrition, hobbies, etc. This framing of self-care limits its applicability to time outside of work, thereby missing an opportunity to integrate self-care into work. The outdated concept of "work–life balance" has similarly fallen out of favor because of the resulting implication that work is always draining and therefore separated from and in opposition to meaningful aspects of life. More recently, approaches have shifted toward the concept of *work-life integration*, recognizing individuals as whole people who have important personal needs both inside and outside of work hours.

A more holistic definition of self-care is needed that incorporates other dimensions of well-being and includes sustaining practices and experiences that can be deployed *during* the workday. The following approach to *strategic self-care* incorporates an evidence-based, multi-dimensional toolkit of strategies (Figure 7.2) that can be personalized,

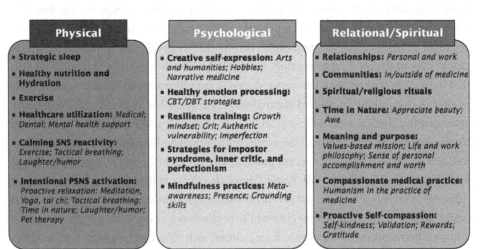

FIGURE 7.2 Strategies to support physical health, psychological and mental health, and relational/spiritual needs.

practiced, and honed. Although this framework organizes self-care strategies into three core domains (physical, psychological, and relational/spiritual), we acknowledge that implementation of the listed strategies will have positive impacts in multiple domains. Strategic self-care is versatile: individuals need a diverse and personalized toolkit characterized by several strategies in each domain that can be utilized with flexibility during busier learning and training periods. This expanded definition of self-care also allows for practices to be integrated during the workday, not just outside of work. Careers in medicine are characterized by intense work commitments and long hours, but also by meaningful moments derived from caring for others, working in teams, belonging to supportive work communities, teaching and/or doing research, and practicing the science and art of medicine. Our framework builds on the concept of work–life integration by encouraging individuals to pay special attention to these positive and rejuvenating moments and count them as part of their own strategic self-care.

In summary, the practice of incorporating restorative strategies with awareness, intention, and commitment in real time throughout the day, both at work *and* outside of work, is the optimal conceptualization of strategic self-care. Such an approach does not "other" self-care activities such that they feel onerous or burdensome, but rather integrates them into work life. On an individual level, prioritizing and practicing self-care with a dedication equal to how we approach our medical education is necessary for the profession's shift toward healthier cultural norms. Organizational buy-in is also necessary: without a shared responsibility philosophy that generates change at the system level, the individual practice of strategic self-care cannot be optimized or integrated into work.

Evidence-Based Strategic Self-Care Practices

An extensive body of literature exists for the many strategies listed in Figure 7.2, and, in the next section, we provide a summary of the evidence behind specific individual health strategies for medical students and GME trainees. Studies that include populations of practicing physicians or non-medical trainees are included only when other data are not available. Strategies are categorized into the same three domains that comprise the Strategic Self-Care Framework: physical, psychological, and relational/spiritual health practices. We discuss the evidence behind each strategy and provide best-practice examples for how training programs and medical schools can facilitate engagement in the specific practice by integrating them creatively into various programmatic structures.

Physical Health Practices

Sleep

Sleep is debatably the most foundational physical self-care strategy for our profession. Despite work-hours reform, sleep deprivation is still a reality in medical training[15,16] and has been associated with autonomic dysfunction,[17] poor neurocognitive performance,[18,19] perceived medical errors,[20] depression,[20–23] a decline in empathy,[24] and burnout.[25] Based on these and many other studies, the American Academy of Sleep Medicine recommends further evaluation of the role of sleep disruption and deprivation and circadian misalignment in physician well-being and burnout.[26]

Interventions aimed at ameliorating sleep deprivation and its consequences have been extensively studied at both the program and system levels. Program-level interventions using protected nap periods for "on-call" residents show increased sleep duration and alertness, though they can be difficult to operationalize practically.[27–29] At the system level, sleep deprivation has been the central driver of Accreditation Council for Graduate Medical Education (ACGME) duty-hour reform since the tragic death of Libby Zion in 1984.[30,31] The focus of this chapter is too broad to adequately discuss the extensive literature on the impact of work-hour limits since 2003; however, we will highlight two recent studies with a focus on their findings on sleep deprivation. The Flexibility in Duty Hour Requirements for Surgical Trainees (FIRST) trial evaluated outcome differences between standard 16-hour shift lengths for surgical interns with flexible shift length without restrictions (meaning shifts could be 24 hours or more).[32] This study showed no significant differences between the study groups on perceived fatigue. A similarly structured study in internal medicine interns, the Individualized Comparative Effectiveness of Models Optimizing Patient Safety and Resident Education (iCOMPARE), evaluated multiple outcomes comparing 16-hour shifts to longer shifts without limits.[33] While there was no difference in burnout, and sleep time per 24 hours was not different when analyzed across 14 days, there were significant differences in sleep length and alertness between the two groups according to shift type that confirmed historical concerns about reduced sleep and alertness during and after extended overnight shifts (e.g., 24 or more hours).[34] These trials and well-being outcomes are described in further detail in Chapters 3 and 7. The current evidence shows that sleep deprivation remains a significant concern despite the 2011 work-hour changes, and larger structural changes are likely needed to optimize sleep hygiene.

Healthy Nutrition

Healthy nutrition is another physical health strategy that warrants attention due to the poor nutritional habits among trainees.[35–38] The drivers of these negative lifestyle changes during training include poor nutrition education,[39,40] lack of time, cost, and high stress levels.[41] Nutrition education electives for preclinical medical students significantly improved self-reported nutritional practices.[42,43] More broadly, a 6-week, 12-hour Healthy Living elective that utilized behavioral goal setting was successful in improving physical self-care practices and was associated with an improved perception of self-reported health status in medical students.[44] For residents and fellows, the main factors contributing to poor nutritional practices include lack of time, overly stringent work ethic, cost of healthy food, and limited choice and/or poor access to healthy food especially during night shifts.[45,46] Providing regular, healthy snacks to working residents showed a positive impact on self-reported cognitive functioning and hypoglycemic symptoms.[47] In summary, training programs and schools can integrate nutrition education into curricula and make healthier nutrition and hydration more accessible during work hours while also targeting unhealthy professional norms (like workaholism) and promoting a culture of self-care that includes regular breaks for nutrition.

Exercise

Exercise has well-established benefits physically, emotionally, and cognitively. Healthy exercise habits have been shown to be associated with a lower prevalence of burnout in GME trainees and practicing physicians.[48-50] Most medical students maintain adequate exercise and fitness levels during medical school, with high stress and lack of time being cited as barriers.[51,52] However, physical activity declines during residency, with lack of time cited as the most common reason for poor exercise habits.[53-55] For these reasons, facilitation of individual engagement in exercise/physical activity has been studied and shows positive impacts. Providing GME trainees multimodal exercise interventions (activity trackers, team-based competitions, free access to fitness resources, etc.) demonstrated improvement in several health outcomes, including systolic blood pressure, HDL cholesterol, and utilization of fitness and nutrition resources.[56,57] Participation in a voluntary, team-based, incentivized exercise program for medical fellows and residents at a large institution, with access to institutional exercise facilities, was associated with significantly increased physical activity, higher median quality of life, and a trend toward decreased burnout.[58] A broader fitness program offered to residents that included multiple activity opportunities with peers as well as exercise testing and group conferences showed good uptake and positive effect on body mass index (BMI) during the intervention.[54] Similarly, participation in a motivational fitness curriculum improved depression, anxiety, stress, and emotional exhaustion scores in family medicine residents post-curriculum.[59] In summary, while exercise is a highly individualized strategy, there are several interventions that training programs and organizations can implement to promote this protective self-care strategy, such as providing access to on-site exercise equipment and incentive programs.

Health Care Utilization

Health care underutilization, or lack of obtaining routine and preventive medical care, by GME trainees and practicing physicians is a long-standing problem. Studies of practicing physicians in the late 1990s and early 2000s show poor health care utilization: only one-third of physicians had identified their own primary care physician,[60] most showed low engagement in preventative services,[61] and few sought medical attention for acute symptoms.[62] Physicians described several reasons that contributed to this phenomenon: some felt pressure to portray an unrealistically healthy image, others did not want to be a burden to colleagues by taking time off to seek medical attention, and many reported alternating states of panic due to knowledge of the worse-case scenario and denial that illness cannot happen to them.[63] Sadly, poor medical health care utilization by GME trainees remains a concerning issue for younger generations as well.[64] Mental health care underutilization across all ages/stages in our profession continues to contribute to the epidemic of poor mental health and burnout. In addition, systemic causes, such as lack of time to attend appointments, are common barriers for GME trainees. Program- and organization-level interventions that facilitate health care utilization by GME trainees include protected time off for appointments, concierge care coordination, facilitated referral support for scheduling appointments, access to telemedicine visits, confidential care without perceived conflicts of interest in the training environment, and co-location of medical and mental health care.[65-68] Ways to improve access to and utilization of mental health care are discussed further in Chapter 9. These program-level interventions address both the time limitations learners generally face and help shift the cultural expectation toward healthy self-care and altruism.

Mind–Body Practices

Mind–body practices calm sympathetic nervous system reactivity, strengthen parasympathetic outflow, and have been shown to be of benefit in medical education. The high stress and fast pace of medical training and its concurrent sleep deprivation have a detrimental impact on autonomic nervous system health.[69,70] *Autogenic training* incorporates visualization or repetitive phrases with the specific goal of activating the parasympathetic nervous system and inducing a state of relaxation. Techniques such as biofeedback, guided imagery, relaxation, meditation, and deep diaphragmatic breathing are all examples of autogenic training. Such interventions have been shown to have a modest positive impact on some clinical conditions including tension headache/migraines, mild-moderate hypertension, pain disorders, anxiety, depression, and functional sleep disorders.[71] Many medical schools have incorporated mind–body courses that teach autogenic training techniques into the academic curriculum, with modest benefits in multiple domains.[72-75] *Tactical breathing* (also known as *box breathing*, *combat breathing*, or *deep diaphragmatic breathing*), for example, is a technique taught by the military and is the cornerstone of biofeedback training used for many symptoms or illnesses.[76] Interventions using this technique in resident physicians showed improved rates of successful simulated intubation in emergency medicine residents[77] and decreased emotional exhaustion in family medicine residents.[78] Other well-established practices to promote autonomic health via parasympathetic outflow augmentation, which we term *intentional relaxation*, include yoga, tai-chi, meditation, acupuncture/acupressure, nature therapy, pet therapy, and laughter/humor. Mindfulness training is discussed in more detail below.

Psychological Health Practices

Creative Self-Expression

Creative self-expression is an established psychological health practice, whether through hobbies such as art, music, writing, or cooking/baking or through engagement in outside-of-medicine interests, including the arts and humanities. For this discussion, we focus on art-based interventions and narrative medicine as two humanities-based examples of individual and group-based activities that can be emphasized during wellness sessions. Art-based interventions in trainees have been shown to improve emotional exhaustion and depersonalization[79] as well as outcomes related to mindfulness, emotional processing, communication, team-building, awareness of personal biases, recognition of personal accomplishments, and tolerance of uncertainty.[80–85] Art-based interventions in a group setting also have been shown to facilitate social connectedness and psychological safety among trainees.[86–87] Narrative medicine has been successfully implemented in medical schools and GME training programs in clinical and educational environments.[88–92] Described as "a rigorous intellectual and clinical discipline . . . to recognize, absorb, interpret, and be moved to action by the stories of others,"[93] these activities allow medical students and GME trainees to externalize their experiences, uncover commonalities and differences, and view encounters through varying perspectives.[94–96] Though standardized assessments remain elusive, data from several systematic reviews and individual studies suggest that narrative medicine shows promise as a strategy for improving medical student and GME trainee reflection, empathy, communication, resilience, and burnout.[97–101]

Healthy Emotion Processing

Healthy emotion processing is a core theme in the approach to strategic self-care (Figure 7.2) and emphasizes developing adaptive coping strategies with the goal of preventing overreliance on maladaptive practices (e.g., substance use, excessive gambling or shopping, etc.). Healthy emotional processing is a foundational component of high emotional intelligence and, as such, is an appropriate longitudinal theme in a wellness curriculum (further described below). By developing their self-regulatory and emotion handling skills, medical students and GME trainees will be better prepared to support and respond to patient emotions, a skill crucial for delivering humanistic and compassionate care. A variety of strategies can be taught to medical students and GME trainees. Although not explicitly studied in resident physicians, specific skills in distress tolerance and emotion regulation from dialectical behavior therapy have shown significant promise in clinical populations.[102] In addition, creative expression, mindfulness techniques, gratitude practice, and growth mindset approaches can also be applied to healthy emotion processing. High emotional intelligence can benefit medical students and GME trainees in many ways. By honing their self-regulatory and emotion handling skills, they will be better prepared to support and manage patient emotions, a skill that is central to the delivery of humanistic and compassionate care. Similarly, because high emotional intelligence is crucial to effective leadership, honing these skills will positively impact team dynamics and any future leadership role that the trainee holds.

Resilience Training

Resilience training refers to the practice of adaptive cognitive strategies that strengthen our ability to process emotions, face adversity, overcome failures, and grow despite challenges that come our way. Ample evidence exists for the many cognitive and behavioral techniques that fit under this definition and enhance a growth mindset, grit, authentic vulnerability, and willingness to embrace imperfection.[103–106] Learning how to healthfully process complex emotions can also be considered part of resilience training, as can positive psychology and mindfulness practices. These concepts and techniques can be integrated into wellness curricula as adaptive strategies that help medical students and GME trainees cope with the challenging experiences that occur during training and beyond (see below).

Strategies to Address Impostor Syndrome and Perfectionism

Strategies to address impostor syndrome and perfectionism are important given how common imposterism and perfectionism are in the medical community. "Imposter syndrome" was first described in the literature as "a self-perceived intellectual or professional phoniness despite evidence to the contrary."[107] This type of negative thought pattern, or cognitive distortion, overlaps with both perfectionism and with having a strong inner critical voice that is harsh and judgmental. Perfectionism is debatably one of the most destructive tendencies commonly found in the medical profession: during medical training and beyond, there is often either internalized or explicit pressure to be perfect, to know everything, to suppress strong emotions and fear, and to never show effort or struggle (be perfect at being perfect). To this point, high perfectionism and impostor syndrome, respectively, were identified in 25% and 32% of first-year medical students in one institution and were associated with high levels of shame, inadequacy, anxiety, and depression.[108] A variety of evidence-based strategies can help medical students and GME trainees reprogram these cognitive distortions as part of a longitudinal curriculum, as described later in the chapter.

Positive Psychology

Positive psychology embraces a strengths-based perspective by building on what is strong rather than just repairing what is wrong.[109] Ample evidence exists outside of the field of medicine for the various benefits of individual-focused positive psychology practices that promote positive emotions and well-being, cultivate positive behaviors and cognitions, and reduce symptoms of depression while enhancing both subjective and measured well-being.[110–113] Examples of positive psychology exercises associated with positive impact on well-being include savoring (replaying mentally) positive experiences, cultivating hope for the future and gratitude for the present, engaging in strengths-based activities, and practicing kindness and humor.[114] By intentionally amplifying positive experiences and emotions, these practices help counteract the inherent negativity bias of the human brain, which allows for easy formation of negative memories as an evolutionarily protective mechanism.[115–117] With repetition, positive psychology techniques harness the neuroplasticity of the human brain to retrain it to actively store positive memories.

The complementary nature of positive psychology and coaching psychology has led to the creation of coaching frameworks that use positive psychology tenets.[118-120] Providing positive psychology training to mentors of internal medicine interns resulted in high satisfaction and decreased emotional exhaustion for the mentees after 1 year, as well as a positive association between coaching program experience and increased coping and relational skills after 3 years.[121,122] A similar positive psychology mentoring program in a community hospital setting resulted in high levels of satisfaction of mentees with the intervention.[123] Interestingly, a larger, multisite study of this same intervention showed positive overall benefit for mentees but detected significant gender and racial differences in well-being and emotional exhaustion following the intervention. In both cases, groups who experience more structural inequality and discrimination (i.e., women and physicians of color) did not experience the same degree of positive impact as their white male peers.[124] This finding highlights the need for further investigation of how mentoring can be best tailored to support trainees from minoritized groups who disproportionately face structural inequality. In summary, the field of positive psychology can benefit medical education through augmenting current models of mentorship as well as by providing concrete practices that can be incorporated into wellness curricula.

Mindfulness Practices

Mindfulness practices help cultivate a specific kind of present-moment awareness: one that is nonjudgmental, compassionate, and encompasses both internal and external experiences. Formal mindfulness training that utilizes the 8-week Mindfulness-Based Stress Reduction (MBSR) course based on the work of Dr. Jon Kabat-Zinn has been shown to have clear well-being benefits in populations of medical students and practicing physicians who choose to participate. In medical students, *voluntary* participation in an MBSR elective increased distress tolerance, decreased burnout, and improved quality of life.[125-128] However, required participation in mindfulness training of an entire cohort of first-year medical students did not show any significant benefits, highlighting the need to offer a variety of strategies to trainees to best fit their temperaments and individual preferences.[129] MBSR training may be even more effective in practicing physicians, where several studies have shown decreased burnout, improved heart rate and blood pressure, increased positive mood states, and enhanced meaningfulness and work satisfaction.[130-139] While no study has been published evaluating the intensive 8-week MBSR intervention in resident physicians, a few have had mixed success with abbreviated interventions.[140-143] A tailored mindfulness-based program offered to a small cohort of residents improved several qualitative perceptions, including the ability to integrate mindfulness into everyday life, self-awareness, equanimity, well-being, and patient interactions.[144] Mindfulness training has clear positive benefits on affective and cognitive functioning for participants who volunteer to participate in such programs. Therefore, mindfulness is an important individual-focused strategy that should be offered in wellness curricula as one example of a proactive self-care strategy.

Relational/Spiritual Strategies

Belonging and Connectivity

A sense of belonging and connectivity are central to one's resilience and well-being.[145] These constructs, when applied to medical education,[146-148] seem to be particularly critical to the well-being of minoritized communities,[149-152] women in medicine,[152] and international graduates.[153] Program interventions that augment a sense of belonging, especially for minority GME trainees, have positive benefits and warrant further evaluation given increasing recognition of the importance of diversity, equity, and inclusion at all levels of our profession. Thus, we emphasize the importance of nurturing relationships and communities (both at work and outside of work) as critical self-care strategies that fall into this third domain.

Opportunities for Spiritual/Religious Practice

Opportunities for spiritual/religious practice are also critical for well-being for many physicians, students, and GME trainees. Emerging evidence in practicing physicians and medical students suggests an association between well-being and spirituality.[154,155] Small cross-sectional studies in internal medicine residents have demonstrated a relationship between spirituality and positive coping throughout training.[156,157] Curricula in spiritual and religious competency have been integrated into GME trainee education in several specialties;[158,159] however, there is a comparative dearth of scholarship exploring the role of secular rituals or spiritual practices in medical student and GME trainee mental health and well-being. Wider hospital system approaches may suggest a role for spiritual or secular rituals in medical education. For example, ICU team implementation of a sacred pause following a patient death has been shown to provide a sense of professional satisfaction, appreciation, and a sense of closure for providers.[160] In particular, palliative care trainees may enjoy particular benefits from engaging in secular or spiritual rituals given the prominence of end-of-life care in their clinical work.[161]

Finding Meaning in Work

Finding meaning in work has been highlighted as a protective self-care strategy in medical education.[162] Adopting a life and work philosophy aligned with core values has also been highlighted as protective in practicing physicians.[163-165] Reflecting on core values, a process known as *self-affirmation*, has several established benefits that may be relevant to medical students and GME trainees, including increased well-being and resilience in non-medical populations.[166,167] This technique can be used to reflect on what is most important in life, and it has been shown to positively impact self-regulation and performance in non-trainee populations.[168] Additionally, studies in practicing physicians as well as medical students have shown a positive association between a sense of greater meaning or personal "calling" and domains associated with increased well-being and diminished burnout.[169,170] Educational interventions have been proposed that support the development and reflection on greater meaning in clinical work.[171] Perhaps the most widely implemented program, the Healer's Art Curriculum, has been utilized in medical schools across the world.[172] This course, which was developed for medical students, provides an opportunity for small-group reflection on themes that include finding a sense of awe in clinical practice as well as caring for oneself through experiences of grief and loss.[173] Studies have shown that, even after completing medical school, the benefits of the curriculum are sustained in subsequent training.[174] There have also been examples of how this curriculum has been adapted for resident trainees: one pediatric program demonstrated that residents experienced a greater sense of belonging and expressed a renewed commitment to patient-centered care after participating in the curriculum.[175]

Enhancing Humanism and Compassion

Humanism and compassion have clear benefits not only for the patients receiving compassion, but also for the caregivers themselves. Caring for patients in a compassionate way benefits patients by improving their health outcomes, increasing engagement in self-care practices, and improving perceived quality of care.[176] Remarkably though, practicing with compassion also clearly benefits clinician well-being. Functional MRI data show that taking actions to relieve someone's suffering stimulates a "reward" pathway in the brain that activates positive emotions and affiliation/connection.[177] Additionally, cross-sectional studies show that high compassion is associated with low burnout and vice-versa.[178] Compassion-based interventions have begun to take root within the medical community.[179] One randomized controlled trial examined how cognitive-based compassion training (CBCT), in an 8- to 10-week course informed by Tibetan Buddhist compassion meditation, improved depression and loneliness and increased compassion in a second-year medical student cohort.[180] Another multiweek course based on Tibetan Buddhist compassion meditation, compassion cultivation training (CCT), showed quantitative improvements in mindfulness as well as qualitative enhancement in stress reduction in medical students.[181,182] Given its potential benefits to both patients and clinicians, offering compassion skills training should be considered as part of longitudinal medical training.

Building Self-Compassion

Self-compassion is a psychological orientation that promotes a warm and compassionate stance toward the self.[183] Self-compassion may have a uniquely protective role against burnout in physicians[184,185] and may be especially important for those who have high perfectionism and impostor syndrome. Several studies have shown that GME trainees and medical students with higher levels of self-compassion experience less burnout.[186-188] An intervention to cultivate self-compassion for health care communities was recently developed by Dr. Kristin Neff and colleagues. Although this intervention has yet to be formally investigated in a medical student or GME trainee cohort, it has shown promise as an intervention to target burnout in the broader health care community.[189] While relatively new as a self-care technique, self-compassion training should also be considered for integration into wellness curricula.

Operationalizing a Longitudinal Wellness Curriculum

Many medical schools and GME training programs have begun to implement longitudinal curricula focused on individual strategies of wellness and resilience. The primary goal of a wellness curriculum is to mitigate training-related empathy loss and burnout and ultimately improve clinician well-being and the clinician–patient relationship through improved communication, quality of care, trust, compassion, and satisfaction.[185–194] A secondary goal is to provide medical students or GME trainees with multiple and diverse examples of adaptive coping strategies to help them expand their definition and practice of self-care and become less reliant on maladaptive strategies. Third, by emphasizing shared experience and vulnerability, sessions can increase awareness of unhealthy cultural norms, foster a sense of belonging, and nurture a culture of safety and resilience.

A strong biological argument exists for teaching self-care strategies to students and GME trainees and encouraging them to practice and hone these new skill sets. Regular practice of key strategies is critical to maintaining their benefits and can be emphasized during curricular sessions by discussing the neuroscience behind repetitive learning (i.e., neuroplasticity) to engender buy-in. Mechanistically speaking, the inherent neuroplasticity of the human brain allows for new learning and skill building. The repetition of any technique leads to axonal pruning, synaptic reorganization, and neural network recruitment, changing the way the brain is "wired," which further facilitates the performance of the technique. Neuroplasticity, however, is not always healthy. Maladaptive coping strategies have been shown to lead to dysfunctional neuroplasticity through strengthening of reward-seeking pathways, while the practice of healthy coping strategies leads to adaptive changes that strengthen cognitive control of the limbic system.[195] The time of greatest neuroplasticity occurs prior to age 30, which is why we advocate for the formal integration of wellness curricula at the medical school and GME levels. Fortunately, brains older than 30 years can be "rewired" with repetitive practice as well, which is why individual-directed interventions have been shown to also benefit practicing physicians as well.[196]

Avoiding Curricular Pitfalls

Although wellness curricula have become ubiquitous in training programs, medical educators frequently encounter generalized pessimism toward these interventions.[197] Wellness sessions are best received by learners when schools and programs embrace a shared accountability philosophy by focusing on efforts to optimize system-level opportunities for student and GME trainee health and engagement while also integrating wellness content into the academic curriculum. In addition, wellness programming must be approached with a growth mindset and strengths-based perspective. Interventions undertaken from a deficiency perspective (i.e., learners are not resilient enough) breed resentment and disengagement by failing to acknowledge that learners enter medical school with higher altruism, lower burnout, and higher physical and emotional health compared to age-matched college graduates.[198] Introduction of the concept of a *growth mindset* (openness to continuous self-improvement and building on strengths) may increase acceptance and uptake of wellness content by framing the importance of self-development in the same way we approach life-long learning to care for others.[87,199] When schools and training programs embrace and operationalize this shared responsibility philosophy and deliver wellness content that is strength-based in its approach, learners are more likely to feel cared for and supported and to be engaged in their own self-care and self-development.

Another pitfall of wellness curricula is that many have limited structure, consistency, and goals. The development and implementation of wellness curricula must be undertaken with the same rigor as other aspects of the formal medical training curriculum. Session facilitators should be trained in wellness techniques and promote instruction through evidence-based approaches. If possible, facilitators should not be in evaluative roles, as such structures may inhibit the cultivation of so-called *sanctuary spaces* where students and GME trainees can share vulnerability openly. Sessions should also be integrated into existing didactic scheduling within protected time in order to limit excess burden on learners, which can increase stress and resentment. Attendance generally should be strongly encouraged, but with an option to opt-out on a case-by-case basis, to emphasize that this training is as important as other aspects of the curriculum. Last, facilitators must continually assess the effectiveness of the curriculum through feedback to adjust the curriculum and include topics and sessions that are requested by learners. Without such approaches, students and GME trainees are likely to become disillusioned by the perceived lack of institutional support and adaptation.

Incorporating Multimodal Techniques and Activities

Given the variability of medical learners' coping strategies, levels of compassion, empathy, and altruism, and attitudes toward self-development, it is imperative that wellness curricula utilize a multimodal approach and highlight an assortment of practices rather than using a "one-size fits all" approach.[200-202] Adult learning theory techniques such as experiential and interactive learning can deliver content in a way that is well-received by learners.[203,204] Highlighting a broad array of wellness strategies helps to ensure that all students and GME trainees are introduced to techniques that are accessible to them and allows them to personalize strategies that are most helpful. We recommend delivering content to small cohorts that can be modeled after traditional Balint groups—small groups with a trained facilitator that are focused on processing emotionally challenging experiences of medical training and caring for patients.[205] Small-group settings are a perfect vehicle to foster belonging and social connectivity between peers and to facilitate community-building through genuine, communal celebrations of successes. They also allow for safer processing of difficult experiences and expressions of vulnerability. The longitudinal continuity of a curriculum delivered in small groups for the duration of school or training allows learners to reflect on their own growth over time, rather than simply exposing self-care deficiencies in a static manner. In the following section, we discuss strategies for implementing each type of activity, although curricular sessions would ideally include a variety of techniques to ensure integration of complementary strategies.

Art and Humanities-Based Activities

Art and humanities-based activities can be integrated into wellness curricula in a variety of ways. *Art-based interventions* typically utilize two approaches: focusing on observational skills and/or integration of art into traditional curricula.[206] Workshops often include guided observations and facilitated discussions of personal responses to works of art[207] led by faculty and/or museum educators. These sessions are often conducted at local art museums, are "designed for peaceful contemplation and close looking" and provide an external and separate learning environment as compared to the hospital.[87,208] Some sessions also utilize experiential activities, such as exploring sculptures and art-making.[80,81] *Narrative medicine* sessions can be conducted through listening, storytelling, and writing. Most narrative medicine sessions include three main components: (1) examination of a work of art (literature, film, music) through close reading, analysis, and reflection; (2) writing a personal response based on the artistic work or a prompt that encourages deeper reflection; and (3) sharing one's writing in pairs or groups.

Positive Psychology

Positive psychology techniques are extremely versatile and can be emphasized throughout a wellness curriculum. One classic practice known as "three good things" encourages participants to record and reflect on three experiences/moments in their day for which they are grateful.[109] This practice helps individuals remember positive moments in their days and, with repetition, can be used to shift the negativity bias of the brain toward neutral or positive. We also find that this strategy can also be helpful for students or GME trainees struggling with imposter syndrome, with the small modification of writing down what they learned, how they improved, or things they did well during the day. Another positive psychology technique focuses on identifying "signature strengths" and utilizing them in new ways in work and leisure. The VIA Survey of Character Strengths measures 24 unique character strengths and provides guidance on how to further develop and utilize them in daily life.[209] This psychometric tool can be self-administered to participants prior to a session to provide content for discussion and sharing. A third technique called "savoring" can be practiced while eating a small piece of food, as participants are cued to notice and lean into the positive emotions and sensations that arise during the experience.[210] Learners can also be encouraged to "savor" a positive memory or success by replaying the memory in their mind or by sharing good news with a trusted confidant who serves as an "amplifier." This positive psychology term denotes a person who celebrates the successes of another person with excitement, thus amplifying the positive energy. Using these various techniques, learners can be encouraged to magnify sustaining experiences that occur during their days. In summary, positive psychology–based education during medical training offers several versatile interventions that can be utilized in a group setting and/or for individual practice.

Mind–Body Calming Practices

Mind–body calming practices, such as guided body scans and tactical breathing, can also be emphasized throughout a wellness curriculum using brief experiential exercises. The bidirectional signaling of the parasympathetic nervous system that is triggered by taking deep, slow breaths allows the body to soothe and regulate the mind and vice versa. This basic technique can be taught through demonstration and with class participation: a slow inspiration through the nose for a count of 4, followed by a 4-second pause, a 4-second slow exhale, and another 4-second pause. Highlighting the physiological mechanism behind this type of slow breathing helps engender buy-in. Tactical breathing can be utilized during a busy workday to calm the body and mind before important events, like rounds/presentations, procedures, and codes/rapid responses, and to assist with better communication when interacting with patients. Medical students and GME trainees can also be encouraged to link this type of breathing to repetitive actions performed throughout the workday to increase utilization (e.g. washing their hands, logging onto computers, waiting for elevators, etc.).

Mindfulness-Based Practices

Mindfulness-based practices include the mind–body techniques listed above as well as different types of meditation: breath (staying focused on the breath), guided (body scan or imagery), mantra (listening to a repetitive sound), movement (staying grounded with the sensations of moving the body), and mindfulness (watching the thoughts as they pass). Two very common misconceptions about meditation are worth emphasizing throughout wellness curricula. To reap the benefits of meditation, one need *not* practice for many minutes/hours at a time. Stressing that even 5 minutes can be beneficial to calming the body's sympathetic outflow when, for example, using tactical breathing, is important for learners who lack free time. Second, and most importantly, meditation does not require keeping one's mind still. The mind will wander with thoughts, commentary, and judgments. The mind's job is to think, feel, and have opinions, and reminding participants of this function can help decrease the frustration some feel during meditation. In fact, intrinsic to the technique of meditation is recognizing when the mind has wandered into the future or past and bringing it back to the present moment with nonjudgmental compassion. By practicing, one becomes more adept at keeping the mind present in critical moments. Other grounding techniques, like using one's senses to come back to the present moment, are additional mindfulness practices that can be highlighted and practiced during curricular sessions.

Choosing Curricular Content Themes

When choosing content for a longitudinal wellness curriculum, it is important to consider appropriate themes, the neurodevelopmental stage of the intended audience, and the integrated multimodal approach described above. Curricular content of each session should ideally include a theme or topic as well as evidence-based, concrete techniques that are pertinent to the specific theme of the session. Importantly, themes covered in wellness curricula must be regularly updated and adapted, particularly based on learner needs and requests. Examples of sessions that can be integrated into wellness curricula are presented below and summarized in Table 7.1.

Strategic Self-Care

Strategic self-care, as discussed in this chapter, should be a core theme within a wellness curriculum. The holistic framework can be introduced to trainees to help them expand their definition of self-care to include multiple domains. Personalization of self-care strategies is encouraged in developing one's multidimensional toolkit, including examples of how to time-adapt key strategies to busier schedules. Incorporating sustaining practices during the workday should be stressed as a critical part of strategic self-care: connecting with patients, teaching peers or team members, practicing the science and art of medicine, and other examples can be highlighted during facilitated discussion and group sharing. Similarly, the importance of taking breaks for hydration, nutrition and team bonding can also be encouraged. Putting all of the above together during a session on strategic self-care may include didactic content, facilitated group discussion, self-reflective writing, and setting a concrete actionable goal, also known as a SMART (specific, measurable, achievable, relevant, and timebound) goal.

Strategic Sleep

Strategic sleep training is an evidence-based[211] and intentional approach for sleep optimization and fatigue management that can be taught to trainees. A session can begin with a short didactic about the biologic impact of shift work on the brain and the strategic use of caffeine, naps, and other fatigue mitigation measures.[212-216] Facilitated group discussion can highlight the importance of recognizing one's own tolerance of sleep deprivation, since sleep needs vary from person to person.[217] Individuals can reflection about how much sleep is needed *minimally* to avoid next day irritability, a surrogate sign of neurocognitive dysfunction from sleep deprivation that is easy to identify, as well as *optimally* to facilitate flow and maximal function. Strategic sleep training includes circadian shift strategies such as (1) light avoidance after a night shift (sunglasses, cell phone dimming, light-blocking curtains), (2) intentional light exposure prior to a night shift using direct sunlight or a light box, and (3) strategic use of melatonin and caffeine. Last, it can be helpful to demonstrate specific mind–body calming practices as they apply to insomnia management and encourage the use of sleep meditation apps and background sound machines.

TABLE 7.1 Operationalizing a wellness curriculum

Session topic	Description of session/ strategies	Multimodal techniques	Timing of session
Strategic self-care	Introduction of framework **Strategies**: • Personalization and optimization strategies • Integration into workday • Growth mindset	Didactic content Facilitated discussion Writing reflection SMART goal setting	Orientation Framework shown at beginning of subsequent sessions
Strategic sleep	Core concepts of strategic sleep **Strategies**: • Night–day transition strategies • Tactical breathing, meditation for insomnia • Sleep apps and sound machines	Didactic content Facilitated discussion Experiential breathing meditation SMART goal setting	Orientation Revisited as needed
Calming the body and mind	Core concept of ANS reactivity **Strategies**: • Tactical breathing • PSNS activation (pets, nature, exercise) • Mindfulness	Didactic content Facilitated discussion Experiential SMART goal setting	Throughout curriculum
Strategies for difficult transitions	Normalize surprises and challenges of recent transition and imposter syndrome **Strategies**: • Growth mindset • Self-compassion • Positive psychology practices (three good things, gratitude)	Facilitated discussion Writing reflection SMART goal setting	Summer of PGY-1 and PGY-2
Imposter syndrome, perfectionism, and the inner critic	Core concept of negativity bias, validation of imposter syndrome **Strategies**: • Growth mindset • Mindfulness • Externalization of self-critical thoughts • Self-compassion	Facilitated discussion Narrative medicine SMART goal setting	Fall of each academic year, all classes
Raising our EQ: Strategies for healthy emotional processing	Recognition/validation of emotions Core concepts of mind–body biochemistry, processing emotions, coping strategies **Strategies**: • Healthy compartmentalization • Naming emotions • Feeling emotions • Cognitive reframing • Intentional forgiveness	Didactic content Group discussion Artistic expression SMART Goal setting	All levels Linked with experiential museum activity

(continued)

TABLE 7.1 Continued

Session topic	Description of session/ strategies	Multimodal techniques	Timing of session
Finding meaning in medicine	Core concepts of "energy tank" and signature strengths **Strategies:** • Positive psychology • Cognitive reframing • Writing "personal oath"	Didactic content Writing reflection Online module Artistic expression	Winter of academic year Art supplies provided
Difficult patient encounters	Core concept of emotionally challenging patient experiences **Strategies:** • Trauma-informed care • Escaping negative thinking traps • Cognitive reframing • Forgiveness	Narrative medicine Facilitated discussion	All levels of training Any time of year
Coping with suffering, death, and dying	Core concept of normalizing grief, sadness, and need for coping around death and dying, narrative medicine **Strategies:** • Boundary setting • Debriefing and support system • Personal rituals • Forgiveness • Formal mental health support	Narrative medicine Facilitated discussion	All levels of training

Healthy Emotion Processing

Healthy emotion processing, as stated above, is foundational to our Strategic Self-Care Framework because this broad group of techniques helps trainees cope with the myriad emotions they experience throughout their lives and careers. We teach this concept through the lens of raising individual emotional intelligence and highlight how this is beneficial not just to our own well-being, but also to how we care for patients and families and how we function in teams. A variety of strategies increase emotional intelligence, and we stress that everyone needs to have their own personalized toolkit (Box 7.1).

Our session begins with a brief didactic on the physiology of the mind–body impact of emotions, biochemically and from an autonomic nervous system perspective. This provides a general understanding of the bodily sensations associated with different emotions. We make the distinction between positive emotions (like awe, joy, gratitude) and negative emotions (like anger, sadness, frustration) and how they activate the parasympathetic and sympathetic nervous systems, respectively. We also briefly review the neurobiological interplay between the limbic system as storage of mostly negative emotions and the prefrontal cortex as higher-level cognitive control. We next reframe coping strategies as active (adaptive), neutral (e.g., distraction via TV or video games),

BOX 7.1 Raising Our EQ: Processing Emotions Healthfully

Didactic Content
- Mind–body physiology
- Body emotion maps
- Neurobiology of emotion regulation: limbic system and prefrontal cortex

Facilitated Discussion Topics
- Reframing strategies as adaptive, neutral, maladaptive
- Healthy compartmentalization of emotional memories

Processing Emotions Framework
- Emotive strategies to feel directly or channel emotion indirectly
- Cognitive strategies to process and grow
- Practice forgiveness (for self and others)
- Intentionally "letting go"

and numbing (maladaptive) strategies to stress the importance of honing *active* coping techniques to prevent overreliance on neutral (unhealthy distraction/avoidance) and maladaptive strategies. Processing emotions is then taught step by step. We introduce a framework of "healthy compartmentalization" to help trainees conceptually organize and store emotional encounters. We highlight the importance of naming emotions as a core technique via a group artistic expression exercise. Next, we encourage trainees to choose an emotional encounter to process. We then highlight *emotive/feeling strategies* that facilitate limbic system unloading, either directly through talking, writing, or focused meditation, or indirectly by channeling the emotion using exercise, music, dance, movies, books, etc. Exercise, especially high-intensity interval training, is very effective for channeling intense emotions like anger and frustration by allowing an already activated limbic system to exert itself. Creative expression (through writing, music, dance, and/or art) can also be utilized to express intense emotions that have activated the limbic system. Other practices like meditation, tactical breathing, spending time in nature, and pet therapy are examples of practices that can also reduce emotional arousal by activating the parasympathetic nervous system. Once the parasympathetic nervous system and prefrontal cortex are activated, *cognitive strategies* that harness prefrontal cortex abstract thinking can be accessed and deployed. Creative expression through writing, music, art, and cooking/baking can be used as a vehicle for deeper reflection by applying cognitive strategies like perspective-taking, reframing, learning the lesson (i.e., growth mindset), and gratitude practice. We highlight two important final steps in healing the emotional memories/scars that sometimes remain trapped in our hippocampi: forgiveness (of self and other) and intentionally "letting go" of the emotional memory after healthfully processing it.

Strategies to Address Impostor Syndrome and Perfectionism

Impostor syndrome, perfectionism, and harsh inner criticism, as discussed above, are very common and destructive cognitive distortions that plague learners and must be addressed in wellness curricula. These thought patterns are especially powerful during times of transitions, when stepping into new roles and learning new skills. Sessions should be scheduled intentionally around such transitions and should include several evidence-based strategies that can help reprogram these destructive thoughts. Because these negative thought patterns are driven partly by cultural/ethnic factors and familial- and self-expectations, these themes can be safely explored through facilitated group discussion. Similarly, these distortions are also driven by the inherent negativity bias of the human brain, which tends to remember, learn, and form impressions more strongly about negative experiences than positive ones.[218] This is a critical concept that trainees must understand to gain awareness of these destructive thought patterns. Furthermore, these cognitive distortions often trigger secondary and tertiary ruminating emotions like self-doubt and self-loathing and can create an internal cascade of limbic system hyperactivation. Learners can be taught various mindfulness practices to gain awareness of the thoughts, as well as autonomic nervous system countermeasures and other mind–body strategies to blunt their negative physiologic impact. Resilience training strategies like growth mindset, with its emphasis on lifelong, dynamic, and constructive learning, is a natural antidote to impostor syndrome. Facilitated discussion about the dangers of perfectionism can include exploring why this is not only an impossible norm in our profession but a harmful one as well. Fear of failing and of making mistakes stifles learning, and avoiding challenges limits opportunities for growth. A culture of perfection breeds isolation, shame, and self-doubt (i.e., impostor syndrome), from both peers but also from "perfect" role models. Sessions can then highlight a variety of adaptive coping strategies that are antidotes to this combination of thought distortions, including growth mindset, mindfulness/awareness of critical inner dialogue, self-compassion techniques, and positive psychology practices like "three good things" and "savoring" the good that we do.

Finding Meaning

Finding meaning is another important longitudinal theme and technique that can be highlighted in a wellness curriculum. To harness the benefit of this technique, learners must gain awareness of what they find meaningful in their education and work. Sessions that address this topic should provide space for deliberate reflection about personal values. We first guide learners through a writing reflection exercise in which they generate a list of activities/interactions they find sustaining in their day-to-day work lives. We prompt with reminders to consider different settings at work that they have enjoyed (different hospital rotations vs. outpatient clinics) as well as different aspects of their responsibilities (patient care, communication, teaching others, learning the science, etc.). We encourage them to be as *concrete* as possible while listing positive experiences, supportive people, and sustaining values. We then encourage sharing of insights using facilitated discussion. Other techniques, especially from positive psychology, can then be taught to help learners *amplify* the positive experiences/memories. We specifically mention "savoring," celebrating with a trusted amplifier, and using the "three good things" technique. Last, another technique to affirm the self through reflection can involve writing about a personal value and its importance in one's life path. Participants can be provided with a list of common values and prompted to explore ways they have exhibited this value in the past (i.e., serving others, caring for family, practicing courage) and ways they intend to express this value in the future. Both of these experiential activities can be augmented by having learners spend the last 10 minutes of the session writing a personal mission statement that expresses their values and incorporates their individual definition of what is meaningful to them.

In summary, several longitudinal themes can be incorporated into wellness sessions (Table 7.1), several of which were described in detail earlier. When designing session content around a theme, consider when themes are most pertinent for the learner to address and time the session appropriately. Multimodal teaching techniques and evidence-based strategies can be highlighted, and sessions should be as interactive as possible. Importantly, themes covered in wellness curricula must be regularly updated and adapted based on trainee needs and requests.

Conclusion

The Shared Responsibility Framework is a call to action: medical systems, schools and training programs, and individual trainees are responsible for interventions that positively impact personal health and well-being. Evidence within the literature demands continued and urgent systematic change to improve harsh work environments and redefine cultural and professional norms to create more supportive, balanced, and positive learning and training experiences. Concurrently, students and GME trainees have a personal responsibility to commit to intentional and strategic self-care to protect and promote their well-being. The central goals of this chapter were to (1) emphasize the importance of the Shared Responsibility Framework (Figure 7.1), which represents simultaneous adaptation and adoption of organizational and individual strategies that promote well-being; (2) introduce an expanded framework for strategic self-care and review the data for many individual-focused strategies that can be utilized by students and GME trainees (Figure 7.2); and (3) provide guidance for the implementation of wellness strategies into meaningful and impactful longitudinal curricula and programmatic structures. When organizations nurture the well-being of individual members by improving system-level drivers of burnout and facilitating individual engagement in strategic self-care, medical students and trainees will feel valued, appreciated, and encouraged to better care for themselves and the populations they serve.

Summary Points

- A shared responsibility approach using organizational and individual strategies is necessary to promote the well-being of GME learners.
- While medical schools and training programs are best suited to impact system-level changes and promote cultural shifts, individuals must also embrace their own responsibility to be as intentional in their self-care practice as they are in their medical training.
- The profession can benefit from a cultural shift toward the concept of Healthy altruism, in which individuals embrace their own self-care as protective, restorative, and essential to lifelong learning and serving others.
- A more holistic definition of self-care organizes evidence-based strategies into three core domains of well-being: physical, psychological, and relational/spiritual. Therefore, the practice of incorporating restorative strategies with awareness, intention, and commitment in real time throughout the day, both at work *and* outside of work, is the optimal conceptualization of strategic self-care, as highlighted in our strategic self-care framework.
- Curricular content should be developed with learner input and session facilitators should utilize several multimodal techniques, such as mindfulness, positive psychology, resilience training, creative expression, reflection-based practices, and facilitated discussions.

Putting It into Practice

For medical educators and well-being champions:

- Adapt the Shared Responsibility Framework to how student and GME trainee well-being needs are being addressed in your program/organization.
- Make a list of well-being interventions that have been launched in the past 2–3 years.
- Categorize them as system-, culture-, mental health-, and/or individual-focused.
- Moving forward, create interventions targeted to each domain.
- Create opportunities to discuss this shared responsibility philosophy.

For curriculum development:

- Perform a needs assessment for topics, themes, and strategies that students and GME trainees feel are most pertinent to their learning experience.
- Develop learning objectives for each session.
- Consider interactive, small-group activities that are best suited to each topic.

- Recruit faculty who are best trained and suited to deliver content.
- Measure session satisfaction; gather and incorporate feedback.

For personal well-being:
- Apply the Strategic Self-Care Framework to your own well-being needs.
- Identify a few "go to" strategies in each of the three domains.
- Time adapt these key strategies to when your schedule allows more or less time for self-care. For example, if exercise is a core strategy, what can you do for exercise if you have (a) 10–15 minutes, (b) 30–45 min, (c) 1–2 hours, or (d) all day?
- Grow your self-care strategy "toolkit": What additional skills do you want to learn/hone over the next 6–12 months? List one skill in each of the three domains. Set SMART goals. Practice.

References

1. Burton J. WHO healthy workplace framework and model. World Health Organization. May 19, 2010. Accessed September 6, 2020. https://www.who.int/publications/i/item/who-healthy-workplace-framework-and-model
2. Bodenheimer T, Sinsky C. From triple to quadruple AIM: care of the patient requires care of the provider. *Ann Fam Med.* 2014;12(6):573–576. doi:10.1370/afm.1713
3. Salyers MP, Bonfils KA, Luther L, et al. The relationship between professional burnout and quality and safety in healthcare: a meta-analysis. *J Gen Intern Med.* 2016;32(4):475–482. doi:10.1007/s11606-016-3886-9
4. Dyrbye LN, Shanafelt TD. Physician burnout: a potential threat to successful health care reform. *JAMA.* 2011;305(19):2009–2010. doi:10.1001/jama.2011.652
5. Oliver D. When "resilience" becomes a dirty word. *BMJ.* 2017;358:j3604. doi:10.1136/bmj.j3604
6. West CP, Dyrbye LN, Erwin PJ, Shanafelt TD. Interventions to prevent and reduce physician burnout: a systematic review and meta-analysis. *Lancet.* 2016;388(10057):2272–2281. doi:10.1016/S0140-6736(16)31279-X
7. De Simone S, Vargas M, Servillo G. Organizational strategies to reduce physician burnout: a systematic review and meta-analysis. *Aging Clin Exp Res.* 2019;33(4):883–894. doi:10.1007/s40520-01901368-3
8. Seelig BJ, Rosof LS. Normal and pathological altruism. *J Am Psychoanal Assoc.* 2001;49(3):933–959. doi.org/10.1177/00030651010490031901
9. Bachner-Melman R, Oakley B. Giving 'til it hurts': eating disorders and pathological altruism. In Latzer Y, Stein D, eds. *Bio-Psycho-Social Contributions to Understanding Eating Disorders.* Springer; 2016:91–103. doi.org/10.1007/978-3-319-32742-6_7
10. Parsa-Parsi RW. The revised declaration of Geneva. *JAMA.* 2017;318(20):1971. doi:10.1001/jama.2017.16230
11. Thomas LR, Ripp JA, West CP. Charter on physician well-being. *JAMA.* 2018;319(15):1541. doi:10.1001/jama.2018.1331
12. Panda M, O'Brien KE, Lo MC. Oath to self-care and well-being. *Am J Med.* 2020;133(2):249–252. doi:10.1016/j.amjmed.2019.10.001
13. Shanafelt TD. Physician well-being 2.0: where are we and where are we going? *Mayo Clin Proc.* 2021:96(10):2682–2693.
14. Wolf R. Wellbeing by generation: Where some thrive, others struggle. Gallup.com. 2021. Accessed September 5, 2021. https://www.gallup.com/workplace/268025/wellbeing-generation-thrive-others-struggle.aspx.

15. Morrow G, Burford B, Carter M, Illing J. Have restricted working hours reduced junior doctors' experience of fatigue? A focus group and telephone interview study. *BMJ Open*. 2014;4(3): e004222. doi:10.1136/bmjopen-2013-004222

16. Basner M, Asch DA, Shea JA, et al. Sleep and alertness in a duty-hour flexibility trial in internal medicine. *N Engl J Med*. 2019;380(10):915–923. doi:10.1056/nejmoa1810641

17. Morales J, Yáñez A, Fernández-González L, et al. Stress and autonomic response to sleep deprivation in medical residents: a comparative cross-sectional study. *PloS One*. 2019;14(4). doi:10.1371/journal.pone.0214858

18. Philibert I. Sleep loss and performance in residents and non-physicians: a meta-analytic examination. *Sleep*. 2005;28(11):1392–1402. doi:10.1093/sleep/28.11.1392

19. Reed DA, Fletcher KE, Arora VM. Systematic review: association of shift length, protected sleep time, and night float with patient care, residents' health, and education. *Ann Intern Med*. 2010;153(12):829–842. doi:10.7326/0003-4819-153-12-201012210-00010

20. Kalmbach DA, Arnedt JT, Song PX, Guille C, Sen S. Sleep disturbance and short sleep as risk factors for depression and perceived medical errors in first-year residents. *Sleep*. 2017;40(2). doi:10.1093/sleep/zsw073

21. Al-Maddah EM, Al-Dabal BK, Khalil MS. Prevalence of sleep deprivation and relation with depressive symptoms among medical residents in King Fahd University Hospital, Saudi Arabia. *Sultan Qaboos Univ Med J*. 2015(1):e78–84

22. Al-Abri MA. Sleep deprivation and depression: a bi-directional association. *Sultan Qaboos Univ Med J*. 2015(1):e4.

23. Kalmbach DA, Fang Y, Arnedt JT, et al. Effects of sleep, physical activity, and shift work on daily mood: a prospective mobile monitoring study of medical interns. *J Gen Intern Med*. 2018;33(6):914–920.

24. Rosen IM, Gimotty PA, Shea JA, Bellini LM. Evolution of sleep quantity, sleep deprivation, mood disturbances, empathy, and burnout among interns. *Acad Med*. 2006;81(1):82–85. doi:10.1097/00001888 200601000-00020

25. Stewart RE, Chambless DL. Cognitive–behavioral therapy for adult anxiety disorders in clinical practice: a meta-analysis of effectiveness studies. *J Consult Clin Psychol*. 2009;77(4):595–606. doi:10.1037/a0016032

26. Kancherla BS, Upender R, Collen JF, et al. Sleep, fatigue and burnout among physicians: an American Academy of Sleep Medicine position statement. *J Clin Sleep Med*. 2020;16(5):803–805. doi:10.5664/jcsm.8408

27. Volpp KG, Shea JA, Small DS, et al. Effect of a protected sleep period on hours slept during extended overnight in-hospital duty hours among medical interns. *JAMA*. 2012;308(21):2208–2217. doi:10.1001/jama.2012.34490

28. Shea JA, Bellini LM, Dinges DF, et al. Impact of protected sleep period for internal medicine interns on overnight call on depression, burnout, and empathy. *J Grad Med Educ*. 2014;6(2):256–263. doi:10.4300/jgme-d-13-00241.1

29. Shea JA, Dinges DF, Small DS, et al. A randomized trial of a three-hour protected nap period in a medicine training program. *Acad Med*. 2014;89(3):452–459. doi:10.1097/acm.0000000000000144

30. Philibert I. New requirements for resident duty hours. *JAMA*. 2002;288(9):1112–1114. doi:10.1001/jama.288.9.1112

31. Nasca TJ, Day SH, Amis ES. The new recommendations on duty hours from the ACGME Task Force. *N Engl J Med*. 2010;363(2):e3–1. doi:10.1056/nejmsb1005800

32. Bilimoria KY, Chung JW, Hedges LV, et al. National cluster-randomized trial of duty-hour flexibility in surgical training. *N Engl J Med*. 2016;374(8):713–727. doi:10.1056/nejmoa1515724

33. Desai SV, Asch DA, Bellini LM, et al. Education outcomes in a duty-hour flexibility trial in internal medicine. *N Engl J Med*. 2018;378(16):1494–1508. doi:10.1056/nejmoa1800965

34. Basner M, Asch DA, Shea JA, et al. Sleep and alertness in a duty-hour flexibility trial in internal medicine. *N Engl J Med*. 2019;380(10):915–923. doi:10.1056/nejmoa1810641

35. Sajwani RA, Shoukat S, Raza R, et al. Knowledge and practice of healthy lifestyle and dietary habits in medical and non-medical students of Karachi, Pakistan. *J Pak Med Assoc*. 2009.

36. Likus W, Milka D, Bajor G, Jachacz-Łopata M, Dorzak B. Dietary habits and physical activity in students from the Medical University of Silesia in Poland. *Rocz Panstw Zakl Hig*. 2013:17–24.

37. Matthews JI, Doerr L, Dworatzek PDN. University students intend to eat better but lack coping self-efficacy and knowledge of dietary recommendations. *J Nutr Educ Behav.* 2016;48(1):12–19. doi:10.1016/j.jneb.2015.08.005

38. Perlstein R, McCoombe S, Macfarlane S, Bell AC, Nowson C. Nutrition practice and knowledge of first-year medical students. *J Biomed Educ.* 2017;2017:1–10. doi:10.1155/2017/5013670

39. Cresci G, Beidelschies M, Tebo J, Hull A. Educating future physicians in nutritional science and practice: the time is now. *J Am Coll Nutr.* 2019;38(5):387–394. doi:10.1080/07315724.2018.1551158

40. Bassin SR, Al-Nimr RI, Allen K, Ogrinc G. The state of nutrition in medical education in the United States. *Nutrition Reviews.* 2020;78(9):764–780. doi:10.1093/nutrit/nuz100

41. Weidner G, Kohlmann C-W, Dotzauer E, Burns LR. The effects of academic stress on health behaviors in young adults. *Anxiety Stress Coping.* 1996;9(2):123–133. doi:10.1080/10615809608249396

42. Crowley J, Ball L, Hiddink GJ. Nutrition in medical education: a systematic review. *Lancet Planet Health.* 2019;3(9): e379–e389. doi:10.1016/s2542-5196(19)30171-8

43. McGrady A, Badenhop D, Lynch D. Effects of a lifestyle medicine elective on self-care behaviors in preclinical medical students. *Appl Psychophysiol Biofeedback.* 2019;44(2):143–149. doi:10.1007/s10484-019-09431-5

44. Kushner RF, Kessler S, McGaghie WC. Using behavior change plans to improve medical student self-care. *Acad Med.* 2011;86(7):901–906. doi:10.1097/acm.0b013e31821da193

45. Lemaire JB, Wallace JE, Dinsmore K, Roberts D. Food for thought: an exploratory study of how physicians experience poor workplace nutrition. *Nutr J.* 2011:10(1):1–8.

46. Hamidi MS, Boggild MK, Cheung AM. Running on empty: a review of nutrition and physicians' well-being. *Postgrad Med J.* 2016;92(1090):478–481. doi:10.1136/postgradmedj-2016-134131

47. Lemaire JB, Wallace JE, Dinsmore K, Lewin AM, Ghali WA, Roberts D. Physician nutrition and cognition during work hours: effect of a nutrition-based intervention. *BMC Health Serv Res.* 2010;10(1):1–9. doi:10.1186/1472-6963-10-241

48. Shanafelt TD, Oreskovich MR, Dyrbye LN, Satele DV, Hanks JB, Sloan JA, Balch CM. Avoiding Burnout: The personal health habits and wellness practices of US surgeons. *Annals of Surgery.* 2012;255(4):625–633. doi:10.1097/SLA.0b013e31824b2fa0

49. Dyrbye LN, Satele D, Shanafelt TD. Healthy exercise habits are associated with lower risk of burnout and higher quality of life among U.S. Medical Students. *Acad Med.* 2017;92(7):1006–1011. doi:10.1097/acm.0000000000001540

50. Olson SM, Odo NU, Duran AM, Pereira AG, Mandel JH. Burnout and physical activity in Minnesota internal medicine resident physicians. *J Grad Med Educ.* 2014;6(4):669–674. doi:10.4300/jgme-d-13-00396

51. Frank E, Galuska DA, Elon LK, Wright EH. Personal and clinical exercise-related attitudes and behaviors of freshmen U.S. medical students. *Res Q Exerc Sport.* 2004;75(2):112–121. doi:10.1080/02701367.2004.10609142

52. Frank E, Tong E, Lobelo F, Carrera J, Duperly J. Physical activity levels and counseling practices of U.S. medical students. *Med Sci Sport Exerc.* 2008;40(3):413–421. doi:10.1249/mss.0b013e31815ff399

53. Williams AS, Williams CD, Cronk NJ, Kruse RL, Ringdahl EN, Koopman RJ. Understanding the exercise habits of residents and attending physicians. *Fam Med.* 2015;47(2):118–123.

54. Rogers LQ, Gutin B, Humphries MC, et al. Evaluation of internal medicine residents as exercise role models and associations with self-reported counseling behavior, confidence, and perceived success. *Teach Learn Med.* 2006;18(3):215–221. doi:10.1207/s15328015tlm1803_5

55. Daneshvar F, Weinreich M, Daneshvar D, et al. Cardiorespiratory fitness in internal medicine residents: are future physicians becoming deconditioned? *J Grad Med Educ.* 2017:9(1):97–101.

56. Thorndike AN, Mills S, Sonnenberg L, et al. Activity monitor intervention to promote physical activity of physicians-in-training: randomized controlled trial. *PLoS One.* 2014;9(6):e100251. doi:10.1371/journal.pone.0100251

57. Schrager JD, Shayne P, Wolf S, et al. Assessing the influence of a Fitbit physical activity monitor on the exercise practices of emergency medicine residents: a pilot study. *JMIR mHealth uHealth.* 2017;5(1):e6239. doi:10.2196/mhealth.6239

58. Weight CJ, Sellon JL, Lessard-Anderson CR, Shanafelt TD, Olsen KD, Laskowski ER. Physical activity, quality of life, and burnout among physician trainees: the effect of a team-based, incentivized exercise program. *Mayo Clin Proc.* 2013;88(12):1435–1442. doi:10.1016/j.mayocp.2013.09.010

59. Nutting R, Grant JT, Ofei-Dodoo S, Runde MS, Staab KA, Richard BR. Increasing resident physician well-being through a motivational fitness curriculum: a pilot study. *Kans J Med.* 2020;13:228–234.

60. Gross CP, Mead LA, Ford DE, Klag MJ. Physician, heal thyself? *Arch Intern Med.* 2000;160(21):3209. doi:10.1001/archinte.160.21.3209

61. Kay MP, Mitchell GK, Del Mar CB. Doctors do not adequately look after their own physical health. *Med J Aust.* 2004;181(7):368–370. doi:10.5694/j.1326-5377.2004.tb06329

62. Pullen D, Cam DE, Doughty MV, Lonie CE, Lyle DM. Medical care of doctors. *Med J Aust.* 1995;162(9):481–484. doi:10.5694/j.1326-5377.1995.tb140011.x

63. Thompson WT, Cupples ME, Sibbett CH, Skan DI, Bradley T. Challenge of culture, conscience, and contract to general practitioners' care of their own health: qualitative study. *BMJ.* 2001;323(7315):728–731. doi:10.1136/bmj.323.7315.728

64. Rangel EL, Castillo-Angeles M, Kisat M, Kamine TH, Askari R. Lack of routine healthcare among resident physicians in New England. *J Am Coll Surg.* 2020;230(6):885–892. doi:10.1016/j.jamcollsurg.2019.11.005

65. Cedfeldt AS, Bower E, Flores C, Brunett P, Choi D, Girard DE. Promoting resident wellness. *Acad Med.* 2015;90(5):678–683. doi:10.1097/acm.0000000000000541

66. Carvour ML, Ayyar BK, Chien KS, Ramirez NC, Yamamoto H. A patient-centered approach to postgraduate trainee health and wellness. *Acad Med.* 2016;91(9):1205–1210. doi:10.1097/acm.0000000000001301

67. Jun TW, Liebert CA, Esquivel M, Cox JA, Trockel M, Katznelson L. A protected time policy to improve dental health among resident physicians. *J Am Dent Assoc.* 2019;150(5):362–368. doi:10.1016/j.adaj.2018.12.016

68. Tan C, Kuhn C, Anderson J, et al. Improving well-being among trainees: A partnership to reduce barriers to primary care services. *J Grad Med Educ.* 2020;12(2):203–207. doi:10.4300/jgme-d-19-00520.1

69. Meerlo P, Sgoifo A, Suchecki D. Restricted and disrupted sleep: effects on autonomic function, neuroendocrine stress systems and stress responsivity. *Sleep Med Rev.* 2008;12(3):197–210. doi:10.1016/j.smrv.2007.07.007

70. Tobaldini E, Cogliati C, Fiorelli EM, et al. One night on-call: Sleep deprivation affects cardiac autonomic control and inflammation in physicians. *Eur J Intern Med.* 2013;24(7):664–670. doi:10.1016/j.ejim.2013.03.011

71. Stetter F, Kupper S. Autogenic training: a meta-analysis of clinical outcome studies. *Appl Psychophysiol Biofeedback.* 2002;27(1), 45–98. doi:10.1023/a:1014576505223

72. Kraemer KM, Luberto CM, O'Bryan EM, Mysinger E, Cotton S. Mind–body skills training to improve distress tolerance in medical students: a pilot study. *Teach Learn Med.* 2016;28(2):219–228. doi:10.1080/10401334.2016.1146605

73. Bond AR, Mason HF, Lemaster CM, et al. Embodied health: the effects of a mind–body course for medical students. *Med Educ Online.* 2013;18(1):20699. doi:10.3402/meo.v18i0.20699

74. Hassed C, de Lisle S, Sullivan G, Pier C. Enhancing the health of medical students: outcomes of an integrated mindfulness and lifestyle program. *Adv Health Sci Educ.* 2008;14(3):387–398. doi:10.1007/s10459-008-9125-3

75. Finkelstein C, Brownstein A, Scott C, Lan Y-L. Anxiety and stress reduction in medical education: An intervention. *Med Educ.* 2007;41(3):258–264. doi:10.1111/j.1365-2929.2007.02685.x

76. HPRC. Tactical breathing for the military. 2020. Accessed January 7, 2022 http://www.hprc-online.org/mental-fitness/sleep-stress/tactical-breathing-military.

77. Grubish L, Kessler J, McGrane K, Bothwell J. Implementation of tactical breathing during simulated stressful situations and effects on clinical performance. *Ann Emerg Med.* 2016;68(4):S115. doi:10.1016/j.annemergmed.2016.08.311

78. Ospina-Kammerer V, Figley CR. An evaluation of the Respiratory One Method (ROM) in reducing emotional exhaustion among family physician residents. *Int J Emerg Ment Health.* 2003;5(1):29–32.

79. Orr AR, Moghbeli N, Swain A, et al. Fostering resilience through art in medical education (FRAME) workshop: a partnership with the Philadelphia Museum of Art. *Adv Med Educ Pract.* 2019;10:361–369. doi:10.2147/amep.s194575

80. Dalia Y, Milam EC, Rieder EA. Art in medical education: a review. *J Grad Med Educ.* 2020;12(6):686–695. doi:10.4300/jgme-d-20-00093.1

81. Jones EK, Kittendorf AL, Kumagai AK. Creative art and medical student development: a qualitative study. *Med Educ.* 2016;51(2):174–183. doi:10.1111/medu.13140

82. Bentwich ME, Gilbey P. More than visual literacy: art and the enhancement of tolerance for ambiguity and empathy. *BMC Med Educ.* 2017;17(1):1–9. doi:10.1186/s12909-017-1028-7

83. Gowda D, Dubroff R, Willieme A, Swan-Sein A, Capello C. Art as sanctuary: a four-year mixed-methods evaluation of a visual art course addressing uncertainty through reflection. *Acad Med.* 2018;93(11S):S8–S13. doi:10.1097/acm.0000000000002379

84. Zarrabi AJ, Morrison LJ, Reville BA, et al. Museum-based education: a novel educational approach for hospice and palliative medicine training programs. *J Palliat Med.* 2020;23(11);1510–1514.

85. Simpkin AL, Schwartzstein RM. Tolerating uncertainty: the next medical revolution? *N Engl J Med.* 2016;375(18):1713–1715. doi:10.1056/nejmp1606402

86. Patel V, Brackman S, Shafi U, et al. Overview of an emergent, arts-based resiliency curriculum to mitigate medical trainee burnout. *Arts Health.* 2020;13(1):98–106. doi:10.1080/17533015.2020.1802608

87. Gooding HC, Quinn M, Martin B, Charrow A, Katz JT. Fostering humanism in medicine through art and reflection. *J Mus Educ.* 2016;41(2):123–130. doi:10.1080/10598650.2016.1169732

88. Kirkland KB, Craig SR. Exploring the surgical gaze through literature and art. *JAMA.* 2018;319(15):1532. doi:10.1001/jama.2018.0396

89. Winkel AF. Narrative medicine: a writing workshop curriculum for residents. *MedEdPORTAL.* 2016;12:10493. doi:10.15766/mep_2374-8265.10493

90. Wesley T, Karam G, Hamer, D. Implementing a narrative medicine curriculum during the internship year: an internal medicine residency program experience. *Perm J.* 2018;22:17–187. doi:10.7812/tpp/17-187

91. Gowda D, Curran T, Khedagi A, et al. Implementing an interprofessional narrative medicine program in academic clinics: feasibility and program evaluation. *Perspect Med Educ.* 2019;8(1):52–59. doi:10.1007/s40037-019-0497-2

92. Chretien KC, Swenson R, Yoon B, et al. Tell me your story: a pilot narrative medicine curriculum during the medicine clerkship. *J Gen Intern Med.* 2015;30(7):1025–1028. doi:10.1007/s11606-015-3211-z

93. Charon R, et al. Introduction. In: Charon R et al, eds. *The Principles and Practice of Narrative Medicine.* Oxford University Press; 2017:1.

94. Milota MM, van Thiel GJ, van Delden JJ. Narrative medicine as a medical education tool: a systematic review. *Med Teach.* 2019;41(7):802–810. doi:10.1080/0142159x.2019.1584274

95. Arntfield SL, Slesar K, Dickson J, Charon R. Narrative medicine as a means of training medical students toward residency competencies. *Patient Educ Couns.* 2013;91(3):280–286. doi:10.1016/j.pec.2013.01.014

96. Charon R, Hermann N, Devlin MJ. Close reading and creative writing in clinical education. *Acad Med.* 2016;91(3):345–350. doi:10.1097/acm.0000000000000827

97. Barber S, Moreno-Leguizamon CJ. Can narrative medicine education contribute to the delivery of compassionate care? A review of the literature. *Med Humanit.* 2017;43(3):199–203.

98. Remein CD, Childs E, Pasco JC, et al. Content and outcomes of narrative medicine programmes: a systematic review of the literature through 2019. *BMJ Open.* 2020;10(1):e031568. doi:10.1136/bmjopen-2019-031568

99. Moss HA, Winkel AF, Jewell A, Musa F, Mitchell L, Speed E, Blank SV. Narrative medicine: using reflective writing workshops to help house staff address the complex and challenging nature of caring for gynecologic oncology patients. *Gynecol Oncol.* 2014;133:73.

100. Birigwa SN, Khedagi AM, Katz CJ. Stop, look, listen, then breathe: the impact of a narrative medicine curriculum on pediatric residents. *Acad Pediatr.* 2017;17(5):e40–e41.

101. Hinyard LJ, Wallace CL, Ohs JE, Trees A. Narrative medicine and reflective practice among providers: connecting personal experiences with professional action for advanced care planning. *J Clin Oncol.* 2018;36(34):S9–9.

102. Linehan, M. *DBT: Skills Training Manual.* Guilford Publications; 2014.

103. Dweck C. *Mindset: The New Psychology of Success.* Random House; 2016.

104. Duckworth A. *Grit: The Power of Passion and Perseverance.* Scribner; 2018.

105. Brown B. *Daring Greatly: How the Courage to Be Vulnerable Transforms the Way We Live, Love, Parent and Lead.* Penguin; 2012.

106. Brown, B. (2010). *The Gifts of Imperfection: Let Go of Who You Think You're Supposed to be and Embrace Who You Are.* Hazelden; 2010.

107. Clance PR, Imes SA. The imposter phenomenon in high achieving women: dynamics and therapeutic intervention. *Psychotherapy: Theory, research & practice.* 1978;15(3):241–247. doi:10.1037/h0086006

108. Hu KS, Chibnall JT, Slavin SJ. Maladaptive perfectionism, impostorism, and cognitive distortions: threats to the mental health of pre-clinical medical students. *Acad Psychiatry.* 2019;43(4):381–385. doi:10.1007/s40596-019-01031-z

109. Seligman ME, Steen TA, Park N, Peterson C. Positive psychology progress: empirical validation of interventions. *Am Psychol.* 2005;60(5):410–421. doi:10.1037/0003-066x.60.5.410

110. Lopez-Gomez I, Chaves C, Hervas G, Vazquez C. Comparing the acceptability of a positive psychology intervention versus a cognitive behavioural therapy for clinical depression. *Clin Psychol Psychother.* 2017;24(5):1029–1039. doi:10.1002/cpp.2129

111. Sin NL, Lyubomirsky S. Enhancing well-being and alleviating depressive symptoms with positive psychology interventions: a practice-friendly meta-analysis. *J Clin Psychol.* 2009;65(5):467–487. doi:10.1002/jclp.20593

112. Seligman MEP, Reivich K, Jaycox K, Gillham, J. *The Optimistic Child.* Houghton Mifflin; 1995.

113. Seligman ME, Csikszentmihalyi M. Positive psychology: An introduction. *Am Psychol.* 2000;55(1):5–14. doi:10.1037/0003-066x.55.1.5

114. Carr A, Cullen K, Keeney C, Canning C, Mooney O, Chinseallaigh E, O'Dowd A. Effectiveness of positive psychology interventions: a systematic review and meta-analysis. *J Posit Psychol.* 2021;16(6):749–769.

115. Hanson R. *Buddha's Brain: The Practical Neuroscience of Happiness, Love & Wisdom.* Harbinger Publications; 2009.

116. Hanson R. *Hardwiring Happiness: The New Brain Science of Contentment, Calm, and Confidence.* Harmony Books; 2016.

117. Green S, Palmer S. *Positive Psychology Coaching in Practice.* Routledge; 2019.

118. Burke J. Conceptual framework for a positive psychology coaching practice. *The Coaching Psychologist.* 2017;14(1):16–25.

119. Castiello D'Antonio A. Coaching psychology and positive psychology in work and organizational psychology. *Psychol Manag J.* 2018;21(2):130–150. doi:10.1037/mgr0000070

120. Kauffman C, Boniwell I, Silberman J. *The Complete Handbook of Coaching.* SAGE Publications Inc; 2010:172–185.

121. Palamara K, Kauffman C, Stone VE, Bazari H, Donelan K. Promoting success: A professional development coaching program for interns in medicine. *J Grad Med Educ.* 2015;7(4):630–637. doi:10.4300/jgme-d-14-00791.1

122. Palamara K, Kauffman C, Chang Y, et al. Professional development coaching for residents: results of a 3-year positive psychology coaching intervention. *J Gen Intern Med.* 2018;33(11):1842–1844. doi:10.1007/s11606-018-4589-1

123. Kakarala R, Smith SJ, Barreto E, Donelan K, Palamara K. When coaching meets mentoring: impact of incorporating coaching into an existing mentoring program at a community hospital. *Cureus.* 2018. doi:10.7759/cureus.3138

124. Palamara K, Chu JT, Chang Y, et al. Who benefits most? A multisite study of coaching and resident well-being. *J Gen Intern Med.* 2022;37(3):539–547. doi:10.1007/s11606-021-06903-5

125. McConville J, McAleer R, Hahne A. Mindfulness training for health profession students—the effect of mindfulness training on psychological well-being, learning and clinical performance of health professional students. *Explore.* 2017;13(1):26–45. doi:10.1016/j.explore.2016.10.002

126. Dobkin PL, Hutchinson TA. Teaching mindfulness in medical school: where are we now and where are we going? *Med Educ.* 2013;47(8):768–779. doi:10.1111/medu.12200
127. Warnecke E, Quinn S, Ogden K, Towle N, Nelson MR. A randomized controlled trial of the effects of mindfulness practice on medical student stress levels. *Med Educ.* 2011;45(4):381–388. doi:10.1111/j.1365-2923.2010.03877.x
128. Rosenzweig S, Reibel DK, Greeson JM, Brainard GC, Hojat M. Mindfulness-based stress reduction lowers psychological distress in medical students. *Teach Learn Med.* 2003;15(2):88–92. doi:10.1207/s15328015tlm1502_03
129. Dyrbye LN, Shanafelt TD, Werner L, Sood A, Satele D, Wolanskyj AP. The impact of a required longitudinal stress management and resilience training course for first-year medical students. *J Gen Intern Med.* 2017;32(12):1309–1314. doi:10.1007/s11606-017-4171-2
130. Dobkin PL, Bernardi NF, Bagnis CI. Enhancing clinicians' well-being and patient-centered care through mindfulness. *J Contin Educ Health Prof.* 2016;36(1):11–16. doi:10.1097/ceh.0000000000000021
131. Amutio A, Martínez-Taboada C, Hermosilla D, Delgado LC. Enhancing relaxation states and positive emotions in physicians through a mindfulness training program: a one-year study. *Psychol Health Med.* 2014;20(6):720–731. doi:10.1080/13548506.2014.986143
132. Asuero AM, Queraltó JM, Pujol-Ribera E, Berenguera A, Rodriguez-Blanco T, Epstein RM. Effectiveness of a mindfulness education program in primary health care professionals: a pragmatic controlled trial. *J Contin Educ Health Prof.* 2014;34(1):4–12. doi:10.1002/chp.21211
133. Fortney L, Luchterhand C, Zakletskaia L, Zgierska A, Rakel D. Abbreviated mindfulness intervention for job satisfaction, quality of life, and compassion in primary care clinicians: a pilot study. *Ann Fam Med.* 2013;11(5):412–420. doi:10.1370/afm.1511
134. Moody K, Kramer D, Santizo RO, et al. Helping the helpers. *J Pediatr Oncol Nurs.* 2013;30(5):275–284. doi:10.1177/1043454213504497
135. Beckman HB, Wendland M, Mooney C, et al. The impact of a program in mindful communication on primary care physicians. *Acad Med.* 2012;87(6):815–819. doi:10.1097/acm.0b013e318253d3b2
136. Goodman MJ, Schorling JB. A mindfulness course decreases burnout and improves well-being among healthcare providers. *Int J Psychiatr Med.* 2012;43(2):119–128. doi:10.2190/pm.43.2.b
137. Irving JA, Dobkin PL, Park J. Cultivating mindfulness in health care professionals: a review of empirical studies of mindfulness-based stress reduction (MBSR). *Complement Ther Clin Pract.* 2009;15(2):61–66. doi:10.1016/j.ctcp.2009.01.002
138. Krasner MS. Association of an educational program in mindful communication with burnout, empathy, and attitudes among primary care physicians. *JAMA.* 2009;302(12):1284. doi:10.1001/jama.2009.1384
139. Oman D, Hedberg J, Thoresen CE. Passage meditation reduces perceived stress in health professionals: a randomized, controlled trial. *J Consult Clin Psychol.* 2006;74(4):714–719. doi:10.1037/0022-006x.74.4.714
140. Gilmartin H, Goyal A, Hamati MC, Mann J, Saint S, Chopra V. Brief mindfulness practices for healthcare providers—a systematic literature review. *Am J Med.* 2017;130(10):1219.e1–1219.e17. doi:10.1016/j.amjmed.2017.05.041
141. Rosdahl JA, Kingsolver K. Mindfulness training to increase resilience and decrease stress and burnout in ophthalmology residents: a pilot study. *Invest Ophthalmol Vis Sci.* 2014;55(13):5579.
142. Goldhagen BE, Kingsolver K, Stinnett SS, Rosdahl JA. Stress and burnout in residents: impact of mindfulness-based resilience training. *Adv Med Educ Pract.* 2015;6:525.
143. Taylor M, Hageman JR, Brown M. A mindfulness intervention for residents: relevance for pediatricians. *Pediatr Ann.* 2016;45(10):e373–e376. doi:10.3928/19382359-20160912-01
144. Aeschbach VM, Fendel JC, Schmidt S, Göritz AS. A tailored mindfulness-based program for resident physicians: a qualitative study. *Complement Ther Clin Pract.* 2021;43:101333. doi:10.1016/j.ctcp.2021.101333
145. Ginsburg KR, Jablow MM. *Building Resilience in Children and Teens: Giving Kids Roots and Wings.* American Academy of Pediatrics; 2020.
146. Roberts LW. Belonging, respectful inclusion, and diversity in medical education. *Acad Med.* 2020;95(5):661–664. doi:10.1097/acm.0000000000003215
147. McKenna KM, Hashimoto DA, Maguire MS, Bynum WE. The missing link: connection is the key to resilience in medical education. *Acad Med.* 2016;91(9):1197–1199. doi:10.1097/acm.0000000000001311

148. Salles A, Wright RC, Milam L, et al. Social belonging as a predictor of surgical resident well-being and attrition. *J Surg Educ.* 2019;76(2):370–377. doi:10.1016/j.jsurg.2018.08.022

149. Walton GM, Cohen GL. A brief social-belonging intervention improves academic and health outcomes of minority students. *Science.* 2011;331(6023):1447–1451. doi:10.1126/science.1198364

150. Strayhorn TL. Exploring the role of race in black males' sense of belonging in medical school: a qualitative pilot study. *Med Sci Educ.* 2020;30(4):1383–1387. doi:10.1007/s40670-020-01103

151. Chandauka RE, Russell JM, Sandars J, Vivekananda-Schmidt P. Differing perceptions among ethnic minority and Caucasian medical students which may affect their relative academic performance. *Educ Prim Care.* 2015;26(1):11–15.

152. Haggins AN. To be seen, heard, and valued: strategies to promote a sense of belonging for women and underrepresented in medicine physicians. *Acad Med.* 2020;95(10):1507–1510. doi:10.1097/acm.0000000000003553

153. Zaidi Z, Dewan M, Norcini J. International medical graduates: promoting equity and belonging. *Acad Med.* 2020;95:12S. doi:10.1097/acm.0000000000003694

154. Salmoirago-Blotcher E, Fitchett G, Leung K, et al. An exploration of the role of religion/spirituality in the promotion of physicians' wellbeing in emergency medicine. *Prevent Med Rep.* 2016;3:189–195. doi:10.1016/j.pmedr.2016.01.009

155. Wachholtz A, Rogoff ML. The relationship between spirituality and burnout among medical students. *J Contemp Med Educ.* 2013;1(2):83. doi:10.5455/jcme.20130104060612

156. Doolittle BR, Windish DM, Seelig CB. Burnout, coping, and spirituality among internal medicine resident physicians. *J Grad Med Educ.* 2013;5(2):257–261. doi:10.4300/jgme-d-12-00136.1

157. Doolittle BR. *Religion and Spirituality for the Healthcare Provider.* Nova Science Publishers, Inc.; 2016.

158. Puchalski CM. The role of spirituality in health care. *Proc (Bayl Univ Med Cent).* 2001;14(4):352–357.

159. Chow HH, Chew QH, Sim K. Spirituality and religion in residents and inter-relationships with clinical practice and residency training: a scoping review. *BMJ Open.* 2021;11(5):e044321. doi:10.1136/bmjopen-2020-044321

160. Kapoor S, Morgan CK, Siddique MA, Guntupalli KK. "Sacred pause" in the ICU: evaluation of a ritual and intervention to lower distress and burnout. *Am J Hosp Palliat Med.* 2018;35(10):1337–1341. doi:10.1177/1049909118768247

161. Montross-Thomas LP, Scheiber C, Meier EA, Irwin SA. Personally meaningful rituals: a way to increase compassion and decrease burnout among hospice staff and volunteers. *J Palliat Med.* 2016;19(10):1043–1050. doi:10.1089/jpm.2015.0294

162. Hipp DM, Rialon KL, Nevel K, Kothari AN, Jardine LDA. "Back to bedside": residents' and fellows' perspectives on finding meaning in work. *J Grad Med Educ.* 2017;9(2):269–273. doi:10.4300/jgme-d-17-00136.1

163. Shanafelt TD, West C, Zhao X, et al. Relationship between increased personal well-being and enhanced empathy among internal medicine residents. *J Gen Intern Med.* 2005;20(7):559–564. doi:10.1007/s11606-005-0102-8

164. Shanafelt TD, Boone S, Tan L, et al. Burnout and satisfaction with work-life balance among us physicians relative to the general US population. *Arch Intern Med.* 2012;172(18):1377. doi:10.1001/archinternmed.2012.3199

165. Weiner EL, Gottlieb M, Wolf B, Swain GR. A qualitative study of physicians' own wellness-promotion practices. *West J Med.* 2001;174(1):19–23. doi:10.1136/ewjm.174.1.19

166. Howell AJ. Self-affirmation theory and the science of well-being. *J Happiness Stud.* 2016;18(1):293–311. doi:10.1007/s10902-016-9713-5

167. Sherman GL. Transformative learning and well-being for emerging adults in higher education. *J Transform Educ.* 2020;19(1):29–49. doi:10.1177/1541344620935623

168. Sherman DK, Cohen GL. The psychology of self-defense: self-affirmation theory. *Adv Exp Soc Psychol.* 2006;38:183–242. doi:10.1016/s0065-2601(06)38004-5

169. Yoon JD, Daley BM, Curlin FA. The association between a sense of calling and physician well-being: a national study of primary care physicians and psychiatrists. *Acad Psychiatry.* 2017;41(2):167–173.

170. Duffy RD, Manuel RS, Borges NJ, Bott EM. Calling, vocational development, and well-being: a longitudinal study of medical students. *J Vocat Behav.* 2011;79(2):361–366. doi:10.1016/j.jvb.2011.03.023

171. Wald HS. Optimizing resilience and wellbeing for healthcare professions trainees and healthcare professionals during public health crises—practical tips for an 'integrative resilience' approach. *Med Teach.* 2020;42(7):744–755. doi:10.1080/0142159x.2020.1768230

172. Remen R, O'Donnell J, Rabow M. The healer's art: education in meaning and service. *J Cancer Educ.* 2008;23(1):65–67. doi:10.1080/08858190701821394

173. Rabow MW, Wrubel J, Remen RN. Authentic community as an educational strategy for advancing professionalism: a national evaluation of the Healer's Art course. *J Gen Intern Med.* 2007;22(10):1422–1428.

174. Jaiswal C, Anderson K, Haesler E. A self-report of the healer's art by junior doctors: does the course have a lasting influence on personal experience of humanism, self-nurturing skills and medical counterculture? *BMC Med Educ.* 2019;19(1):1–9. doi:10.1186/s12909-019-1877-3

175. Lader M, Burke AE, Stolfi A, Andarsio E, Hanson C, Boreman C. A program's experience with Healer's Art: fostering compassionate healing and human connection. *Acad Pediatr.* 2018;18(5):e33. doi:10.1016/j.acap.2018.04.091

176. Trzeciak S, Mazzarelli A. *Compassionomics: The Revolutionary Scientific Evidence That Caring Makes a Difference.* Studer Group; 2019.

177. Klimecki OM, Leiberg S, Ricard M, Singer T. Differential pattern of functional brain plasticity after compassion and empathy training. *Soc Cogn Affect Neurosci.* 2013;9(6):873–879. doi:10.1093/scan/nst060

178. Wilkinson H, Whittington R, Perry L, Eames C. Examining the relationship between burnout and empathy in healthcare professionals: a systematic review. *Burn Res.* 2017;6:18–29. doi:10.1016/j.burn.2017.06.003

179. Conversano C, Ciacchini R, Orrù G, Di Giuseppe M, Gemignani A, Poli A. Mindfulness, compassion, and self-compassion among health care professionals: What's new? A systematic review. *Front Psychol.* 2020;11:1683. doi:10.3389/fpsyg.2020.01683

180. Mascaro JS, Kelley S, Darcher A, et al. Meditation buffers medical student compassion from the deleterious effects of depression. *J Posit Psychol.* 2016;13(2):133–142. doi:10.1080/17439760.2016.1233348

181. Weingartner LA, Sawning S, Shaw MA, Klein JB. Compassion cultivation training promotes medical student wellness and enhanced clinical care. *BMC Med Educ.* 2019;19(1):1–11. doi:10.1186/s12909-019-1546-6

182. Gurfein EG. *Enhancing Empathy and Emotion Regulation to Decrease Burnout: A Pilot Study of Compassion Cultivation for Physicians in Training.* ProQuest Dissertations Publishing; 2017.

183. Neff KD. The development and validation of a scale to measure self-compassion. *Self Identity.* 2003;2(3):223–250. doi:10.1080/15298860309027

184. Mills J, Chapman M. Compassion and self-compassion in medicine: self-care for the caregiver. *Australas Med J.* 2016;9(5):87–91.

185. Quinn, MA, Grant LM, Sampene E, Zelenski AB. A curriculum to increase empathy and reduce burnout. *West Med J.* 2020;119(4):258–262.

186. Olson K, Kemper KJ, Mahan JD. What factors promote resilience and protect against burnout in first-year pediatric and medicine-pediatric residents? *J Evid Based Complementary Altern Med.* 2015;20(3):192–198. doi:10.1177/2156587214568894

187. Kemper KJ, Schwartz A, Wilson PM, et al. Burnout in pediatric residents: three years of national survey data. *Pediatrics.* 2020;145(1):e20191030. doi:10.1542/peds.2019-1030

188. Godthelp J, Muntinga M, Niessen T, Leguit P, Abma T. Self-care of caregivers: self-compassion in a population of Dutch medical students and residents. *MedEdPublish.* 2020;9(1). doi:10.15694/mep.2020.000222.1

189. Neff KD, Knox MC, Long P, Gregory K. Caring for others without losing yourself: an adaptation of a mindful self-compassion program for healthcare communities. *J Clin Psychol.* 2020;76(9):1543–1562. doi:10.1002/jclp.23007

190. Weng H-C, Hung C-M, Liu Y-T, et al. Associations between emotional intelligence and doctor burnout, job satisfaction and patient satisfaction. *Med Educ.* 2011;45(8):835–842. doi:10.1111/j.1365-2923.2011.03985.x

191. Derksen F, Bensing J, Lagro-Janssen A. Effectiveness of empathy in general practice: a systematic review. *Br J Gen Pract.* 2013;63(606):e76–84. doi:10.3399/bjgp13x660814

192. Dyrbye LN, West CP, Satele D, et al. Burnout among U.S. medical students, residents, and early career physicians relative to the general U.S. population. *Acad Med*. 2014;89(3):443–451. doi:10.1097/acm.0000000000000134

193. Bellini LM, Shea JA. Mood change and empathy decline persist during three years of internal medicine training. *Acad Med*. 2005;80(2):164–167. doi:10.1097/00001888-200502000-00013

194. Riess H, Kelley JM, Bailey RW, Dunn EJ, Phillips, M. Empathy training for resident physicians: a randomized controlled trial of a neuroscience-informed curriculum. *J Gen Intern Med*. 2012;27(10):1280–1286.

195. Cabib S, Campus P, Conversi D, Orsini C, Puglisi-Allegra S. Functional and dysfunctional neuroplasticity in learning to cope with stress. *Brain Sci*. 2020;10(2):127. doi:10.3390/brainsci10020127

196. Thomas L, et al. Evidence-based interventions for medical student, trainee, and practicing physician well-being: A CHARM annotated bibliography. Tomescu O, ed. Alexandria, VA: Alliance for Academic Internal Medicine; published online November 2017. Accessed February 9, 2022. https://www.im.org/resources/wellness-resiliency/charm/best-practice-group

197. Meeks LM, Ramsey J, Lyons M, Spencer AL, Lee WW. Wellness and work: mixed messages in residency training. *J Gen Intern Med*. 2019;34(7):1352–1355. doi:10.1007/s11606-019-04952-5

198. Brazeau CMLR, Shanafelt T, Durning SJ, et al. Distress among matriculating medical students relative to the general population. *Acad Med*. 2014;89(11):1520–1525. doi:10.1097/acm.0000000000000482

199. Theard MA, Marr MC, Harrison, R. The growth mindset for changing medical education culture. *EClinicalMedicine*. 2021;37:100972.

200. Gleichgerrcht E, Decety J. Empathy in clinical practice: how individual dispositions, gender, and experience moderate empathic concern, burnout, and emotional distress in physicians. *PLoS ONE*. 2013;8(4):e61526. doi:10.1371/journal.pone.0061526

201. van Ryn M, Hardeman RR, Phelan SM, et al. Psychosocial predictors of attitudes toward physician empathy in clinical encounters among 4732 1st year medical students: a report from the changes study. *Patient Educ Couns*. 2014;96(3):367–375. doi:10.1016/j.pec.2014.06.009

202. Williamson K, Lank PM, Lovell EO, Emergency Medicine Education Research Alliance (EMERA). Development of an emergency medicine wellness curriculum. *AEM Educ Train*. 2018;2(1):20–25.

203. Mahan JD, Stein DS. Teaching adults—best practices that leverage the emerging understanding of the neurobiology of learning. *Curr Probl Pediatr Adolesc Health Care*. 2014;44(6):141–149. doi:10.1016/j.cppeds.2014.01.003

204. Reed S, Shell R, Kassis K, et al. Applying adult learning practices in medical education. *Curr Probl Pediatr Adolesc Health Care*. 2014;44(6):170–181. doi:10.1016/j.cppeds.2014.01.008.

205. Yazdankhahfard M, Haghani F, Omid A. The Balint group and its application in medical education: A systematic review. *J Educ Health Promot*. 2019;8:124. doi:10.4103/jehp.jehp_423_18. eCollection 2019.

206. Mukunda N, Moghbeli N, Rizzo A, Niepold S, Bassett B, DeLisser HM. Visual art instruction in medical education: a narrative review. *Med Educ Online*. 2019;24(1):1558657. doi:10.1080/10872981.2018.1558657

207. Gaufberg E, Williams R. Reflection in a museum setting: the personal responses tour. *J Grad Med Educ*. 2011;3(4):546–549. doi:10.4300/jgme-d-11-00036.1

208. Miller A, Grohe M, Khoshbin S, Katz JT. From the galleries to the clinic: applying art museum lessons to patient care. *J Med Humanit*. 2013;34(4):433–438.

209. Ruch W, Niemiec RM, McGrath RE, Gander F, Proyer RT. Character strengths-based interventions: open questions and ideas for future research. *J Posit Psychol*. 2020;15(5):680–684. doi:10.1080/17439760.2020.1789700

210. Smith JL, Bryant FB. Savoring and well-being: mapping the cognitive-emotional terrain of the happy mind. In: MD Robinson, M Eid, eds. *The Happy Mind: Cognitive Contributions to Well-Being*. Springer, Cham; 2017:139–156. doi:10.1007/978-3-319-58763-9_8

211. Redeker NS, Caruso CC, Hashmi SD, Mullington JM, Grandner M, Morgenthaler TI. Workplace interventions to promote sleep health and an alert, healthy workforce. *J Clin Sleep Med*. 2019;15(04):649–657. doi:10.5664/jcsm.7734

212. Wright KP, Bogan RK, Wyatt JK. Shift work and the assessment and management of shift work disorder (SWD). *Sleep Med Rev*. 2013;17(1):41–54. doi:10.1016/j.smrv.2012.02.002

213. Avidan AY. Sleep and fatigue countermeasures for the neurology resident and physician. *Continuum.* 2013;19(1):204–222. doi:10.1212/01.con.0000427205.67811.08
214. Tassi P, Muzet A. Sleep inertia. *Sleep Med Rev.* 2000;4(4):341–353. doi:10.1053/smrv.2000.0098
215. Van Dongen PA, Price NJ, Mullington JM, Szuba MP, Kapoor SC, Dinges DF. Caffeine eliminates psychomotor vigilance deficits from sleep inertia. *Sleep.* 2001;24(7):813–819. doi:10.1093/sleep/24.7.813
216. Smith MR, Eastman CI. Shift work: health, performance and safety problems, traditional countermeasures, and innovative management strategies to reduce circadian misalignment. *Nature and Science of Sleep.* 2012;4:111–132. doi:10.2147/nss.s10372
217. Van Dongen PA, Baynard MD, Maislin G, Dinges DF. Systematic interindividual differences in neurobehavioral impairment from sleep loss: evidence of trait-like differential vulnerability. *Sleep.* 2004;27(3):423–433. doi:10.1093/sleep/27.3.423
218. Baumeister RF, Bratslavsky E, Finkenauer C, Vohs KD. Bad is stronger than good. *Rev Gen Psychol.* 2001;5(4):323–370. doi:10.1037/1089-2680.5.4.323

8

System-Level Interventions

Mariah A. Quinn, Lauren Banaszak,
Kathleen McFadden, and Kerri Palamara McGrath

What Is a System-Level Intervention to Support Well-Being?

Interventions to improve the well-being for physicians-in-training generally can be categorized into those that are aimed at individuals or those that are aimed at "the system" or "the institution/organization." The system could include *places* such as the health system or an individual institution, such as a hospital or medical school, in which learners engage in clinical learning and service, as well as smaller units therein, such as departments or training programs. It also could consist of *processes:* for instance, how clinical work is structured and functions, or how and what kind of mentorship learners receive. System-level interventions have the potential to modify the experience of many or most learners rather than a single learner. In broad strokes, systems-level interventions influence workload, workflow, and/or culture and meaning in work.

System-level interventions often provide structural or policy support to address specific individual-level needs and can be operationalized through individuals. Table 8.1 provides a list of examples organized by domains of culture, workload, and learning climate, as well as mental health support. Because the systems in which we work are complex, with many interrelated components, an intervention designed to support a specific individual need may impact multiple domains. For instance, consider a suicide risk reduction program utilizing an online cognitive behavioral therapy program.[1] When such a program is provided to all learners as a standard part of a curriculum, regardless of perceived risk, it not only supports the individual who may be at risk, but it also could shift the conversation around mental health, help-seeking,

TABLE 8.1 Examples of individual needs with aligned system interventions

Domain	Individual need	Aligned system intervention
Culture, learning climate	Time for recuperation and bonding after childbirth or adoption	Parental leave policies, such as ACGME VI.C.2[119]
	Time to attend appointments to attend to personal health	ACGME VI.C.1.d).(1) "Residents must be given the opportunity to attend medical, mental health, and dental care appointments, including those scheduled during their working hours."[119]
	Being free of harassment and discrimination	Confidential reporting, policies against learner mistreatment[85,86]
	Safe learning climate	Training all teaching faculty in setting safe learning climate[28,97,101,102]
	Reduction of competition	Pass–fail grading[29-21]
Workload	Adequate sleep and time away from work	Duty-hour limitations, service size caps, such as ACGME VI.F.1[119]
	Reduction of time spent preparing for exams	Pass–fail grading of ACGME Step Exams
Mental health	Easy access to confidential, free or low-cost, high-quality mental health care	Embedded well-resourced mental health support within a school or medical center[2]
	Suicide prevention	Computer-based suicide prevention program for all learners[1]

and suicide in the entire community of learners, thereby impacting the culture more broadly. Developing a robust mental health care infrastructure at an institution may similarly have multifaceted impacts.[2]

As we review evidence surrounding systems-level interventions and make recommendations, we emphasize that medical schools, health systems, and regulatory bodies all have important roles to play. The ownership of the problem—and solutions—must be shared, as articulated in the CHARM Charter on Well-Being.[3]

Why Systems-Level Interventions?

As described in Chapter 3, those who enter medical school begin with high resilience, low burnout, and high empathy, all of which move in a disturbing direction over time.[4,5] The fact that a highly resilient group experiences a negative trajectory in well-being over training suggests that the system of training itself requires examination and intervention rather than focusing solely on individual interventions and self-care. While individual-level interventions do have importance, when high-quality interventions specifically targeting residents have been assessed, systems-facing interventions were found to be more effective in reducing burnout.[6-10] Considering interventions directed at the individual or the system is a case of "both-and," wherein neither can be ignored.

Systems-Level Interventions Focused on Workload

Ways to Measure and Defined Workload Holistically

Workload is a critical concept in designing systems that enhance or maintain well-being. In general, it is common to think of workload as a list of tasks to be completed. However, more holistic ways of understanding workload include measurements of the effect of the work on the worker. Measures in this category can include physiologic data (e.g., heart rate variability, eye movement tracking) or survey-based measurements.[11,12] The NASA Task-Load Index is the most common of these tools and is widely validated across industries. The NASA Task-Load Index includes domains of mental and physical demands, time pressure, effort required, degree of performance, and frustration.[13] The Physician Task Load Index, illustrated in Figure 8.1, was derived from the NASA Task-Load Index.[14]

The demands of one's work can be counterbalanced or supported by resources, a concept captured in the Demands-Resources model introduced in Chapter 1.[15] Demands include all tasks, whether clinical or nonclinical, including curriculum and training experiences or research. Resources include teaching, mentoring, and support from faculty, as well as other environmental and cultural resources.[11] Perception of effort, as captured in the Physician Task Load Index, could be influenced by factors external to the medical school or health system, such as the commute to work or weather conditions. These external factors can influence medical student or graduate medical education (GME) trainee metrics of workload. All of these considerations should be kept in mind when tallying the holistic workload placed on the student and GME trainee when designing the learning or work environment in a way that mitigates excessive work.

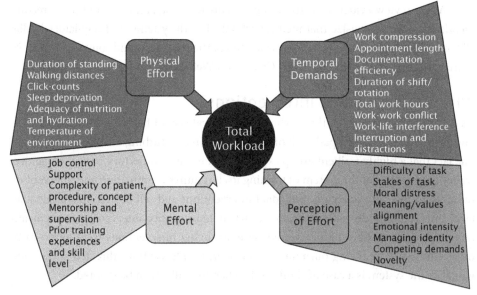

FIGURE 8.1 Physician Task Load Index domains with examples.

Physician workload, for practicing physicians and physicians-in-training alike, includes demands and tasks with high emotional valence as well as those that may reduce meaning in work. For example, giving bad news to a patient or a patient's family, experiencing negative clinical outcomes, or working with a patient who is abusive requires expending emotional effort. That emotional work itself is just that—work. Additionally, work tasks may be inherently meaningful (such as taking a patient history or counseling a patient in one's field of specialization) or may reduce meaning in work. For instance, time spent documenting in the medical record or sending faxes to obtain medical records serve a clinical purpose but do not carry the same sense of value for most physicians or physicians-in-training as the aforementioned tasks. Even tasks that are meaningful to one physician may seem less so to another. Learning itself is also work—cognitive load requiring time and attention. The work of learning a task, concept, skill, etc. is also modulated by one's preexisting skill, the match between teaching and learning style, interest, learner confidence, and other factors related to the learner's identity and personal factors. Finally, all of these tasks are done in work environments that shape student and GME trainee tasks through policies, culture, attitudes, and observed behaviors. Therefore, it is critical to incorporate an understanding of the work of learning itself into any model of workload for medical students, residents, or fellows and to consider factors unique to each individual that modify workload.

The Relationship Between Meaning in Work and Workload

Meaning and purpose support engagement and creativity and can buffer against the detrimental effects of stress and high workload.[16] Many physicians report a strong sense of calling to their work, a finding associated with greater levels of meaning in life.[17,18] Meaning in work reduces burnout.[19-21] All work activities do not carry the same sense of meaning for most physicians and physicians-in-training. A higher burden of administrative tasks, including greater use of the electronic health record (EHR), is associated with higher levels of burnout.[22-24]

Team-based care can be an important way to reduce the administrative burden experienced by physicians-in-training.[25,26] Dedicated time for learning and reflection is also a critical element of designing clinical learning experiences for medical students, residents, and fellows. As discussed in Chapter 1, medical students and GME trainees learn and function in complex adaptive systems in which change impacting one group may have unanticipated or somewhat unpredictable consequences for another group. Other clinical professions, such as nursing, also experience substantial association between meaning in work and well-being.[27] When utilizing team-based care models as a systems-level intervention to shift administrative burden to other health professionals, the risk of undermining the well-being of another group is real, so should be undertaken with care. Ways to avoid these types of zero-sum traps (making well-being worse for one group as a result of interventions to improve another group's well-being) are described further in Chapter 11.

Work-Load Interventions and Well-Being in Undergraduate Medical Education

Medical students face different workload stressors depending on whether they are in their preclinical or clinical years, and interventions have sought to address workload at both stages. A large cross-sectional study of medical students found that being on hospital ward rotations or rotations involving overnight call were both associated with burnout. Factors such as call frequency, number of inpatients cared for per day or admitted per week, ambulatory rotation visit volume, or consult service volume were not found to be associated with burnout.[28,29]

Another major source of workload for students is studying for examinations, particularly if the stakes for exams are high for determining class standing or residency prospects. Pass–fail grading, particularly in the first 2 years of medical school, reduces distress and does not reduce performance or residency attainment among cohorts of students.[29-31] This gain in well-being may relate specifically to the lower workload of testing itself or to lower stress and modifications in the environment, with reduced competition and greater collaboration. The US Medical Licensing Examination (USMLE) exams are a considerable ongoing source of workload and cost for medical students. The 2020 pause and subsequent elimination of the Step 2 Clinical Skills exam in the setting of the COVID-19 pandemic has been widely celebrated by students who "saw it as a source of stress with little actual value."[32] Close attention to test frequency and evaluation rubrics for preclinical students as well as the rotation structure for clinical students are central systems-level interventions to consider at the medical school level.

Work-Load Interventions and Well-Being in Graduate Medical Education

As described in Chapter 4, for GME trainees, measures of workload such as work hours and frequency of overnight call have been shown to be associated with burnout in some studies but not others.[33-38] In sum, studies of GME trainee cohorts do not demonstrate a consistent relationship between work hours, call frequency, or self-reported workload and burnout.[39-41] In addition, efforts to further limit protracted shift length have not shown consistent benefit as it relates to measures of well-being.[38,41-43] Given the lack of clarity about whether shift-length limitations, such as those mandated by the Accreditation Council for Graduate Medical Education (ACGME) 2011 work-hour rules, the I-COMPARE and FIRST study trials were performed to test the impact on education, well-being, and patient outcomes in the setting of more flexible duty hours.[44,45]

The I-COMPARE study was a cluster randomized trial involving 63 internal medicine programs. In the study, 32 programs were allowed flexibility to waive the maximum shift length and minimum duration of time off between shifts. Researchers compared educational and patient safety outcomes in these programs, with the 31 programs adhering to the 2011 work-hour shift length limitations. Both groups were still bound by the ACGME 80-hour maximum. This trial utilized time-motion observations, surveys, and In Training

Exam (ITE) scores to assess educational outcomes and well-being. When comparing the "flexible" and standard duty-hour programs, there was no significant change in the amount of time interns spent in direct patient care, no significant difference in ITE scores between programs, and no significant differences in burnout between programs. However, while validated assessments of burnout did not differ significantly, burnout in both groups was high, and interns in "flexible" programs reported greater dissatisfaction with work hours and scheduling as well as a number of important drivers of well-being, such as time for rest with concordant concern about fatigue's impact on personal and patient safety, time with family and friends, and time for hobbies. Participants in the flexible duty hours study arm also perceived a negative impact on health, morale, and well-being. Importantly, because the work hours limit for both groups was 80 hours per week, the study reflected efforts to structure shifts rather than reduce overall work hours.[44]

The FIRST trial was a cluster-randomized trial of 117 general surgery residency programs in which 58 programs were granted shift length flexibility (as described in the I-COMPARE trial above) versus 59 that were asked to adhere to the 2011 duty- ours, with both groups bound by the 80-hour per week limit. The primary patient care outcomes were 30-day rates of postoperative death or serious complications. Primary resident outcomes were resident perceptions and satisfaction regarding their well-being and education. No significant differences were found in patient care outcomes between the flexible and standard duty-hour programs. Overall satisfaction with well-being and education were also not significantly inferior in flexible versus standard programs.[45] A follow-up study utilizing semi-structured interviews with seven program directors, two attending physicians, and five residents who had experienced both standard and flexible duty hours (interns were excluded) found that program directors and attending physicians typically considered the flexible duty hours schedule to be helpful in reducing transitions of care. Residents also reported on the benefits of waiving shift length limitations and protected sleep periods between shifts in the flexible arm by allowing them to advance from internship to the next year of residency with skill acquisition, progressive responsibility, and better skills to manage sleep in a way that would help them in the future. They also felt that, in the flexible arm, they more routinely had a full post-call day off, which allowed them greater ability to attend to personal commitments.[46]

Understanding Why Workload Measures May Not Relate Consistently to Well-Being Measures

There are several possible explanations of why limitations in measures of workload, as exemplified by duty-hour limitation metrics, may not make a clear difference on student and GME trainee well-being. The impact of expecting the same amount of work in less time—also called *work compression*—is one possible explanation because such compression may increase time pressure.[11] Additionally, learners may feel—due to their own experiences or the formal or informal messaging received from their instructors—that they are less well prepared for their clinical tasks.[47] An intervention that reduced patient volume for learners and faculty supervisors alike appeared to improve both learning and patient outcomes.[48] As elucidated in the qualitative analysis following the FIRST trial, there also may be unintended consequences from specific types of duty hour limits; for instance, residents in this small study would prefer to work a longer shift in order to have a full post-call day off because this allowed them greater flexibility during that post-call day.[46] Finally, it is possible that the work hours restrictions (which still cap work at 80 hours per week) have not yet reduced the number of hours of week to a threshold that can optimally support well-being. Population-level data, for example, suggest an increased burden of stress-associated illness in groups working longer than 55–60 hours per week.[49]

In an environment in which regulatory requirements could lead to compression of a work day, the resources available to complete the work become even more critical. Additional protected time to complete administrative tasks that need to occur outside of direct clinical work has been found to be beneficial, since those who spend more time on administrative tasks may in turn experience higher rates of burnout.[50-51] Medical students and GME trainees enact many of the same strategies that attending physicians do to complete these tasks, such as working at home on the EHR in order to meet the demands of their work. Interventions to improve efficiency for GME trainees have often focused on enhancing the work of the interprofessional team. For instance, an intervention in which pharmacy trainees, supervised by a pharmacist, performed medication histories and reconciled medication lists on hospital admissions for general medicine patients improved burnout among residents on those services.[25] Team-based care models such as these have been shown to improve well-being in practicing physicians as well as residents.[26,52] These interventions lower workload by off-loading tasks and potentially by modifying the culture of the clinical learning environment.[52]

Systems-Level Interventions Focused on Culture

While the formal curriculum plays out in the planned and delivered curricular content, the "hidden curriculum" (the unintended lessons in behaviors, skills, and attitudes conveyed implicitly in the clinical learning environment) is omnipresent and active in the course of work across learning environments. Messages conveyed implicitly through the hidden curriculum can be either positive (e.g., role-modeled interactions with patients) or negative. For learners, the hidden curriculum influences the culture of the clinical learning environment and affects learning and performance. For example, in a simulation study where rudeness was the experimental variable, teams' diagnostic and procedural performance declined due to reduced information-sharing and help-seeking when an observer was rude.[53] The impact of incivility and microaggressions on well-being is discussed in greater detail below. These negative events likely contribute to increased emotional workload by increasing the overall cognitive load of work.

In the next section, we first describe the role of promoting an inclusive culture as a critical aspect of supporting well-being in the learning environment. Then we describe additional interventions to enhance a culture of well-being for medical students and GME trainees.

Promoting an Inclusive Culture in Graduate and Undergraduate Medical Education

Nearly all trainees will experience or witness bias in their careers, yet few report this bias and many may not know how to respond. Promoting an inclusive culture begins first with understanding the drivers of bias, discrimination, and harassment and having a grounding belief that there is opportunity for growth. It is imperative that involvement in these efforts is wide and motivated by leadership's commitment to an inclusive culture. Individual and systemic factors must be considered through intentional efforts to identify and eliminate practices that are exclusionary and sustain inequities within institutions.[54-56] The American Association of Medical Colleges (AAMC) describes the vision for this state: "when every person can attain their full potential and no one is disadvantaged from achieving this potential by their social position, group identity, or any other socially determined circumstance."[57]

The Impact of Bias and Discrimination on the Learning Environment

Understanding the spectrum of the "isms"—a term comprising the attitudes, actions, or organizational structure that oppress an individual based on which group they belong to or identify as part of—is critical in ensuring that inclusion efforts are focused broadly.[58] Examples of "isms" are oppression due to color of skin (racism), gender (sexism), economic status (classism), older age (ageism), religion (e.g., anti-Semitism), sexual orientation (heterosexism), and language/immigrant status (xenophobism).[58] Table 8.2 outlines additional terms that one should be familiar with when engaging in this work.

Once definitions are understood, the next step is to consider the impact of "isms" on learners, their well-being, and the learning environment. These impacts can be broken down into (1) the negative experiences themselves, (2) isolation resulting from silence and lack of action or response, and (3) differences in learner performance and evaluation over time due to these experiences. Additionally, it is helpful to consider the multidirectionality by which medical students and GME trainees can be victims of "isms": directed from patients and their families, supervisors, colleagues, other learners, peers, or other health care workers in the clinical and learning environments.[54]

Every component of well-being is affected by microaggressions and bias behavior. Such experiences can create a hostile and invalidating learning climate and work environment that interferes with one's ability to focus, learn, creatively problem-solve, process information, and develop teamwork and trust.[66,67] While each experience might be low impact in the short term, repeated microaggressions and incivilities amount to an accumulative "wear and tear" effect (also known as *allostatic load*), which is associated with increased stress, lower well-being, impaired coping, and increased burnout, cynicism,

TABLE 8.2 Key terms for addressing bias and "isms" in the learning environment

Terms impacting how humans think/feel/act	
Bias	A conscious or unconscious (implicit) attitude or preference in favor of or against individuals, groups, or beliefs.[59]
Stereotypes	Fixed belief impression of a group.[60]
Prejudice	Preference, attitude, belief, or inclination for one group over another that interferes with impartiality.[61-63]
In-group Favoritism	Tendency to respond more positively to people from one's ingroups than to people from outgroups.[64]
Privilege	A right that only some people have access or availability to because of their majority/dominant group membership.[61-63]
Terms that are the product of thoughts/feelings/acts	
Discrimination	Unequal treatment of individuals and groups based on race, gender, social class, sexual orientation, physical ability, religion, etc.[61-63]
Harassment	The use of comments or actions that can be offensive, embarrassing, humiliating, demeaning, and unwelcome.[63]
Microaggression	Everyday verbal, nonverbal, and environmental slights, snubs, or insults (intentional or unintentional), which communicate hostile, derogatory, or negative messages to persons based solely upon their marginalized group membership.[62,63,65]
Incivility	Rude and discourteous behavior in violation of workplace norms for mutual respect.[66]
Structural Inequality	Systemic disadvantage(s) of one social group compared to other groups, rooted and perpetuated through discriminatory practices (conscious or unconscious) that are reinforced through institutions, ideologies, representations, policies/laws, and practices.[62,63]
Intersectionality	The fluid and interconnected social categorizations such as race, class, and gender as they apply to a given individual or group, creating overlapping and interdependent systems of discrimination or disadvantage.[62,63]
Terms to guide institutional efforts	
Diversity	All the characteristics that make one individual or group different from another.[61-63]
Inclusion	Authentically bringing traditionally excluded individuals and/or groups activities, and decision/policy making in a way that shares power.[61-63]
Equity	The condition that would be achieved if one's identity or group membership no longer predicted how one fares.[61-63]
Terms to guide individual efforts	
Ally	An individual who supports a group other than one's own (such as race, gender, age, ethnicity, sexual orientation, religion, etc.). An ally acknowledges oppression and actively commits to reducing their own complicity, investing in strengthening their own knowledge and awareness of oppression.[61-63]
Upstander	A person who speaks or acts in support of an individual or cause, particularly someone who intervenes on behalf of a person being harassed, discriminated against, or treated unfairly.[67]

anxiety, and depression.[66,68,69] A lifetime of these stressful experiences can lead to other chronic health conditions such as hypertension, insomnia, substance use disorder, and posttraumatic stress disorder.[54,66,68–70] The negative ruminations and reduced sense of self-worth, meaning, and purpose that result from microaggressions, bias, and incivility can lead to distraction, avoidance of the offending person or environment, impaired performance and evaluation of performance, lower productivity, lower job satisfaction, and interprofessional challenges.[71–74] As performance is affected, so are opportunities for promotion, advancement, funding, and earning over time.[55]

The culture of the learning environment and psychological safety—defined as an "individual's sense of being able to show and employ oneself without fear of negative consequences to self-image, status or career"—are significantly impacted by the presence of "isms," the structural inequalities that predispose to inequality, and the isolation that occurs when bias is inappropriately handled. In particular, when we consider competencies of practice-based learning and systems-based practice, we need to also ask: How we can fairly evaluate one learner against another when the system itself is laden with inequality?[72–74] Those who experience bias may feel that they have less access to resources, role models, future opportunities, and mentors. Lack of response to mistreatment, bias, or incivility can contribute to a sense of isolation and loneliness for the victim.[75] Those who witness bias can also experience moral distress when unsure of how to respond.[76] Last, when medical students or GME trainees witness or experience bias in the learning environment, there may be an erosion altruism, empathy, and enthusiasm for the profession, which can later impact the quality of care they deliver and further promote an unsupportive hidden curriculum.[77] Due to all of these consequences, as well as the moral imperative to support vulnerable groups such as learners, interventions to address bias and mistreatment are therefore critical components of a systems approach to supporting well-being.

Trauma-Informed Medical Education

Trauma-informed medical education (TIME) is one framework that has been suggested to both examine institutional bias, address the hidden curriculum, educate those in the learning environment, and support those who have witnessed or experienced bias.[69] TIME assumes that all systems have bias that exposes learners to trauma, and it advocates for the individual- and system-level change that must happen to prevent further trauma. This strategy includes *four Rs* (Figure 8.2).[69]

Realize

An important first step is to create clear policies that are communicated transparently to all employees, faculty, staff, learners, and students detailing that "isms" of any kind will not be tolerated.[54,55,57,75,77–79] Leaders must examine local institutional bias and culture, particularly with regard to processes such as awards, evaluations, nominations, hiring, recruitment, grants, and leadership opportunities.[77,80]

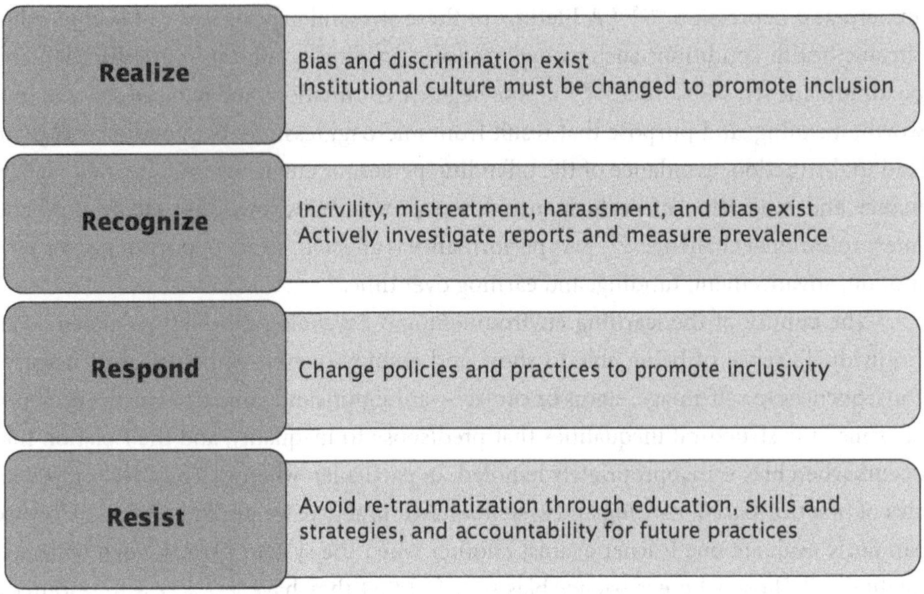

Realize	Bias and discrimination exist Institutional culture must be changed to promote inclusion
Recognize	Incivility, mistreatment, harassment, and bias exist Actively investigate reports and measure prevalence
Respond	Change policies and practices to promote inclusivity
Resist	Avoid re-traumatization through education, skills and strategies, and accountability for future practices

FIGURE 8.2 Approach to trauma-informed medical education (TIME).

Developing transparent and equitable processes using criterion-based metrics can begin to eliminate potential individual and structural bias.[80] Efforts to increase diversity among learner cohorts are an important first step but must also be accompanied by approaches that foster equity and inclusion as well as efforts to enhance diversity among faculty who will serve as mentors and role models for their learners.[80–82]

Recognize

The ability to investigate reports necessitates the existence of a reporting system that holds the victim's psychological safety as paramount.[55,56,77,78,83] Eliminating the fear of retaliation and lowering the effort and burden associated with reporting can help increase the likelihood that when mistreatment and bias occurs, it will be reported.[84] One way to address this concern is to create alternative reporting options for those who fear reporting.[85] Examples could be through an ombudsperson or other anonymous confidential reporting mechanisms separate from the learner's direct chain of supervision. Every report should be investigated, and, as investigations occur, transparency and accountability should be made clear, with the results of the investigation ultimately being shared with the victim.[77] A restorative justice framework, repairing and preventing harm caused by mistreatment by incorporating input for solutions from all stakeholders, is one approach successfully used by some organizations. With this approach, the victim, perpetrator (which can be an individual or institution), and the learning community collectively identify areas for improvement while examining the experience from multiple perspectives.[82]

Respond

Creating community and support for those who experience and witness bias is an empathic leadership response to trauma in the learning environment. Examples of response approaches were introduced in Chapter 6 and further described in Chapter 7; these include dialogue groups and reflection sessions, access to mental health services and counseling, stress management resources and groups, and support for work-life stress through an employee assistance program or other student and resident mental health services.[55,56,82,86,87]

Synergistic efforts between appointed leaders in diversity and well-being (chief diversity and wellness officers, designated institutional officials, program directors, deans) can improve well-being and reduce burnout for minority or marginalized groups through programming and data analysis.[87] Together, these leaders can sponsor joint programming to improve the experience for marginalized groups, such as mentoring initiatives, grant-writing workshops, connectivity groups, speaker series, interview and presentation skills, and medical writing and editorial assistance.[88] Additionally, examining well-being measures stratified by demographic group, such as EHR burden and workload data, quality and safety data, and burnout metrics, can help to identify domains that may be disproportionately impacting certain groups. Together, diversity and wellness leadership can subsequently identify areas for improvement at the institutional level.

Resist

Many training programs, curricula, case-based discussions, and retreat models exist in the literature for addressing bias within an organization.[55,56,67,81,89–93] A framework for educational interventions to resist retraumatization is as follows: (1) create a safe space in which to learn; (2) raise awareness of prevalence and impact of bias; (3) promote self-awareness of personal implicit bias (e.g., use Implicit Association Test [IAT]) and how to overcome implicit bias;[81,88–92] (4) provide skills to recognize and address implicit bias, inequities, microaggressions, and discrimination; provide language to be an ally and upstander;[67,91–93] and (5) encourage individuals to set goals and self-monitor behavior and practices.[81]

These systematic interventions to combat bias and microaggressions while supporting a learning environment that ensures well-being must start early in training. By instituting evidence-based changes starting at the medical student level, institutions can ensure more successful and supported learners during a long training process. If established early, these behaviors will become an inherent part of a learner's toolkit, traveling with them from medical school into residency. Organizations that invest systematically in supporting the well-being of their faculty, GME trainees, and students can create a self-fulfilling environment and promote professional fulfillment.

Medical Student Culture and Learning Environment

The Learning Environment

The culture and environment of the workplace and learning space are critical for medical student well-being and education. Whereas *environment* refers to the overarching "feel" of a particular institution, *culture* refers to the institution's shared values, traditions, and expectations. Medical students are often eager to assimilate into or feel like a valued member of their learning environment from early stages of education. This is particularly true during the clerkship years, when students are surrounded by GME trainees and attending physicians who will serve as role models for their future clinical practice. Students report stress associated with attempting to be liked—the greatest factor they perceive as driving their clerkship grades.[94] These are also the years during which students begin to endorse concerns about losing control of personal and professional factors in their own lives and eventual loss of well-being.[28,36,95] Overnight call for medical students has been significantly associated with burnout, while pass–fail curricula also have been correlated with reduced symptoms of burnout and increased general well-being in training.[28,30,96,97] As previously mentioned, patterns of distress begin early in medical school, so identifying opportunities to intervene early on can have a significant effect on the subsequent burnout trajectory.[98–100]

The Hidden Curriculum and Formation of Professional Identity

As medical students assimilate into their learning environment, they also quickly internalize the values they see embodied in everyday work. In addition to structured curricula (lectures and clerkship rotations) and informal curriculum ("chalk talks" and impromptu teaching on the wards), most acknowledge a hidden curriculum which is carried out through the behaviors, professionalism, and practice patterns of those whom trainees seek to emulate. The "hidden curriculum" of medicine drives the formation of professional identity, is the foundation of patient interactions, and leads to the establishment of role models for trainees.[96] Interventions that address these "implicit messages" in the culture may therefore have multilayered impacts. Removing implicit and explicit biases in clerkship evaluations may help foster positive professional identity formation, although this change will involve significant culture change and faculty development.[30] Having dedicated mental health, therapy, and mind–body integration programs was associated with less suicidal ideation and depression, with some of this effect likely due to a culture change prioritizing the mental health and well-being of medical students.[96] Ideally, the creation of systems-level program interventions to address the hidden curriculum, bias, and culture of the learning environment can holistically improve the well-being of an organization and those who work within it. However, research in this area is limited and additional robust and high-quality medical education research to identify successful strategies.[96]

Role of Graduate Medical Education Trainees in the Medical Student Learning Environment

GME trainees have a significant role in the medical student experience, as described in Chapter 5. When surveyed across multiple academic centers, medical students' exposure to cynicism expressed by supervising residents strongly correlates with negative perceptions of the learning environment.[98,101] Some students detailed this cynicism as one of the strongest negative impacts on the learning environment, more so than the level of faculty supervision or rotational organization.[28] Support from residents and faculty supervision together are clearly drivers of medical student well-being. Proposed intervention strategies could include explicit orientation of GME trainees to successful models of medical student supervision with concomitant systems-level interventions to build faculty–student relationships and support well-being of the entire clinical team.[28,96,100]

Role of Faculty Professionalism

Faculty role-modeling of professional behavior—including treatment of colleagues, clinical encounters, and language used to discuss patients—is crucial in the reduction of student burnout.[100,101] In a survey-based assessment of medical students, a supportive learning environment and empathic support from faculty leaders led to reduced burnout when working in the professional environment.[100] While students showed resilience to patient suffering and death, those who were mistreated by superiors had increased depression and stress.[101] Specifically, witnessed lapses in professionalism exhibited by role models was associated with a less supportive learning environment and, by association, reduced student support.[98] When surveyed, pre-clerkship students noted that the most frequent lapses included arrogance, breach of confidentiality, lack of cultural or religious sensitivity, or impairment.[98,101] Recognizing the impact of these behaviors and actions can serve as specific targets for training and faculty development efforts.

Learner Mistreatment and Neglect

Overt learner mistreatment is defined by the AAMC as overt abuse, harassment, discrimination based on race, gender, or sexual orientation, and any behavior which diminishes the dignity of a learner. Such actions are relatively rare in student surveys.[98,101] These may be either intentional or unintentional actions that can prevent a learner from achieving their full potential and, though relatively rarely reported in student surveys, are detrimental to well-being.[77,98,101] However, many more behaviors exhibited in the learning environment can negatively affect medical student well-being aside from frank mistreatment. These practice patterns may instead reflect learner neglect, which can be more subtle, including such actions as purposefully excluding or preventing a learner from contributing to a team, referring to a student by anything other than their name, failing to acknowledge the student, and deferring feedback.[98,101,102] Systems-level training to ensure that faculty are cognizant of these behaviors is imperative in ensuring student success.[55,101,102] Chapter 10 also describes some of the regulatory requirements related to mistreatment that can be leveraged to build supportive systems to prevent and address student mistreatment.

Mentorship and Community

Learners and professionals at all levels find meaning in community—particularly in the ability to share and discuss difficult experiences in a nonjudgmental environment. Interventions designed to increase community may therefore benefit well-being. For example, the presence of learning communities has been investigated as a pre-clerkship curricular intervention designed to reduce stress, improve connectivity among peers, and augment students' perspectives of their learning environment.[97,99,103] In 24 ACGME-accredited institutions, 18 of which had learning communities, students' responses to the 18-item Medical Student Learning Environment Survey (MLES) were significantly higher in learning-community institutions compared with those schools without learning communities. Notably, clinical performance improved along with a sense of belonging, connection with leadership, and relationship with peers.[103] Other comprehensive medical school curriculum revisions have shown substantial growth in the well-being and happiness of students as part of a redesigned well-being focused learning community.[99] Students also endorse benefit from humanities-, ethics-, and communication-focused curricular models when compared to more traditional didactic models. Additionally, focused attention on topics increasingly of importance to many trainees, such as social and global medicine, can increase the quality of the learning environment.[97]

The most effective learning communities include robust mentoring or coaching at both faculty and peer-to-peer levels. Coaching is another systems-level intervention which improves the overall learning environment, and GME trainees who undergo dedicated coaching with a positive psychology framework endorse better programmatic satisfaction.[104–106] Longitudinal faculty mentorship is crucial to seeing improvements in burnout.[96] This mentorship also fosters a sense of well-being, support, and belonging during critical years of training as the professional identity of the developing physician is solidified.[107]

GME Culture and Learning Environment

The Overall Learning Environment and Team Dynamics

The culture and environment of an institution are also critical for resident and fellow well-being and professional success. Residents and fellows are subject to the environment and culture of multiple entities, including those of the medical team, residency or fellowship program, institution, and even health care system. Because GME trainees work within multiple distinct but interconnected environments, system-wide interventions that target well-being must find the appropriate balance of specificity, adaptability, and pervasiveness in order to be effective.

The Job Demands-Resources Model is a useful framework to understand the effect of workplace environment on employee satisfaction and productivity.[14] This model has been found to be applicable to the GME trainee. In a survey of surgical training programs, job satisfaction was significantly predicted by workplace climate and was also associated with increased perceived organizational support and decreased burnout.[108] Other studies have also found a relationship between overall workplace/learning climate and work engagement, job satisfaction, and rates of burnout.[34,109]

The day-to-day job responsibilities of residents and fellows and their interactions with other staff play a large role in shaping the workplace climate.[110] Some of the team-based factors having a positive correlation to resident job satisfaction include all team members working to their full potential, nurses having empathy and appreciation for resident work, perceived appreciation from the nurses, supportive social networks within the residency program, and perceived appreciation from attending physicians. Other workload factors associated with job satisfaction include clear job expectations and boundaries, appropriate balance of teaching and patient care tasks, and increasing hours of sleep within the last 24 hours. Interestingly, the factor shown to have the *strongest* association with job satisfaction is resident perception of patients receiving high-quality care. These findings suggest that resident and fellow well-being can be strongly influenced by systems-level initiatives and policies that support a positive workplace environment through training and education of nurses and other ancillary staff, clear delineation of duties and expectations, and the enforcement of work-hour restrictions. It is also clear that GME trainee well-being can be supported by the creation of a culture of gratitude, which can be facilitated through frequent recognition for a job well done, provision of emotional support systems, and enhancing connections with colleagues and patients.[111]

Team dynamics in particular can affect workplace climate.[112] A multi-institutional study in the Netherlands found a positive association between teamwork effectiveness and the overall learning climate.[113] Aspects critical to the identity of an effective team include having mutual respect for one another, clinical teachers willing to discuss opinions honestly and address problems adequately, residents feeling empowered to ask questions and seek guidance, and clarification of resident expectations and how they are to be assessed. Conversely, dissatisfaction with emotional support from supervisors has been found to be a significant predictor of GME trainee burnout and emotional exhaustion.[114] The residency learning climate has also been found to affect the patient experience, with the overall learning environment being positively associated with physician communication and a feeling of safety.[115] Thus, promotion of positive teamwork dynamics can be fostered at the institutional level by faculty development and teamwork interventions, as well as by supporting an environment where clear communication and feedback is encouraged. These interventions are not only beneficial to trainees, but also may lead to better patient care.

In addition to interventions at the systems level, residencies and fellowships can also enact policies at the program-level to create a positive learning environment and enhance the perceived support of the organizational climate. For example, the provision of academic support through stipends for academic resources, formal access to board review questions, or formal on-site board preparation courses have all been associated with lower rates of burnout, greater job satisfaction, greater perceived organizational support, less work–life strain, and a greater proportion of high performers on the ITE.[116] Additionally, both faculty–trainee and near-peer mentorship programs have been associated with decreased rates of burnout and higher levels of both workplace and personal satisfaction.[117,118]

System Impacts of Wellness Programs and Curricula

In 2017, the ACGME developed requirements which recognized that training programs have a role in enacting policies and programs that encourage resident and fellow well-being.[119] Subsequently, an unprecedented number of wellness programs and curricula have been implemented at training institutions across the country. These curricula have been variable in regard to structure, perception by trainees, and effectiveness in reducing burnout.

Many institutions have enacted longitudinal wellness curricula that provide education on the identification of burnout, skills to improve resilience, and mindfulness techniques.[120-123] In essence, these curricula are a systematic implementation of interventions that seek to modify individual attributes and coping mechanisms. Institutions have also tried to promote a healthier work environment through interventions such as healthy cooking demonstrations, the provision of healthier food in the cafeteria, workplace gym space or exercise classes, and funding to promote trainee participation in local sports leagues.[124,125] While many of these wellness curricula and interventions have been positively perceived by trainees, the mitigation of burnout has not been reliably demonstrated across all settings and intervention types. As previously described, individually focused interventions are ultimately limited in scope since they do not address the systems-level drivers of burnout.

Some institutions have chosen to implement established individually focused wellness initiatives from other disciplines. In particular, Coping with Work and Family Stress, an evidence-based workplace mental health and substance abuse preventive intervention, has been shown to be effective in the GME setting. Residents who participated in the curriculum reported decreased or similar levels of perceived job stress and family stress post-intervention, compared to increased levels of stress over time experienced in the control group, and greater reductions in anxiety, depression, and alcohol consumption during the study period.[126] As another example, an emergency medicine residency assessed the implementation of The Happiness Practice, a corporate wellness program consisting of monthly didactic sessions led by two former business executives.[127] Interestingly, the intervention was associated with a paradoxical trend toward a slight increase in overall burnout, emotional exhaustion, and depersonalization. The residents were highly dissatisfied with the program, citing frustration in that the instructors had a poor understanding of residency stressors and that the program lacked relevance to the trainee experience. These experiences suggest that corporate wellness initiatives must be implemented with caution in the medical education setting because this population experiences a unique constellation of stressors that may be inadequately addressed by programs intended for the general public.

Many programs instead have opted to develop a retreat model to promote well-being among their trainees in response to the ACGME mandate, either in lieu of or as a complement to longitudinal curricula. These retreats typically consist of 1-day trainings focused on topics such as team-building and bonding, empathy, guided reflection, burnout assessment, effective communication, and personal strategies for developing resilience.[128,129] While these curricula have been received positively by residents, data are lacking on whether such interventions actually lead to a reduction in burnout or the acquisition of resiliency skills, and it is difficult to measure the impact of such programs in a dynamic environment in which stresses to well-being are frequently evolving. Despite the lack of quantitative data for both longitudinal and retreat-based wellness curricula, the development of such initiatives requires few resources and can offer leadership opportunities for GME trainees such that their implementation should be encouraged. Additionally, if implemented with resident input into content, such programs may have a positive effect on the perceived support by leadership, thus enhancing a culture of wellness.

The "Wellness Infrastructure": Supports for Self-Care and Community-Building

Many programs have systematized creative interventions to normalize mental health care and a supportive culture. One residency program created an initiative to introduce trainees to counseling services and facilitated attendance at their initial consultation by scheduling an appointment for all residents and relieving them of clinical responsibilities during that time.[130] Prior to this program, many residents were unaware of how to schedule a consultation. Most residents accepted the offer for a scheduled counseling session, perceived the consultation as positive, and said they would likely seek counseling services in the future. Of note, the study authors noted that scheduling appointments during usual work hours and excusing residents from their clinical responsibilities during this time was critical to promoting a workplace culture of support and normalizing the need for counseling services among medical professionals.

GME trainees often experience difficulty in scheduling medical, mental, or dental care appointments due to their busy clinical schedules. Some training programs have protected time for such appointments, using a "wellness day" or "personal day" model. One program provided all residents with up to 5 wellness days with the goal of promoting flexibility when scheduling these important self-care activities.[131] Most residents thought that the enactment of wellness days had a positive impact on their experience, and there was a trend toward decreased rates of burnout among residents who used these days. There was also a statistically significant reduction in the use of sick days during the year that this initiative was implemented, although the causal relationship between wellness days and use of sick time requires further study.

The nature and tone of the trainee evaluation process can also have a large impact on wellness, self-confidence, and resiliency. One program sought to redesign the resident assessment process by integrating personalized advising and the voice of the learner.[132] The intervention included the creation of a resident assessment facilitation team (RAFT), consisting of a program director, advisor, medical educator, and the resident. The RAFT assessment process started with a short narrative provided by the resident followed by a conversation among all committee members encompassing resident self-assessment, educational planning, and need for further support or assistance. The resident then developed several goals and considerations for ways that others could support their achieving those goals. A post-intervention survey found stable measures of well-being in the RAFT group compared to a downward trend during residency in others.

Development of a "wellness infrastructure" through interventions such as coaching, peer support programs, and establishment of wellness champions may also enhance an overall culture of well-being. In one institution, a coaching program to practice self-reflection and seek guidance from faculty in a non-evaluative capacity was positively perceived and resulted in less emotional exhaustion and burnout than in a historical cohort.[133] Many institutions are now beginning to enact peer support programs for both trainees and faculty, consisting of trained clinician peers who provide one-on-one support to individuals following emotionally stressful events through reflective listening, validation of emotions, discussion of coping strategies, and the provision of organizational resources for additional help. Evaluative data on the impacts on well-being outcomes for such programs are currently lacking, though these support systems have thus far been perceived favorably.[134] Similarly, the presence of official wellness champions was associated with decreased rates of burnout and depression among surgical residents and fellows. These individuals identify ways to improve program structure through implementation of wellness initiatives, but their presence may have a positive effect on the culture by indicating leadership support for prioritizing well-being.[135]

Conclusion

Interventions at the system level intended to promote trainee well-being have the potential to be more impactful than those that only address individual factors, as illustrated in Figure 8.3. First and foremost, each institution must strive to create an inclusive culture that ameliorates bias, harassment, and discrimination. Second, systemic policies that promote a positive learning climate and best optimize learner workload for education and well-being, such as developing a pass–fail curricula, enforcing work-hour restrictions, minimizing "scutwork" when appropriate, and creating relevant faculty development programs, have the potential to be most effective. In addition, structural changes

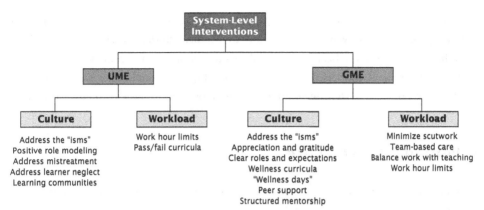

FIGURE 8.3 Summary of approach to system-level interventions in undergraduate medical education (UME) and graduate medical education (GME) programs.

to implement programs that support positive individual attributes, foster professional development, normalize self-care, and enhance community also have value. Such initiatives can include wellness curricula, learning communities, novel assessment systems, formalized coaching, peer support programs, and establishing wellness champions. Many of the sentiments expressed in this chapter are also articulated in the Charter on Well-Being, which can serve as a guide to policymakers, organizations, and individual physicians striving to promote well-being by improving system supports for workload and workflow, protecting opportunities for self-care, and enhancing a trustworthy culture of medicine.[3] Given the enormous influence of the system on physician well-being, institutions and programs should prioritize positively shaping the environment in which students learn and GME trainees work to facilitate their professional growth and personal development.

Summary Points

- System-level interventions can modify the experience of many learners and have been shown to be more effective at reducing burnout than individually targeted interventions.
- An association between workload and burnout among learners has not been reliably demonstrated; however, interventions to improve efficiency and promote team-based care have been shown to improve GME trainee well-being.
- Understanding and addressing the "isms" (e.g. racism, sexism, ageism, etc.) and their effect on learners is critical to ensuring an inclusive culture and learning environment; institutions should develop policies, strategies, and educational practices to promote inclusivity, mitigate bias, and prevent trainee mistreatment.
- Resident supervisory practices and faculty role modeling contribute to the "hidden curriculum" and play a large role in shaping medical students' professional development and well-being.

- Well-being curricula have inconsistently demonstrated an effect on burnout but are often perceived positively by GME trainees. Medical student learning communities, dedicated time for medical and mental health appointments, holistic and resident-driven assessment models, formalized mentorship and coaching, and peer support programs are other system-level interventions shown to promote trainee well-being.

Putting It Into Practice

- Consider the demands-resources model for learners to address both sources of workload and aligned efficiencies and resources.
- Consider using the trauma informed medical education (TIME) framework to examine institutional bias, address the hidden curriculum, improve the learning environment, and support those who have witnessed or experienced bias.
- Explore opportunities for faculty to improve addressing learner mistreatment and neglect.
- Consider instituting pass–fail curricula and learning communities for medical students that have focused programs dedicated to mentoring, coaching, and mental health resources.
- Medical schools, residency programs, and fellowship programs can consider interventions such as a "wellness day" (or half-day) so that learners can attend medical, dental, and mental health appointments.
- Consider using an opt-out mental health consultation scheduled for the learner, during which time they are excused from learning or clinical duties.

References

1. Guille C, Frank E, Zhao Z, et al. Work-family conflict and the sex difference in depression among training physicians. *JAMA Intern Med.* 2017;177(12):1766. doi:10.1001/jamainternmed.2017.5138
2. Ey S, Moffit M, Kinzie JM, Brunett PH. Feasibility of a comprehensive wellness and suicide prevention program: a decade of caring for physicians in training and practice. *J Grad Med Educ.* 2016;8(5):747–753. doi:10.4300/JGME-D-16-00034.1
3. Thomas LR, Ripp JA, West CP. Charter on physician well-being. *JAMA.* 2018;319(15):1541. doi:10.1001/jama.2018.1331
4. Dyrbye LN, West CP, Satele D, et al. Burnout among U.S. medical students, residents, and early career physicians relative to the general U.S. population: *Acad Med.* 2014;89(3):443–451. doi:10.1097/ACM.0000000000000134
5. Bellini LM, Baime M, Shea JA. Variation of mood and empathy during internship. *JAMA.* 2002;287(23):3143–3146.
6. Panagioti M, Panagopoulou E, Bower P, et al. Controlled interventions to reduce burnout in physicians: a systematic review and meta-analysis. *JAMA Intern Med.* 2017;177(2):195. doi:10.1001/jamainternmed.2016.7674
7. Busireddy KR, Miller JA, Ellison K, Ren V, Qayyum R, Panda M. Efficacy of interventions to reduce resident physician burnout: a systematic review. *J Grad Med Educ.* 2017;9(3):294–301. doi:10.4300/JGME-D-16-00372.1

8. Goitein L, Shanafelt TD, Wipf JE, Slatore CG, Back AL. The effects of work-hour limitations on resident well-being, patient care, and education in an internal medicine residency program. *Arch Intern Med.* 2005;165(22):2601–2606. doi:10.1001/archinte.165.22.2601

9. Gopal R, Glasheen JJ, Miyoshi TJ, Prochazka AV. Burnout and internal medicine resident work-hour restrictions. *Arch Intern Med.* 2005;165(22):2595. doi:10.1001/archinte.165.22.2595

10. Martini S. Burnout comparison among residents in different medical specialties. *Acad Psychiatry.* 2004;28(3):240–242. doi:10.1176/appi.ap.28.3.240

11. Committee on Systems Approaches to Improve Patient Care by Supporting Clinician Well-Being, National Academy of Medicine, National Academies of Sciences, Engineering, and Medicine. *Taking Action Against Clinician Burnout: A Systems Approach to Professional Well-Being.* National Academies Press; 2019:25521. doi:10.17226/25521

12. Weinger MB, Reddy SB, Slagle JM. Multiple measures of anesthesia workload during teaching and nonteaching cases [published online May 2004]. *Anesth Analg.* 2004:1419–1425. doi:10.1213/01.ANE.0000106838.66901.D2

13. Hart SG, Staveland LE. Development of NASA-TLX (Task Load Index): results of empirical and theoretical research. In: AP Hancock, A Meshkati, eds. *Advances in Psychology.* Vol 52. Elsevier; 1988:139–183. doi:10.1016/S0166-4115(08)62386-9

14. Harry E, Sinsky C, Dyrbye LN, et al. Physician task load and the risk of burnout among US physicians in a national survey. *Jt Comm J Qual Patient Saf.* 2021;47(2):76–85. doi:10.1016/j.jcjq.2020.09.011

15. Demerouti E, Bakker AB, Nachreiner F, Schaufeli WB. The job demands-resources model of burnout. *J Appl Psychol.* 2001;86(3):499–512.

16. Rushton CH, ed. *Moral Resilience.* Vol 1. Oxford University Press; 2018. doi:10.1093/med/9780190619268.001.0001

17. Steger MF. Meaning in life. In: Lopez SJ, Snyder CR, eds. *The Oxford Handbook of Positive Psychology.* Oxford University Press; 2009:678–688. doi:10.1093/oxfordhb/9780195187243.013.0064

18. Tak HJ, Curlin FA, Yoon JD. Association of intrinsic motivating factors and markers of physician well-being: a national physician survey. *J Gen Intern Med.* 2017;32(7):739–746. doi:10.1007/s11606-017-3997-y

19. Ben-Itzhak S, Dvash J, Maor M, Rosenberg N, Halpern P. Sense of meaning as a predictor of burnout in emergency physicians in Israel: a national survey. *Clin Exp Emerg Med.* 2015;2(4):217–225. doi:10.15441/ceem.15.074

20. Shanafelt TD, West CP, Sloan JA, et al. Career fit and burnout among academic faculty. *Arch Intern Med.* 2009;169(10):990. doi:10.1001/archinternmed.2009.70

21. Tak HJ, Curlin FA, Yoon JD. Association of intrinsic motivating factors and markers of physician well-being: a national physician survey. *J Gen Intern Med.* 2017;32(7):739–746. doi:10.1007/s11606-017-3997-y

22. Rao SK, Kimball AB, Lehrhoff SR, et al. The impact of administrative burden on academic physicians: results of a hospital-wide physician survey. *Acad Med.* 2017;92(2):237–243. doi:10.1097/ACM.0000000000001461

23. Shanafelt TD, Dyrbye LN, Sinsky C, et al. Relationship between clerical burden and characteristics of the electronic environment with physician burnout and professional satisfaction. *Mayo Clin Proc.* 2016;91(7):836–848. doi:10.1016/j.mayocp.2016.05.007

24. Domaney NM, Torous J, Greenberg WE. Exploring the association between electronic health record use and burnout among psychiatry residents and faculty: a pilot survey study. *Acad Psychiatry.* 2018;42(5):648–652. doi:10.1007/s40596-018-0939-x

25. Hillmann W, Hayes BD, Marshall J, et al. Improving burnout through reducing administrative burden: a pilot of pharmacy-driven medication histories on a hospital medicine service [published online July 29, 2020]. *J Gen Intern Med.* doi:10.1007/s11606-020-06066-9

26. Sinsky CA, Bodenheimer T. Powering-Up Primary care teams: advanced team care with in-room support. *Ann Fam Med.* 2019;17(4):367–371. doi:10.1370/afm.2422

27. Ziedelis A. Perceived calling and work engagement among nurses. *West J Nurs Res.* 2019;41(6):816–833. doi:10.1177/0193945918767631

28. Dyrbye LN, Thomas MR, Harper W, et al. The learning environment and medical student burnout: a multicentre study. *Med Educ.* 2009;43(3):274–282. doi:10.1111/j.1365-2923.2008.03282.x

29. Reed DA, Shanafelt TD, Satele DW, et al. Relationship of pass/fail grading and curriculum structure with well-being among preclinical medical students: a multi-institutional study: *Acad Med.* 2011;86(11):1367–1373. doi:10.1097/ACM.0b013e3182305d81

30. Spring L, Robillard D, Gehlbach L, Moore Simas TA. Impact of pass/fail grading on medical students' well-being and academic outcomes: Impact of pass/fail grading on student outcomes. *Med Educ.* 2011;45(9):867–877. doi:10.1111/j.1365-2923.2011.03989.x

31. Bloodgood RA, Short JG, Jackson JM, Martindale JR. A change to pass/fail grading in the first two years at one medical school results in improved psychological well-being. *Acad Med.* 2009;84(5):655–662. doi:10.1097/ACM.0b013e31819f6d78

32. Weiner S. What the elimination of a major medical licensing exam—Step 2 CS—means for students and schools. Published April 2, 2021. Accessed April 6, 2021. https://www.aamc.org/news-insights/what-elimination-major-medical-licensing-exam-step-2-cs-means-students-and-schools

33. Sargent MC, Sotile W, Sotile MO, Rubash H, Barrack RL. Stress and coping among orthopaedic surgery residents and faculty. *J Bone Jt Surg-Am Vol.* 2004;86(7):1579–1586. doi:10.2106/00004623-200407000-00032

34. van Vendeloo SN, Godderis L, Brand PLP, Verheyen KCPM, Rowell SA, Hoekstra H. Resident burnout: evaluating the role of the learning environment. *BMC Med Educ.* 2018;18(1):54. doi:10.1186/s12909-018-1166-6

35. Golub JS, Weiss PS, Ramesh AK, Ossoff RH, Johns MM. Burnout in residents of otolaryngology--head and neck surgery: a national inquiry into the health of residency training: *Acad Med.* 2007;82(6):596–601. doi:10.1097/ACM.0b013e3180556825

36. Dyrbye L, Shanafelt T. A narrative review on burnout experienced by medical students and residents. *Med Educ.* 2016;50(1):132–149. doi:10.1111/medu.12927

37. Fletcher KE, Reed DA, Arora VM. Patient safety, resident education and resident well-being following implementation of the 2003 ACGME duty hour rules. *J Gen Intern Med.* 2011;26(8):907–919. doi:10.1007/s11606-011-1657-1

38. Krug MF, Golob AL, Wander PL, Wipf JE. Changes in resident well-being at one institution across a decade of progressive work hours limitations. *Acad Med.* 2017;92(10):1480–1484. doi:10.1097/ACM.0000000000001675

39. Campbell J, Prochazka AV, Yamashita T, Gopal R. Predictors of persistent burnout in internal medicine residents: a prospective cohort study. *Acad Med.* 2010;85(10):1630–1634. doi:10.1097/ACM.0b013e3181f0c4e7

40. Ripp J, Babyatsky M, Fallar R, et al. The incidence and predictors of job burnout in first-year internal medicine residents: a five-institution study. *Acad Med.* 2011;86(10):1304–1310. doi:10.1097/ACM.0b013e31822c1236

41. Ripp JA, Bellini L, Fallar R, Bazari H, Katz JT, Korenstein D. The impact of duty hours restrictions on job burnout in internal medicine residents: a three-institution comparison study. *Acad Med.* 2015;90(4):494–499. doi:10.1097/ACM.0000000000000641

42. Reed DA, Fletcher KE, Arora VM. Systematic review: association of shift length, protected sleep time, and night float with patient care, residents' health, and education. *Ann Intern Med.* 2010;153(12):829–842. doi:10.7326/0003-4819-153-12-201012210-00010

43. Parshuram CS, Amaral ACKB, Ferguson ND, et al. Patient safety, resident well-being and continuity of care with different resident duty schedules in the intensive care unit: a randomized trial. *Can Med Assoc J.* 2015;187(5):321–329. doi:10.1503/cmaj.140752

44. Desai SV, Asch DA, Bellini LM, et al. Education outcomes in a duty-hour flexibility trial in internal medicine. *N Engl J Med.* 2018;378(16):1494–1508. doi:10.1056/NEJMoa1800965

45. Bilimoria KY, Chung JW, Hedges LV, et al. National cluster-randomized trial of duty-hour flexibility in surgical training. *N Engl J Med.* 2016;374(8):713–727. doi:10.1056/NEJMoa1515724

46. Kreutzer L, Dahlke AR, Love R, et al. Exploring qualitative perspectives on surgical resident training, well-being, and patient care. *J Am Coll Surg.* 2017;224(2):149–159. doi:10.1016/j.jamcollsurg.2016.10.041

47. Ludmerer KM. Redesigning residency education — moving beyond work hours. *N Engl J Med.* 2010;362(14):1337–1338. doi:10.1056/NEJMe1001457

48. McMahon GT, Katz JT, Thorndike ME, Levy BD, Loscalzo J. Evaluation of a redesign initiative in an internal-medicine residency. *N Engl J Med*. 2010;362(14):1304–1311. doi:10.1056/NEJMsa0908136

49. Pega F, Náfrádi B, Momen NC, et al. Global, regional, and national burdens of ischemic heart disease and stroke attributable to exposure to long working hours for 194 countries, 2000–2016: a systematic analysis from the WHO/ILO Joint Estimates of the Work-related Burden of Disease and Injury. *Environ Int*. 2021;154:106595. doi:10.1016/j.envint.2021.106595

50. Stevens K, Davey C, Lassig AA. Association of weekly protected nonclinical time with resident physician burnout and well-being. *JAMA Otolaryngol--Head Neck Surg*. 2020;146(2):168–175. doi:10.1001/jamaoto.2019.3654

51. Eckleberry-Hunt J, Lick D, Boura J, et al. An exploratory study of resident burnout and wellness. *Acad Med J Assoc Am Med Coll*. 2009;84(2):269–277. doi:10.1097/ACM.0b013e3181938a45

52. Hamama L, Hamama-Raz Y, Stokar YN, Pat-Horenczyk R, Brom D, Bron-Harlev E. Burnout and perceived social support: the mediating role of secondary traumatization in nurses vs. physicians. *J Adv Nurs*. 2019;75(11):2742–2752. doi:10.1111/jan.14122

53. Riskin A, Erez A, Foulk TA, et al. The impact of rudeness on medical team performance: a randomized trial. *Pediatrics*. 2015;136(3):487–495. doi:10.1542/peds.2015-1385

54. Fnais N, Soobiah C, Chen MH, et al. Harassment and discrimination in medical training: a systematic review and meta-analysis. *Acad Med*. 2014;89(5):817–827. doi:10.1097/ACM.0000000000000200

55. Hill KA, Samuels EA, Gross CP, et al. Assessment of the prevalence of medical student mistreatment by sex, race/ethnicity, and sexual orientation. *JAMA Intern Med*. 2020;180(5):653. doi:10.1001/jamainternmed.2020.0030

56. de Bourmont SS, Burra A, Nouri SS, et al. Resident physician experiences with and responses to biased patients. *JAMA Netw Open*. 2020;3(11):e2021769. doi:10.1001/jamanetworkopen.2020.21769

57. AAMC. AAMC statement on gender equity. Published January 2020. Accessed March 20, 2021. https://www.aamc.org/what-we-do/equity-diversity-inclusion/aamc-statement-gender-equity

58. The Institute for Democratic Renewal. A community builder's tool kit. Accessed March 12, 2021. https://www.google.com/url?sa=t&rct=j&q=&esrc=s&source=web&cd=&ved=2ahUKEwixmvPirb_vAhVLmuAKHYmHDqAQFjAAegQIBBAD&url=http%3A%2F%2Forganizingforpower.files.wordpress.com%2F2009%2F06%2Fcommunity-builders-tool-kit.pdf&usg=AOvVaw3SkPiHKMfyn00evuTxLsQO

59. Bias. *Oxford Online Dictionary*. Accessed March 12, 2021. https://www.oxfordlearnersdictionaries.com/us/definition/english/bias_1

60. Stereotype. *Oxford Online Dictionary*. Accessed March 12, 2021. https://www.oxfordlearnersdictionaries.com/us/definition/english/stereotype_1

61. W. K. Kellogg Foundation. Racial resource guide. April 15, 2014. Accessed March 12, 2021. http://www.racialequityresourceguide.org/about/glossary

62. Potapchuk M, Leiderman S, et al. Racial equity tools glossary. Center for Assessment and Policy Development; July 2022. Accessed December 22, 2022. https://www.racialequitytools.org/glossary

63. University of Washington College of the Environment. Diversity, equity and inclusion glossary. September 2021. Accessed December 22, 2022. https://environment.uw.edu/about/diversity-equity-inclusion/tools-and-additional-resources/glossary-dei-concepts/

64. Jhangiani R, Tarry H, Stangor C. Stereotypes, prejudice, and discrimination. In R Jhangiani, H Tarry, C Stangor. *Principles of Social Psychology*. 1st International H5P ed. Accessed March 12, 2021. https://opentextbc.ca/socialpsychology/chapter/ingroup-favoritism-and-prejudice/

65. Sue DW. Microaggressions: more than just race. November 17, 2010. Accessed March 12, 2021. https://www.psychologytoday.com/us/blog/microaggressions-in-everyday-life/201011/microaggressions-more-just-race

66. Zurbrügg L, Miner KN. Gender, Sexual orientation, and workplace incivility: who is most targeted and who is most harmed? *Front Psychol*. 2016;7. doi:10.3389/fpsyg.2016.00565

67. Ho CP, Chong A, Narayan A, et al. Mitigating Asian American bias and xenophobia in response to the coronavirus pandemic: how you can be an upstander. *J Am Coll Radiol*. 2020;17(12):1692–1694. doi:10.1016/j.jacr.2020.09.030

68. Siller H, Tauber G, Komlenac N, Hochleitner M. Gender differences and similarities in medical students' experiences of mistreatment by various groups of perpetrators. *BMC Med Educ.* 2017;17(1):134. doi:10.1186/s12909-017-0974-4

69. McClinton A, Laurencin CT. Just in TIME: trauma-informed medical education. *J Racial Ethn Health Disparities.* 2020;7(6):1046–1052. doi:10.1007/s40615-020-00881-w

70. Sue DW, Alsaidi S, Awad MN, Glaeser E, Calle CZ, Mendez N. Disarming racial microaggressions: microintervention strategies for targets, white allies, and bystanders. *Am Psychol.* 2019;74(1):128–142. doi:10.1037/amp0000296

71. Miner KN, Diaz I, Wooderson RL, McDonald JN, Smittick AL, Lomeli LC. A workplace incivility roadmap: Identifying theoretical speedbumps and alternative routes for future research. *J Occup Health Psychol.* 2018;23(3):320–337. doi:10.1037/ocp0000093

72. Klein R, Julian KA, Snyder ED, et al. Gender bias in resident assessment in graduate medical education: review of the literature. *J Gen Intern Med.* 2019;34(5):712–719. doi:10.1007/s11606-019-04884-0

73. Klein R, Ufere NN, Rao SR, et al. Association of gender with learner assessment in graduate medical education. *JAMA Netw Open.* 2020;3(7):e2010888. doi:10.1001/jamanetworkopen.2020.10888

74. Ross DA, Boatright D, Nunez-Smith M, Jordan A, Chekroud A, Moore EZ. Differences in words used to describe racial and gender groups in medical student performance evaluations. Gold JA, ed. *PLoS One.* 2017;12(8):e0181659. doi:10.1371/journal.pone.0181659

75. Osseo-Asare A, Balasuriya L, Huot SJ, et al. Minority resident physicians' views on the role of race/ethnicity in their training experiences in the workplace. *JAMA Netw Open.* 2018;1(5):e182723. doi:10.1001/jamanetworkopen.2018.2723

76. Wheeler M, de Bourmont S, Paul-Emile K, et al. Physician and trainee experiences with patient bias. *JAMA Intern Med.* 2019;179(12):1678. doi:10.1001/jamainternmed.2019.4122

77. Pradhan A, Buery-Joyner SD, Page-Ramsey S, et al. To the point: undergraduate medical education learner mistreatment issues on the learning environment in the United States. *Am J Obstet Gynecol.* 2019;221(5):377–382. doi:10.1016/j.ajog.2019.04.021

78. Dzau VJ, Johnson PA. Ending sexual harassment in academic medicine. *N Engl J Med.* 2018;379(17):1589–1591. doi:10.1056/NEJMp1809846

79. Boatright D, O'Connor PG, E. Miller J. Racial privilege and medical student awards: addressing racial disparities in alpha omega alpha honor society membership. *J Gen Intern Med.* 2020;35(11):3348–3351. doi:10.1007/s11606-020-06161-x

80. Boatright D, O'Connor PG, E. Miller J. Racial privilege and medical student awards: addressing racial disparities in Alpha Omega Alpha honor society membership. *J Gen Intern Med.* 2020;35(11):3348–3351. doi:10.1007/s11606-020-06161-x

81. Mark S, Link H, Morahan PS, Pololi L, Reznik V, Tropez-Sims S. Innovative mentoring programs to promote gender equity in academic medicine. *Acad Med J Assoc Am Med Coll.* 2001;76(1):39–42. doi:10.1097/00001888-200101000-00011

82. Boatright D, Berg D, Genao I. A roadmap for diversity in medicine during the age of COVID-19 and George Floyd [published online January 19, 2021]. *J Gen Intern Med.*s11606-020-06430-06439. doi:10.1007/s11606-020-06430-9

83. Ross PT, Abdoler E, Flygt L, Mangrulkar RS, Santen SA. Using a modified A3 lean framework to identify ways to increase students' reporting of mistreatment behaviors. *Acad Med.* 2018;93(4):606–611. doi:10.1097/ACM.0000000000002033

84. DiBrito SR, Lopez CM, Jones C, Mathur A. Reducing Implicit Bias: Association of Women Surgeons #HeForShe Task Force Best Practice Recommendations. *J Am Coll Surg.* 2019 Mar;228(3):303–309. doi:10.1016/j.jamcollsurg.2018.12.011. Epub 2019 Jan 4. PMID: 30611895; PMCID: PMC7170165.

85. Dzau VJ, Johnson PA. Ending sexual harassment in academic medicine. *N Engl J Med.* 2018;379(17):1589–1591. doi:10.1056/NEJMp1809846

86. Bergman D, Liljefors I, Palm K. The effects of dialogue groups on physicians' work environment: a matter of gender? Albin TJ, ed. *Work.* 2015;52(2):407–417. doi:10.3233/WOR-152105

87. Ackerman-Barger K, Boatright D, Gonzalez-Colaso R, Orozco R, Latimore D. Seeking inclusion excellence: understanding racial microaggressions as experienced by underrepresented medical and nursing students. *Acad Med.* 2020;95(5):758–763. doi:10.1097/ACM.0000000000003077

88. Yanagihara R, Berry MJ, Carson MJ, et al. Building a diverse workforce and thinkforce to reduce health disparities. *Int J Environ Res Public Health*. 2021;18(4):1569. doi:10.3390/ijerph18041569

89. Perdomo J, Tolliver D, Hsu H, et al. Health equity rounds: an interdisciplinary case conference to address implicit bias and structural racism for faculty and trainees. *MedEdPORTAL*. 2019;15(1):10858. doi:10.15766/mep_2374-8265.10858

90. Lehr S, Banaji M. Implicit Association Test (IAT). November 29, 2011:9780199828340–0033. doi:10.1093/obo/9780199828340-0033

91. Carnes M, Devine PG, Baier Manwell L, et al. The effect of an intervention to break the gender bias habit for faculty at one institution: a cluster randomized, controlled trial. *Acad Med*. 2015;90(2):221–230. doi:10.1097/ACM.0000000000000552

92. Sukhera J, Watling C. A framework for integrating implicit bias recognition into health professions education: *Acad Med*. 2018;93(1):35–40. doi:10.1097/ACM.0000000000001819

93. Chary A, Molina M, Dadabhoy F, Manchanda E. Addressing racism in medicine through a resident-led health equity retreat. *West J Emerg Med*. 2021;22(1):41–44. doi:10.5811/westjem.2020.10.48697

94. Bullock JL, Lai CJ, Lockspeiser T, et al. In pursuit of honors: a multi-institutional study of students' perceptions of clerkship evaluation and grading. *Acad Med*. 2019;94:S48–S56. doi:10.1097/ACM.0000000000002905

95. Dyrbye LN, Thomas MR, Huntington JL, et al. Personal life events and medical student burnout: a multicenter study. *Acad Med J Assoc Am Med Coll*. 2006;81(4):374–384. doi:10.1097/00001888-200604000-00010

96. Wasson LT, Cusmano A, Meli L, et al. Association between learning environment interventions and medical student well-being: a systematic review. *JAMA*. 2016;316(21):2237. doi:10.1001/jama.2016.17573

97. Zgheib NK, Dimassi Z, Arawi T, Badr KF, Sabra R. Effect of targeted curricular reform on the learning environment, student empathy, and hidden curriculum in a medical school: a 7-year longitudinal study. *J Med Educ Curric Dev*. 2020;7:2382120520953106. doi:10.1177/2382120520953106

98. Hendelman W, Byszewski A. Formation of medical student professional identity: categorizing lapses of professionalism and the learning environment. *BMC Med Educ*. 2014;14(1):139. doi:10.1186/1472-6920-14-139

99. Drolet BC, Rodgers S. A comprehensive medical student wellness program: design and implementation at Vanderbilt School of Medicine: *Acad Med*. 2010;85(1):103–110. doi:10.1097/ACM.0b013e3181c46963

100. Brazeau CMLR, Schroeder R, Rovi S, Boyd L. Relationships between medical student burnout, empathy, and professionalism climate. *Acad Med*. 2010;85:S33–S36. doi:10.1097/ACM.0b013e3181ed4c47

101. Cook AF, Arora VM, Rasinski KA, Curlin FA, Yoon JD. The prevalence of medical student mistreatment and its association with burnout. *Acad Med*. 2014;89(5):749–754. doi:10.1097/ACM.0000000000000204

102. Buery-Joyner SD, Ryan MS, Santen SA, Borda A, Webb T, Cheifetz C. Beyond mistreatment: learner neglect in the clinical teaching environment. *Med Teach*. 2019;41(8):949–955. doi:10.1080/0142159X.2019.1602254

103. Smith SD, Dunham L, Dekhtyar M, et al. Medical student perceptions of the learning environment: learning communities are associated with a more positive learning environment in a multi-institutional medical school study. *Acad Med J Assoc Am Med Coll*. 2016;91(9):1263–1269. doi:10.1097/ACM.0000000000001214

104. Palamara K, Kauffman C, Chang Y, et al. Professional development coaching for residents: results of a 3-year positive psychology coaching intervention. *J Gen Intern Med*. 2018;33(11):1842–1844. doi:10.1007/s11606-018-4589-1

105. Nimmons D, Giny S, Rosenthal J. Medical student mentoring programs: current insights. *Adv Med Educ Pract*. 2019;10:113–123. doi:10.2147/AMEP.S154974

106. Palamara K, Chu JT, Chang Y, et al. Who benefits most? A multisite study of coaching and resident well-being [published online June 7, 2021]. *J Gen Intern Med*. doi:10.1007/s11606-021-06903-5

107. Frei E, Stamm M, Buddeberg-Fischer B. Mentoring programs for medical students—a review of the PubMed literature 2000–2008. *BMC Med Educ*. 2010;10(1):32. doi:10.1186/1472-6920-10-32

108. Appelbaum NP, Lee N, Amendola M, Dodson K, Kaplan B. Surgical resident burnout and job satisfaction: the role of workplace climate and perceived support. *J Surg Res*. 2019;234:20–25. doi:10.1016/j.jss.2018.08.035

109. Lases LSS, Arah OA, Busch ORC, Heineman MJ, Lombarts KMJM. Learning climate positively influences residents' work-related well-being. *Adv Health Sci Educ Theory Pr*. 2019;24(2):317–330. doi:10.1007/s10459-018-9868-4

110. Davenport DL, Henderson WG, Hogan S, Mentzer RM, Zwischenberger JB. Study P in the WC of SR and Q of C: surgery resident working conditions and job satisfaction. *Surgery*. 2008;144(2):332–338. e5. doi:10.1016/j.surg.2008.03.038

111. Kasman DL, Fryer-Edwards K, Iii CHB. Educating for professionalism: trainees' emotional experiences on IM and pediatrics inpatient wards. *Acad Med*. 2003;78(7):12.

112. Wallace JE, Lemaire J. On physician well being-you'll get by with a little help from your friends. *Soc Sci Med*. 2007;64(12):2565–2577. doi:10.1016/j.socscimed.2007.03.016

113. Jansen I, Silkens MEWM, Stalmeijer RE, Lombarts KMJM. Team up! Linking teamwork effectiveness of clinical teaching teams to residents' experienced learning climate. *Med Teach*. 2019;41(12):1392–1398. doi:10.1080/0142159X.2019.1641591

114. Prins JT, Hoekstra-Weebers JE, Gazendam-Donofrio SM, et al. The role of social support in burnout among Dutch medical residents. *Psychol Health Med*. 2007;12(1):1–6. doi:10.1080/13548500600782214

115. Smirnova A, Arah OA, Stalmeijer RE, Lombarts KMJM, van der Vleuten CPM. The association between residency learning climate and inpatient care experience in clinical teaching departments in the Netherlands. *Acad Med*. 2019;94(3):419–426. doi:10.1097/ACM.0000000000002494

116. Lee N, Appelbaum N, Amendola M, Dodson K, Kaplan B. Improving resident well-being and clinical learning environment through academic initiatives. *J Surg Res*. 2017;215:6–11. doi:10.1016/j.jss.2017.02.054

117. Zhang H, Isaac A, Wright ED, Alrajhi Y, Seikaly H. Formal mentorship in a surgical residency training program: a prospective interventional study. *J Otolaryngol Head Neck Surg*. 2017;46(1):13. doi:10.1186/s40463-017-0186-2

118. Fischer J, Alpert A, Rao P. Promoting intern resilience: individual chief wellness check-ins. *MedEdPORTAL*. 2019;15:10848. doi:10.15766/mep_2374-8265.10848

119. ACGME. ACGME Common Program Requirements, VI. The learning and working environment. Published online 2017. Accessed December 22, 2022. https://www.acgme.org/globalassets/PFAssets/ProgramRequirements/CPRs_Section-VI_with-Background-and-Intent_2017-01.pdf

120. Aggarwal R, Deutsch JK, Medina J, Kothari N. Resident wellness: an intervention to decrease burnout and increase resiliency and happiness. *MedEdPORTAL*. 2017;13:10651. doi:10.15766/mep_2374-8265.10651

121. Parsons M, Bailitz J, Chung AS, et al. Evidence-based interventions that promote resident wellness from the Council of Emergency Residency Directors. *West J Emerg Med*. 2020;21(2):412–422. doi:10.5811/westjem.2019.11.42961

122. Williams-Karnesky RL, Greenbaum A, Paul JS. Surgery resident wellness programs: the current state of the field and recommendations for creation and implementation. *Adv Surg*. 2020;54:149–171. doi:10.1016/j.yasu.2020.05.005

123. Quinn MA, Grant LM, Sampene E, Zelenski AB. A curriculum to increase empathy and reduce burnout. *WMJ Off Publ State Med Soc Wis*. 2020;119(4):258–262.

124. Mari S, Meyen R, Kim B. Resident-led organizational initiatives to reduce burnout and improve wellness. *BMC Med Educ*. 2019;19(1):437. doi:10.1186/s12909-019-1756-y

125. Watson DT, Long WJ, Yen D, Pichora DR. Health promotion program: a resident well-being study. *Iowa Orthop J*. 2009;29:83–87.

126. Saadat H, Snow DL, Ottenheimer S, Dai F, Kain ZN. Wellness program for anesthesiology residents: a randomized, controlled trial. *Acta Anaesthesiol Scand*. 2012;56(9):1130–1138. doi:10.1111/j.1399-6576.2012.02705.x

127. Hart D, Paetow G, Zarzar R. Does implementation of a corporate wellness initiative improve burnout? *West J Emerg Med*. 2019;20(1):138–144. doi:10.5811/westjem.2018.10.39677

128. Haber MA, Gaviola GC, Mann JR, et al. Reducing burnout among radiology trainees: a novel residency retreat curriculum to improve camaraderie and personal wellness: 3 strategies for success. *Curr Probl Diagn Radiol.* 2020;49(2):89–95. doi:10.1067/j.cpradiol.2019.09.001
129. Castillo J, Chang BP, Choe J, Carter WA. Trainees and faculty healing together: a resident—and faculty-directed wellness initiative for emergency medicine residents. *AEM Educ Train.* 2018;2(4):334–335. doi:10.1002/aet2.10122
130. Broxterman J, Jobe A, Altenhofen D, Eck L. Promoting resident well-being through programmatic scheduled wellness consultation. *J Gen Intern Med.* 2019;34(5):659–661. doi:10.1007/s11606-019-04877-z
131. Mendoza D, Holbrook A, Bertino F, Theriot D, Ho C. Using wellness days to mitigate resident burnout. *J Am Coll Radiol.* 2019;16(2):221–223. doi:10.1016/j.jacr.2018.09.005
132. Foster E, Biery N, Dostal J, Larson D. RAFT (Resident Assessment Facilitation Team): supporting resident well-being through an integrated advising and assessment process. *Fam Med.* 2012;44(10):731–734.
133. Palamara K, Kauffman C, Stone VE, Bazari H, Donelan K. Promoting success: a professional development coaching program for interns in medicine. *J Grad Med Educ.* 2015;7(4):630–637. doi:10.4300/JGME-D-14-00791.1
134. Shapiro J, Galowitz P. Peer support for clinicians: a programmatic approach. *Acad Med.* 2016;91(9):1200–1204. doi:10.1097/ACM.0000000000001297
135. Bui AH, Ripp JA, Oh KY, et al. The impact of program-driven wellness initiatives on burnout and depression among surgical trainees. *Am J Surg.* 2020;219(2):316–321. doi:10.1016/j.amjsurg.2019.10.027

9

Raising Awareness and Ensuring Access to Mental Health Resources

Carol A. Bernstein, Claire Haiman, and Laurel E. S. Mayer

Introduction: The Case for Well-Being Includes Mental Health

Over the past two decades, there has been a significant increase in awareness of the prevalence, vulnerabilities, and substantial impact of both burnout[1,2] and depression[3] in physicians, medical students, and graduate medical education (GME) trainees. The relationship between burnout and depression is a topic of some debate but is critical to understand so that appropriate solutions and treatments in both areas can be developed and implemented.

Well-being, as a modern concept relevant to health and medicine, was described by Halbert L. Dunn.[4] In it, he refers to a World Health Organization (WHO) description of health as "a state of complete physical, mental, and social well-being and not merely the absence of disease and infirmity." Dunn further argues that conditions require that the medical field shift its perspective from "disease and death" to a more positive "good health" approach that views well-being not as an "uninteresting area of 'unsickness' but rather a fascinating and ever-changing panorama of life itself, inviting exploration of its every dimension."[4] Further, he elaborates that "it is essential to shift from considering sickness and wellness as a dichotomy toward thinking of disease and health as a graduated scale."[4] As such, it is necessary to consider the following: (1) whether the relationship between well-being and mental health, focusing primarily on burnout and depression, is best appreciated as a dichotomy or along a spectrum or continuum; (2) the stressors unique to medical training and the range of mental health concerns that can arise; (3) the models of care and mental health resources recommended to fully support the medical student and GME trainee during the long process of training; and (4) common barriers that inhibit medical students and GME trainees from accessing mental health support and treatment. Through this exploration, we can consider implications for organizational efforts, programming, and interventions to promote well-being, alleviate distress, and treat pathology.

The Relationship Between Burnout and Stress

As described in earlier chapters, the medical literature is replete with articles describing burnout in health care. Many studies have specifically focused on the burnout experience of medical students and GME trainees. However, failure to distinguish between symptoms of burnout and those of mental health disorders (especially depression) could lead to both inadequate treatment of psychiatric conditions and neglect of the systemic issues which contribute to burnout.[5] Burnout has been characteristically described as having three components: emotional exhaustion, feelings of depersonalization and cynicism, and a sense of ineffectiveness or lack of perceived personal accomplishment.[6] Depression, on the other hand, is a psychiatric disorder with symptoms that can cause significant distress or impairment in social, occupational, or other important areas of functioning and therefore may easily be confused with burnout. This finding raises the question: Do burnout and depression lie on a continuum, or are they distinct entities that often co-occur (like obesity and hypertension)? Given that making a diagnosis will likely inform the treatment approach, it is important to more fully understand the relationship between burnout and depression.

Burnout, Depression, and the Stress Continuum

Stress as a general response to difficult situations happens to everyone, every day, and most people develop coping mechanisms to get through the experience. *Distress* occurs when life is, at times, harder than expected; for example, after the unexpected death of a patient. Distress may tax someone's usual coping strategies and often requires (and responds well) to additional supportive strategies. For example, following the unexpected death of a patient, deliberately taking time to reflect and mourn the loss may be useful. If distress persists, additional support strategies may include intentionally building in breaks, increasing mindfulness opportunities, and seeking additional support from family, friends, or work colleagues. Some may engage in brief therapy or take medications to help get through the rough patch. At the far end of the stress continuum are *mental health disorders* (e.g., depression, anxiety, posttraumatic stress disorder [PTSD]). These are medical illnesses that are best assessed and treated by behavioral health clinicians who have the expertise to employ evidence-based psychotherapy and medications as needed.

The Relationship Between Stress and Burnout

Job stress can be defined as the harmful physical and emotional responses that occur when the requirements of the job do not match the capabilities, resources, or needs of the worker.[7] Burnout is considered a consequence of prolonged exposure to stressors at work[6] and was initially described among workers in service industries (e.g., health care, law enforcement, education). Codified by the WHO in 2019, burnout is described as an "occupational phenomenon" and not a medical condition. Thus, along the stress continuum described above, burnout could fall within the "distress" range, where usual coping strategies are less effective and require augmentation or additional support. As described in prior chapters, the professional and personal impacts of burnout are now well-established. Removing oneself from the work environment should, therefore, alleviate many symptoms of burnout. However, as conditions that induce burnout are widespread within the health care system, moving to another position may not alleviate these symptoms. Furthermore, leaving one's position may be anathema to physicians who pride themselves on putting patient care first and abnegating their own needs.

The Relationship Between Stress and Depression

Depression, on the other hand, is a psychiatric disorder and is anchored at the far end of the stress continuum. Depression is characterized in part by low or sad mood, diminished interest or loss of pleasure in almost all activities, fatigue or loss of energy, feelings of worthlessness, and a diminished ability to think or concentrate. These symptoms may cause significant distress or impairment in social, occupational, or other important areas of functioning.[8] Affective illnesses such as depression run in families,[9] suggesting a genetic vulnerability to developing depression, although intense or prolonged stress (including work stress) can precipitate depression even in those without a family history. Depression requires treatment by a trained medical or mental health professional and may include medication.

The Relationship Between Burnout and Depression

Although stress, distress, burnout, and depression are presented above as constructs that potentially exist along a spectrum, some argue that burnout and depression are categorically different.[6,10-12] Those who support burnout as separate and distinct from depression argue that burnout is not a disease, is situation-specific, and is driven by a demanding work environment characterized by insufficient resources to complete one's job.[11] Depression, in contrast, has well-defined diagnostic criteria and, most importantly, occurs "context-free," although it can be precipitated by stress. Some recent data suggest little overlap between factors contributing to symptoms of depression and burnout.[13] However another study[14] reported 7 of 8 risk factors were associated with both burnout and depression, and some studies that have examined burnout and depression among physicians note that individuals with higher burnout scores on the Maslach Burnout

Inventory, for example, frequently also meet screening criteria for depression.[13,15] This finding can be interpreted in several ways: burnout may be a precursor of, risk factor for,[14,16,17] or independent from—though sometimes comorbid with—depression.[11,13]

Why Does the Relationship Between Burnout and Depression Matter?

Given the importance of making a diagnosis to help guide treatment and interventions, the relationship between burnout and depression is critical to elucidate. Those in the "burnout is not depression" camp argue that, since burnout is related to the work environment, interventions must be directed at the system level to be effective in decreasing burnout.[1] Therefore, relying solely on individual approaches to address burnout (e.g., enhancing personal resilience or mindfulness) without addressing the system is akin to recommending acetaminophen for a fever without prescribing antibiotics to treat the underlying infection. Additionally, when burnout is not seen as a mental illness because its origins are external to the individual, some may feel that there is less stigma associated with having burnout compared with having a psychiatric diagnosis such as depression. In fact, with the increased awareness of burnout's pervasiveness across many specialties,[18] acknowledging that one suffers from burnout may now be normalized as an area of camaraderie with others experiencing the consequences of working in an ineffective system. Being part of a community, even if burnout is the entry point, may also serve at least in part to provide a sense of support and belonging to counteract the feelings of being overwhelmed and isolated which often accompany burnout. The continued stigma around being diagnosed with or seeking support for mental illness, despite burnout becoming less stigmatized, therefore illustrates that there remains value in distinguishing between burnout and depression so that people can avail themselves of the full menu of treatments that may help them.

Stressors in Medical Student and GME Training

The Model of Medical Education

Although clinical experience is recommended prior to applying to medical school, many students may not matriculate with the sophisticated, fully developed coping skills necessary in the hospital environment.[19] The process of becoming a successful physician requires tremendous dedication, resilience, and consistent academic excellence. Motivated by a strong commitment to help others in distress and a belief that the patient's needs outweighs one's own, medical students and GME trainees are repeatedly challenged to contend with the emotional demands of this intense, sometimes high-stakes environment. It is perhaps this commitment to help others in at times "life-or-death" settings that reveals both personal strength and individual vulnerability to burnout. In addition, the stresses of this environment may precipitate depression in vulnerable individuals.

Stress at the Individual Level

The very traits that contribute to academic success in the classroom—high achievement orientation, obsessional attention to detail, perfectionism—may become maladaptive[20] during clinical training experiences and thus contribute to a source of stress and anxiety. While the volume of information taught during the preclinical years is greater when compared to undergraduate education and often more rigorous, medical students know how to be successful students, and mistakes or failures primarily impact them as individuals (affecting their self-esteem). However, in the clinical setting, the increased responsibility of caring for patients means that errors and mistakes impact not only the individual student but also the patient. To minimize potential harm to patients, medical students are closely supervised. For individuals who have been previously successful and rewarded largely due to their own efforts, close supervision may be perceived as a lack of trust and confidence in one's abilities. This may be exemplified by the rising rates of burnout among medical students significantly seen during the clinical years.[15]

Increased responsibility for patient care and patient outcomes intensifies further with the transition from medical student to resident physician. In fact, transitions to each postgraduate year are often accompanied by an increase in anxiety, largely related to feelings of (in)competence and responsibility and the ambivalence of balancing increased independence with the need for continued supervision.[21] In addition, in circumstances where, despite the trainee's best efforts, a poor patient outcome or patient death occurs, GME trainees may experience significant distress and decreased self-efficacy. Frustration with failed medical efforts may sometimes be expressed as "anger at the system." Or, conversely, for those already sensitive to negative interactions, the conflation of outcome and professional self-worth can be devastating. Additionally, limits to flexibility and autonomy resulting from medical education and training leave little opportunity for control, independence, and time to process, and these can be additive to the above experiences.

One can readily imagine a number of scenarios that may present quite similarly as a result of these circumstances. For example, consider a GME trainee with self-doubt and low self-esteem who experiences fatigue and irritability in the context of a particularly grueling clinical stint with crushing hours. A patient dies, and the supervising attending physician is demeaning and critical. In one instance, the GME trainee has a history of depression in college; in another, the trainee has no significant mental health history. While either may develop depression, the person in the first example may be more likely to experience depression due to prior history. Nevertheless, both system- and individual-level interventions would be of benefit to both trainees.

When considering how to address stresses, burnout, and depression in training, it may be helpful to consider the mantra of "medicine is a marathon not a sprint" and develop a long-term strategy to manage the stress. Perhaps an even more apt analogy is to liken medical education to high-intensity interval training: bursts of sustained high activity followed by brief recovery periods—and the need for recovery to occur quickly.

This conceptualization is in keeping with the *affect regulation model*,[22-24] which posits individuals possess a window of tolerance in which they experience a delicate balance between the sympathetic and parasympathetic branches of the autonomic nervous system that facilitates an optimal state in which they can tolerate ambiguity, reflect on their experiences, and attend to the tasks at hand. High-intensity situations or stressors require shifts out of the window of tolerance into action-oriented sympathetic-dominant states, followed by a quick return to baseline within the window of tolerance. This model for health prizes elasticity and the flexibility to respond to the needs of the situation while resting and relaxing when the opportunity presents itself.[22] How to find opportunities for rest and relaxation within an increasingly taxed health care system can be a challenge, leading to chronic stress which may reset one's baseline, effectively upregulating one into a sympathetic-dominant physiological state that shares much in common with anxiety, or alternately, downregulating into a parasympathetic-dominant state that is akin to depression.[23,24]

Stress at the Interpersonal Level

While medical care is based on a team approach, medical education has historically functioned as a hierarchy. Medical students enter at the bottom and progressively advance through medical school, residency, and fellowship to the attending physician level. This hierarchy can make students and GME trainees vulnerable to mistreatment, compounding normal interpersonal stressors of the workplace. Furthermore, the classic apprenticeship model of medical education relies on seniority, experience, and respect for this hierarchy. While generational differences have always existed,[25] the current generations in training (Millennials and now Gen Z) may be less tolerant of hierarchy and more demanding of an equal role in decision-making.[26] Moreover, the current pace of technological advances in diagnosis, assessment, and treatment, may favor those who are younger and more adept with these changes.[26] Simultaneously, technology may also contribute to a change in the prominence and perceived usefulness of historically valued aspects of medical care (e.g., rather than examine the patient to diagnose appendicitis, a CT scan is ordered prior to conducting a thorough clinical exam). Such generational preferences, coupled with an apparent decreased valuing of expertise based on seniority and experience, may contribute to a perception by the older generation that the younger generation is entitled or unappreciative, while trainees may feel that their supervisors are out of touch. The resulting culture clash may contribute to a sense of lack of validation of and appreciation for all team members, leading to an increase in tension within the learning environment.

Tensions related to hierarchy and individual versus team goals may be even more intense for GME trainees. Medical students are active learners whose goal is to acquire knowledge. The GME trainee, however, is both an employee and learner and must provide service as well as obtain an education. The learning environment thus becomes characterized by the tension between the education and service balance and frequently leads to a conflict between the two.

Stressors from the Health Care System

Some of the stresses experienced by the current generation of medical students and GME trainees may be understood by the paradox of having to achieve at a higher level than their predecessors (higher Medical College Admissions Test scores, higher undergraduate grades, authorship on research publications, etc.)[27] to get a seat at the table, only to find that the professional world they are entering is increasingly in disrepair. They are expected to be near perfect to be accepted into medical school, only to enter a world of clinical practice that is increasingly harried, disjointed, overridden by paperwork, driven by concerns regarding malpractice, and influenced by productivity drivers that minimize job satisfaction. Simultaneously, they often experience reduced opportunities for significant meaningful patient contact and the ability to feel that one is making a difference in the lives of one's patients. For trainees and physicians oriented toward caring for others, these mismatched expectations may be the most damaging challenge to their own mental health, prompting an "existential vacuum" in which their lives have diminished meaning.[28,29]

The distinction between burnout and depression underpins the question of "What is broken?"—the individual or the system—but may be less relevant when viewed through the lens of the stress-diathesis model, [30,31] in which stress can trigger pathological responses in individuals with vulnerabilities. Those with more underlying individual vulnerabilities may require less stress to trip this wire, and, similarly, exposure to more stress may set off pathological responses even in those with little to no underlying vulnerability. Regardless of where one enters this system, a feedback loop quickly takes hold where stress leads to exhaustion and depletion, which in turn leads to depressive symptoms (low self-esteem, negative cognitions, hopelessness) that produce a lower capacity for tolerating stress and so on. Similarly, as per the clinical affect regulation model[22,23] individuals vary in terms of the width of their window of tolerance (i.e., how much stress they can tolerate). Defining factors, including temperament as well as trauma, enable some individuals to tolerate more stress for more time before shifting outside the window of tolerance. However, enough stress over a long enough period of time will push just about anyone into either a sympathetic-/anxiety-like or parasympathetic-/depression-like dominant mode of coping.

When the question of "What is broken?" is instead reframed as "What is helpful?" it seems obvious enough that those struggling with either burnout or depression (or from some combination of the two, depending on how you choose to frame it) benefit from systems-level interventions that increase access to resources and decrease demands, as well as individual-level interventions that address depressive symptoms (e.g., cognitive distortions, feelings of helplessness) and build resilience through solutions-focused, evidence- and mindfulness-based treatments and practices. Ultimately, what may be most important is that viewing burnout and depression along a continuum has the potential to more effectively highlight both the contextual and individual factors at work and in turn inform the comprehensive set of solutions most likely to be effective at reducing overall psychological symptom burden.

Barriers to Treatment-Seeking for Trainees

There are many known barriers to treatment-seeking by medical students and GME trainees. They include and are perhaps not limited to time (and the lack thereof), cost, concern for impact on their career/professional advancement, and stigma.[32]

Time

For the GME trainee in particular, the 80-hour work week often precludes trainees from accessing medical care during "regular business hours." The Accreditation Council for Graduate Medical Education (ACGME) has attempted to address this problem by mandating that programs make provisions to allow GME trainees time to go to medical (including mental health) or dental appointments.[33] GME training programs have begun to implement structural changes to their scheduling, for example, including "wellness days" during which GME trainees are encouraged to make health care appointments. However, training requirements as well as patient care responsibilities often impinge on these arrangements. The increased availability of telehealth both for mental health and routine medical visits may offset time challenges by making access to care more feasible.

Cost

Cost, as a barrier to treatment, remains significant for both medical students and GME trainees. Many mental health providers do not participate on insurance panels because of long-standing unfavorable reimbursement rates or are simply closed to taking new patients. Medical students and GME trainees still maintain considerable debt, and GME trainee salaries may not be sufficient to support out-of-pocket costs for regular treatment. Even when connecting with a provider who does accept the trainee's insurance, the recurrent co-pays can add up and become a financial stressor.

Concern for Impact on Career and Professional Advancement

While services provided at comprehensive campus-based mental health centers are confidential, and protected under the Family Educational Rights and Privacy Act (FERPA) and the Health Insurance Portability and Accountability Act (HIPAA), for some, confidentiality concerns remain paramount, such that GME trainees may preferentially request treatment outside of their home institutions.

Medical students and GME trainees also function as treatment providers themselves and therefore occupy a different category from other students at campus-based treatment centers. Furthermore, medical student and GME trainee impairment has the potential to directly impact patient care. As a result, questions of impairment may lead to the need for drug screening and/or a "fitness for duty" evaluation, particularly for GME trainees. It is essential that fitness for duty evaluations be provided by clinicians other than those participating in the treatment of trainees. Having treating clinicians participate in fitness for duty evaluations has a chilling effect on treatment-seeking and makes treatment a sham in which students and trainees must "perform" well as opposed to freely discussing their struggles so that they might receive appropriate care.

For some, confidentiality concerns may be due to being treated by one's own psychiatry colleagues—a clinician with whom they might work or "run into in the hallway." Under no circumstances is it appropriate for any medical student or GME trainee to be treated by someone who might also concurrently serve in a supervisory or evaluative role within their training. This circumstance may serve as a deterrent to seeking treatment, especially in smaller training settings.

Other confidentiality concerns extend to worries about information subject to disclosure that may have a career impact. Medical students and GME trainees are frequently concerned about questions on licensure or credentialing applications which inquire about histories of treatment for psychiatric disorders. Fortunately, the Federation of State Medical Boards has been working actively to advocate that states eliminate questions about history of medical or mental health diagnosis and treatment and only ask about current impairment to practice, and many states have revised their licensure questions accordingly.[34] Elimination of such questions on hospital credentialing applications will hopefully soon follow suit.

Stigma

Related to the confidentiality concerns for career advancements, stigma still persists (even among physicians) with having a mental health diagnosis. Medical students and GME trainees express concern that patients would not want them as their doctor and that colleagues would not trust them to care for their patients if it were revealed that they had a mental health issue.[35] Additional concerns about potentially damaging inferences in faculty letters of recommendation and/or promotion also exist.

Some reduced treatment-seeking among Asian, Asian American, Black, and Latinx communities may be associated with underrepresentation of mental health treatment providers in the field who "look like me" and "get it." Among those who identify as Black, Indigenous, and Persons of Color (BIPOC) there has been an observed decreased inclination to seek or continue in treatment with a racially non-concordant clinician.[36,37] In addition, stigma about mental illness may sometimes be greater within some communities, further affecting treatment-seeking.[38,39]

Personality Traits

Possessing traits characteristic of the archetypal "physician personality"[20]—being high achieving, obsessional, and perfectionistic—may serve as a powerful barrier to treatment. Perfectionism, as related to high achievement, often confuses being driven to succeed with being perfect. Perfectionists worry that others will value them only if they are perfect, and thus they are less likely to reveal their "mistakes" or "failures." For those who work hard to be as close to perfect as possible and are used to achieving what they set out to do, the experience of uncertainty and lack of control can feel like a failure, particularly when viewed through the lens of the medical model in which they are schooled. Built around pathology, the medical model focuses on what is wrong—the disorder— rather than on the person with the disorder. Difficulties may be experienced as pathologies that overshadow all that is good about the person. Compounding this, the "secret omnipotence" of physicians may lead them to think that they are personally responsible for everything that happens to a patient, disregarding and overlooking that the practice of medicine involves teams and collaborations. Treatments may not go as planned, and expected (side effects) and unexpected outcomes occur that are beyond the physician's control. Nevertheless, the physician feels guilt and self-reproach about possible mistakes or misjudgments, especially if the patient dies. In addition, the "total-surround" aspects of medical education and training in which all aspects of one's performance are intensely scrutinized, evaluated, and ranked may lead to internalization and an intense self-consciousness that furthers the excoriating self-criticism described above.[40] Students and GME trainees are not used to making mistakes or "failing." They have enormous personal strength and therefore can often "compensate" for feelings that they do not really belong or worry about being "exposed." This capacity can make it difficult to identify those who are struggling and obscure their need for assistance, which only ends up making them feel more isolated and alone since no one really knows how they feel.

As a result, we may see a personality interacting with the environment (again, the stress-diathesis model) that prompts the question: Does the culture of medicine take high-achieving, perfectionistic students and GME trainees and, by putting them in high-stakes environments (in which grades become intensely consequential in terms of life choices, given the competitiveness of the field and where death is a possible outcome in any number of clinical encounters) with an overwhelming focus on pathology and intense scrutiny, promote reliance on primitive psychological defenses of dissociation, splitting, compartmentalization, and the like (because failure is not an option and/or cannot be tolerated) that ultimately weaken overall coping strategies or well-being? This question in some ways highlights the gift of not viewing wellness and pathology as a dichotomy; rather, by expanding the spectrum to include well-being, students and trainees are offered the opportunity to consider their experiences absent the lens of pathology.

Models of Mental Health Care and Access to Treatments

Mental health issues such as major depression, generalized anxiety disorder, or bipolar disorder and their psychiatric treatments are best managed by behavioral health experts (e.g., trained counselors, social workers, psychiatric nurse practitioners, psychologists, and psychiatrists). In addition to licensed mental health clinicians, many groups and organizations within health care systems have also developed programs that focus more broadly on wellness and well-being, though the language used to describe such programs is often imprecise. For example, an "Office of Work-Life," perhaps organized through a human resources department, may offer what are referred to as "mental health promotion events" and include "steps challenges" to encourage exercise, individual coaching to achieve personal physical health goals, webinars or toolkits to promote healthy sleep habits, and more. Many organizations offer screening events for both physical health (e.g., blood pressure) and mental health (e.g., screening for depression) under the umbrella of wellness. Given the variety of offerings, frequent lack of coordination across departments and services, and confusion that often exists around marketing how these resources are intended to meet certain specific needs, developing mental health services and resources to connect students and GME trainees to the appropriate care can be challenging and often requires targeted resource investment.

Mental Health Care for Medical Students

A variety of models exist for medical student mental health services, ranging from consultation and referral services, which aim to quickly link students with providers in the community, to the quasi-group practice, in which treatment providers from the community act as affiliates of an institution, provide care to students on site, and then transition those requiring longer-term care to their own private practice settings. Increasingly prevalent are comprehensive campus-based mental health centers, which offer short-term treatment as well as outreach and prevention efforts and often operate in tandem with on-site medical service providers under the umbrella of a student health center. Although there is a growing trend toward the formation of these comprehensive centers, student body size and resource constraints, such as salaries and space, are important considerations and potential budgetary barriers.

Rising levels of symptom acuity and utilization of services at campus-based mental health centers over the past two decades[41] have contributed to a shift toward the comprehensive model. These comprehensive campus-based mental health centers are usually staffed by salaried clinicians and often offer 24/7 access for urgent needs, rapid triage, and disposition, as well as short-term psychotherapy, psychiatric evaluation, and treatment. In addition, the importance of lowering barriers to care has been underscored by research about low rates of treatment-seeking among students with suicidal ideation,[42] as well as additional studies which suggest that only about half of those students in need of mental health care actually seek the help they need.[35,41,43,44] Numbers accessing care drop even further when considering students from historically marginalized communities, such as Black, Latinx, Asian/Asian American, and international students and GME trainees.[43,45,46]

These trends have shifted models of care from individual interventions with learners who present for care in various stages of distress, toward a model that promotes moving upstream to intervene earlier. This includes expanding outreach efforts to medical students as well as working with institutional partners across campus on the shared responsibility of building communities that promote belonging and well-being, rather than simply identifying at-risk individuals earlier in the disease process. One good example is the social-ecological approach detailed by the Jed Foundation and their campus-based suicide prevention work,[47] which reframes suicide prevention on campus as the responsibility of the entire campus community, rather than simply the provenance of the mental health service. Various spokes of this wheel include restricting access to means, promoting social connectedness, developing crisis management protocols, and offering substance use interventions, as well as increasing early identification of students in distress and increasing help-seeking behavior.

Ideally, "many hands make light the work" and reduce the burden of care for the well-being of medical students. However, as a result of increased awareness and the decreased stigma of help-seeking, one impact is that traditional mental health services/counseling centers are increasingly challenged to offer a wide range of treatment services to accommodate students in all states of distress. The combination of higher symptom acuity and increased utilization of services has resulted in the dilution of traditional weekly psychotherapy, greater intervals between appointments, shorter treatments, and increased reliance on referral to off-campus community providers.[48,49]

One potential positive development from the COVID pandemic has been a rapid transition to more telepsychiatry offerings,[50] which has lowered barriers to care, providing more convenient, private access.[48] The ability to access telepsychiatric care without the "time wasted" of commuting to and from the treatment site is a boon to many tightly scheduled medical students and GME trainees. This option is particularly relevant during demanding periods of education or training (e.g., major clinical year), when utilization tends to drop off as it becomes difficult for students to free up time to attend sessions, particularly during business hours. Additionally, accessing care off-campus leads to cost and time burdens for medical students because of travel and/or copays. Having telepsychiatry options available through no-cost campus-based mental health centers may facilitate increased help-seeking during particularly vulnerable periods.

Mental Health Care for GME Trainees

Although considered trainees in the eyes of program directors and faculty, residents and clinical fellows are considered employees from the perspective of the hospital system. As employees, medical (including mental health) services are provided by the institution, and GME trainees are eligible for these as hospital employees, with options often including an employee assistance program (EAP; either on- or off-site) and health insurance mental health benefits. However, the unique employee status of the GME trainee, nonstandard work hours, high clinical demands, and constraints of the training environment can present significant barriers to GME trainees interested in seeking mental health care. Unfortunately, many human resources programs frown on the provision of special services for target populations within an organization, which could be construed as discriminatory (Section 3:Title VII).[51] Furthermore, an EAP that operates Monday to Friday, during daytime hours without evening or weekend availability, may be of limited use and benefit to GME trainees, especially if the EAP is located off site. EAPs tend to be designed for short-term (e.g., five or fewer session) interventions, such as grief counseling, stress management, and parenting guidance, and they frequently lack the resources for longer-term care. Additionally, psychopharmacology services are not typically included with EAPs since most are staffed by social workers or psychologists and do not include prescribing physicians within their panels. Thus, many EAPs do not have clinicians who are able to treat those GME trainees who suffer from a host of mental health conditions, such as attention-deficit hyperactivity disorder (ADHD), bipolar disorder, or others requiring specialized expertise such as eating disorders or substance abuse.

Mental health treatment of GME trainees through community referral can similarly be challenging due to the frequently irregular or unpredictable nature of the GME trainee's schedule, which may result in cancellation of visits due to unexpected clinical obligations or emergencies. Referrals to community providers can also be limited by the many community mental health providers who are out-of-network on many GME trainee insurance plans, either due to the associated cost and/or time spent in submitting or following-up on claims for out-of-network benefits.

Increasingly, some GME offices are moving toward the establishment of internal comprehensive mental health services for their GME trainees.[52] Like medical school student mental health services, such programs provide GME trainees with access to a psychologist or psychiatrist for evaluation and short-term treatment. GME trainees are typically eligible for a certain number of sessions at no cost to them and then referred out if longer-term treatment is required. Alternatively, in some models, insurance claims are billed directly for services. When properly staffed, these internal models offer more convenient, rapid access to behavioral health clinicians who are familiar with the hospital environment and culture and the unique issues facing GME trainees. Limitations of this model include reliance on clinicians who may be known to, or even supervise, the GME trainees seeking treatment; concerns about true confidentiality when clinical visit notes are documented within the hospital EHR (which could lead to reluctance for residents to use this service); and the remaining need for community referral when longer-term treatment is indicated or preferred.

In addition to mental health treatment access, the ACGME mandates that institutions offer self-screening. However, screening in the absence of the provision of available services may be complicated at best and dangerous at worst as it can decrease trust in institutional processes and future endeavors.[53] Therefore, organizations should deploy self-screening measures that align with available resources. Targeted routing to online resources is often a first step that organizations can take when on-site resources to respond to individual screening responses are limited, but, ideally, screening tools should be aligned with ability to respond to positive screens locally.

Additional Considerations and Next Steps
Awareness and Destigmatization

Even while stigma remains an issue, treatment-seeking, particularly among younger generations, has increased dramatically across almost all demographic groups. Generation Z is the least likely among recent generations to report being in good mental health and the most likely to report seeking mental health treatment,[54] and campus-based counseling centers have seen a steady increase in service utilization. Between Fall 2009 and Spring 2015, counseling center utilization increased by an average of 30–40%. Some of this increased use of mental health services may also be due to increased pathology as these data also suggest an increase in the acuity of symptoms over recent years, with an increased number of students presenting for treatment with lifetime histories of threat-to-self.[49] It is likely, though, that some of the increased utilization is, at least in part, reflective of the decades-long efforts to normalize mental health concerns and reduce stigma about seeking treatment.

As efforts to destigmatize mental health and treatment have grown, they have also become more nuanced. Whereas previously "awareness days" and self-screening may have represented the gold standard, current models include curricular changes that bring mental health awareness content directly to students and GME trainees who might otherwise not have engaged in self-learning had the information not been incorporated into academic coursework.[55] For example, "Let's Talk,"[56] pioneered at Cornell University, offers satellite offices in which a student can "drop in" for an anonymous visit with a clinician, thereby eliminating the "paper trail" and enhancing more convenient access. Other efforts work to meet communities where they are in order to normalize treatment-seeking and lower barriers to care, rather than relying on a one-size-fits-all approach; these focus on relationship-building with vulnerable populations that underutilize services.

Preventing Well-Being from Becoming Another Performance Metric

As well-being becomes more recognized as necessary for sustainable practice, there is a paradoxical risk of making "well-being" simply another check box on a long list of "to-do items" that students and GME trainees are required to address. Students and GME trainees may end up "performing well-being" (as when clinicians are tasked with fitness for duty evaluations, described above), rather than benefiting from these efforts.

Studies have shown that, compared to students without burnout, students with burnout experience greater lapses in professionalism.[57,58] Thus, an increased effort is being made to conceptualize well-being as a curricular element necessary to achieve professionalism. The ACGME core competency that calls for physicians to be self-sacrificing and put the patient's need first is being clarified so that this concept does not come at the expense of the GME trainee's health.[59] This is now often referred to as "the oxygen mask principle"; in other words, just as during an in-flight emergency, individuals should secure their own oxygen supply before assisting others, clinicians need to attend to their own needs in order to be able to best care for patients.

Another strategy to integrate well-being into one's professional ethos links the promotion of physician well-being to improved patient well-being. Akin to earlier campaigns on smoking cessation, efforts to encourage physicians to educate patients about the negative effects of smoking (e.g., lung cancer, etc.) were largely ineffective until the education was directly targeted to physicians who smoked. When doctors themselves stop smoking, they are more likely to counsel their patients about the benefits of smoking cessation.[60–62] Similarly, physicians who regularly exercise are more likely to discuss exercise with their patients.[63,64] Thus, to best help patients establish their own healthy behaviors, physicians must be counseled about being "well." Maintaining one's own healthy lifestyle will both improve one's quality of life and help one provide better care to one's patients. Students and GME trainees may be most helped by being educated in systems and by physicians who practice what they preach and are themselves models of "well-being."

Responding to Tragedy

The response to local tragedies, such as the death of a colleague, can be enormously complex and challenging. While death can and does occur due to accident or illness, here we discuss the death of a medical student, GME trainee, or colleague due to suicide.

Being a physician comes with an increased risk for death by suicide.[65] The known neurobiology of suicide[66] suggests a stress-diathesis model, with affected individuals being generally unaware of having a genetic vulnerability to suicide until suicidal ideation develops. Approximately 90% of individuals who die by suicide have a diagnosable mental health condition.[67] However, only 45% had contact with a primary care provider 1 month before death by suicide, and 24% had contact with a mental health clinician in the year prior to the suicide.[68] Rates of suicidal ideation in medical students and GME trainees have been reported as high as 11%.[3,69] Returning to the burnout–depression relationship, depression is a known risk factor for suicidal ideation and suicide. The relationship between burnout and suicidal ideation is less clear. An early study[69] suggested that burnout carried an increased risk of suicidal ideation independent of the presence of depression, although more recent data from the same group[13] did not replicate that association: the risk for suicide was carried by the presence of depression, not burnout. Clearly, this has significant implications for screening, interventions, and treatment.

Responding to suicide requires sensitivity and discretion. As the deceased is always a family member as well as a colleague, it is the family that should direct what may and may not be communicated about the cause of their loved one's death. This often manifests as a tension between the needs of students and GME trainees and the wishes of the family. Detailed information is often not disclosed at the request of the family or because it has not been confirmed. This may be perceived by students and GME trainees as the institution withholding information, which may contribute to anger and frustration, often directed at the program or hospital. Often, the lack of acknowledgment of the cause of death is itself an inferred communication by many that the death was a suicide no matter the actual cause.

In addition, suicide contagion is a real phenomenon, and important guidelines exist to guide media communications[70,71] to minimize this risk. The American Foundation for Suicide Prevention and the Higher Education Mental Health Alliance[72] have published postvention toolkits to help guide institutions in the aftermath of a student[73] or GME trainee[74] death by suicide. An important aspect of these guidelines is offering tailored support for impacted individuals and communities that avoids large-scale public memorials which may spark contagion. Support is the responsibility of the whole campus or institution—not simply the mental health service—and leadership and communication during crises and in response to tragedies can significantly impact the community's reaction to and trajectory of the aftermath.[75]

The COVID-19 Pandemic Has Changed How We Talk About Mental Health and Burnout

The COVID-19 pandemic has had an important impact on the consideration of emotional symptoms not previously highlighted in the burnout and mental health literature for the health care workforce. The pervasiveness and intensity of anxiety, fear, and uncertainty, particularly in the early months of the pandemic, contributed to a normalization of these symptoms. Stigma related to mental health concerns may have decreased.[76] Shanafelt and colleagues, known for their significant contributions to the burnout literature, published an early piece on "understanding and addressing sources of anxiety" among health care workers.[77] Given the known consequences of previous pandemics[78,79] on the mental health of individuals, the mental health and well-being of first responders and the broader health care workforce rose to national importance through commentaries and publications in top medical journals[80-89] as well as in the lay press. Early rates of depressive symptoms in front-line physicians, nurses, and GME trainees ranged from 25% to 50%,[81-83,90] anxiety and "distress" ranged from 20% to 71%,[81-83] and acute and posttraumatic stress reactions were markedly elevated (50–57%).[82,83]

Increases in burnout in GME trainees beyond baseline levels, however, did not immediately materialize,[91-93] perhaps due to the intense sense of meaning, purpose,[91] and teamwork that physicians found in their work. For the first time in the more than 10 years of the Intern Health Study, the rate of depression among first-year GME trainees significantly decreased in the first quarter of 2020 (although it was back to baseline levels by the next quarter).[94] Rates of anxiety, depression, and PTSD among health care professionals remained high,[83,90] although may be improving.[75,95] Burnout, however, seems to be more prevalent and prominent than ever[96] in the COVID era, perhaps exemplified by the observation that one in five health care workers are considering leaving the field.[97,98]

The silver lining to these observed psychological impacts of COVID is that the national conversation around the importance of the well-being *and* mental health of the health care professional workforce remains strong. There is greater acknowledgment of and commitment to developing interventions at both individual and system levels.[1,79,99] Despite the changes in the landscape related to the COVID pandemic, ongoing discussions regarding the relationship of burnout and stress to psychiatric diagnosis remain important to our understanding of the stresses and challenges faced by trainees as they navigate the medical education system.

Conclusion

There has been increasing awareness of the pervasiveness and depth of stress experienced in the process of becoming a physician, manifesting along a continuum as distress, burnout, depression, and other mental health diagnoses. This has contributed to increased awareness of the need to address both individual and systemic vulnerabilities so that appropriate remedies across the spectrum can be developed and implemented to promote well-being, alleviate distress, and treat pathology. Maintaining one's own healthy lifestyle will both improve one's quality of life and help one provide better care to one's patients. To this end, students and GME trainees will benefit from modeling of good self-care, boundary-setting, and work–life integration from physicians who practice what they preach and are themselves models of "well-being." And yet, amid growing strain on the health care system, highlighted and amplified by the COVID-19 pandemic, maintaining a healthy lifestyle is a challenge for students, GME trainees, and practicing physicians. Having easy no- or low-cost access to support, whether these be explicit treatment services or one-off debriefing groups is essential given the multiple demands on the medical student's and GME trainee's time. Finally, psychoeducation for students and GME trainees about these issues using a systems-level framework may be most helpful in normalizing their difficulties, lowering barriers to care, and enhancing access to treatment so that whether or not they choose to identify themselves as grappling with "burnout" or "depression," help is easily accessible.

Summary Points

- Well-being, as a modern concept relevant to health and medicine, is described as "a state of complete physical, mental, and social well-being and not merely the absence of disease and infirmity."

- Stress, distress, burnout, and depression are important constructs that potentially exist along a wellness to illness spectrum.
- To fully achieve well-being, it is critical to consider both individual- and system-level approaches to address mental health issues across the continuum from medical student to GME trainee to attending.
- Reducing known barriers that impede trainees from seeking help and facilitating access to quality mental health care must become a priority at our academic institutions.
- Physicians who are themselves models of "well-being" will provide better care to their patients.

Putting It into Practice

- Identify the current status of mental health resources for residents and medical students at your institution.
- Identify key sources of stress and well-being for health care workers at your institution.
- Identify and approach partners, outside of mental health treatment providers, who might share the responsibility for building a culture of well-being at your institution.
- Survey trainees to identify obstacles to treatment.
- Establish an ongoing process to evaluate both the well-being and mental health needs of staff as well as systems-level issues that foster, or hamper, a culture of well-being.

References

1. Shanafelt TD. Physician well-being 2.0: Where are we and where are we going? *Mayo Clin Proc.* 2021;96(10):2682–2693. doi:10.1016/j.mayocp.2021.06.005
2. Shanafelt TD, Noseworthy JH. Executive leadership and physician well-being: nine organizational strategies to promote engagement and reduce burnout. *Mayo Clin Proc.* 2017;92(1):129–146. doi:10.1016/j.mayocp.2016.10.004
3. Rotenstein LS, Ramos MA, Torre M, et al. Prevalence of depression, depressive symptoms, and suicidal ideation among medical students: a systematic review and meta-analysis. *JAMA.* 2016;316(21):2214–2236. doi:10.1001/jama.2016.17324
4. DUNN HL. High-level wellness for man and society. *Am J Public Health Nations Health.* 1959;49(6):786–792. doi:10.2105/ajph.49.6.786
5. Oquendo MA, Bernstein CA, Mayer LES. A key differential diagnosis for physicians-major depression or burnout? *JAMA Psychiatry.* 2019;76(11):1111–1112. doi:10.1001/jamapsychiatry.2019.1332
6. Maslach C, Leiter MP. Understanding the burnout experience: recent research and its implications for psychiatry. *World Psychiatry.* 2016;15(2):103–111. doi:10.1002/wps.20311
7. DHHS (National Institute for Occupational Safety and Health (NIOSH)). DHHS Publication Number 99-101, STRESS . . . At Work. 1999. Accessed December 21, 2022. https://www.cdc.gov/niosh/docs/99-101/default.html

8. American Psychiatric Association. *Diagnostic and Statistical Manual of Mental Disorders*. 5th ed. American Psychiatric Association: 2013.

9. Flint J, Kendler KS. The genetics of major depression [published correction appears in Neuron. 2014 Mar 5;81(5):1214]. *Neuron*. 2014;81(3):484–503. doi:10.1016/j.neuron.2014.01.027

10. Leiter M and Durup J. The discriminant validity of burnout and depression: a confirmatory factor analytic study. *Anxiety, Stress and Coping*. 1994;7:357–373. doi: 10.1080/10615809408249357.

11. Melnick ER, Powsner SM, Shanafelt TD. In reply-defining physician burnout, and differentiating between burnout and depression. *Mayo Clin Proc*. 2017;92(9):1456–1458. doi:10.1016/j.mayocp.2017.07.005

12. Summers RF. The elephant in the room: what burnout is and what it is not. *Am J Psychiatry*. 2020;177(10):898–899. doi:10.1176/appi.ajp.2020.19090902

13. Menon NK, Shanafelt TD, Sinsky CA, et al. Association of physician burnout with suicidal ideation and medical errors [published correction appears in JAMA Netw Open. 2021 May 3;4(5):e2115436]. *JAMA Netw Open*. 2020;3(12):e2028780. doi:10.1001/jamanetworkopen.2020.28780

14. Rotenstein LS, Zhao Z, Mata DA, Guille C, Sen S. Substantial overlap between factors predicting symptoms of depression and burnout among medical interns. *J Gen Intern Med*. 2021;36(1):240–242. doi:10.1007/s11606-020-05664-x

15. Dyrbye LN, West CP, Satele D, et al. Burnout among U.S. medical students, residents, and early career physicians relative to the general U.S. population. *Acad Med*. 2014;89(3):443–451. doi:10.1097/ACM.0000000000000134

16. Ahola K, Honkonen T, Kivimäki M, et al. Contribution of burnout to the association between job strain and depression: the health 2000 study. *J Occup Environ Med*. 2006;48(10):1023–1030. doi:10.1097/01.jom.0000237437.84513.92

17. Bianchi R, Schonfeld IS, Laurent E. Burnout-depression overlap: a review. *Clin Psychol Rev*. 2015;36:28–41. doi:10.1016/j.cpr.2015.01.004

18. Shanafelt TD, West CP, Sinsky C, et al. Changes in burnout and satisfaction with work-life integration in physicians and the general US working population between 2011 and 2017. *Mayo Clin Proc*. 2019;94(9):1681–1694. doi:10.1016/j.mayocp.2018.10.023

19. Jordan RK, Shah SS, Desai H, Tripi J, Mitchell A, Worth RG. Variation of stress levels, burnout, and resilience throughout the academic year in first-year medical students. *PLoS One*. 2020;15(10):e0240667. doi:10.1371/journal.pone.0240667

20. Gabbard GO. The role of compulsiveness in the normal physician. *JAMA*. 1985;254(20):2926–2929. doi:10.1001/jama.1985.03360200078031

21. Strohbehn GW, Levy K, Tsao PA, Cronin DT, Heidemann LA, Del Valle J. The 'July effect' in supervisory residents: assessing the emotions of rising internal medicine PGY2 residents and the impact of an orientation retreat. *Med Educ Online*. 2020;25(1):1728168. doi:10.1080/10872981.2020.1728168

22. Hill D. *Affect Regulation Theory. A Clinical Model* (Norton Series on Interpersonal Neurobiology). W.W. Norton & Co; 2015.

23. Corrigan FM, Fisher JJ, Nutt DJ. Autonomic dysregulation and the Window of Tolerance model of the effects of complex emotional trauma. *J Psychopharmacol*. 2011;25(1):17–25. doi:10.1177/0269881109354930

24. Siegel DJ. *The Developing Mind*. Guilford Press; 1999.

25. Twenge JM. Generational changes and their impact in the classroom: teaching Generation Me. *Med Educ*. 2009;43(5):398–405. doi:10.1111/j.1365-2923.2009.03310.x

26. Hopkins L, Hampton BS, Abbott JF, et al. To the point: medical education, technology, and the millennial learner. *Am J Obstet Gynecol*. 2018;218(2):188–192. doi:10.1016/j.ajog.2017.06.001

27. Kratzke I, Kapadia MR, Egawa F, Beaty JS. Medical student selection. *Surg Clin North Am*. 2021;101(4):635–652. doi:10.1016/j.suc.2021.05.010

28. Frankl VE. *Man's Search for Meaning: An Introduction to Logotherapy* (4th ed.) (I. Lasch, Trans.). Beacon Press; 1992.

29. Yalom ID. *Existential Psychotherapy*. Basic Books; 1980.

30. Robins CJ, Block P. Cognitive theories of depression viewed from a diathesis-stress perspective: evaluations of the models of Beck and of Abramson, Seligman, and Teasdale. *Cogn Ther Res*. 1989;13:297–313.

31. Oquendo MA, Sullivan GM, Sudol K, et al. Toward a biosignature for suicide. *Am J Psychiatry.* 2014;171(12):1259–1277. doi:10.1176/appi.ajp.2014.14020194

32. Aaronson AL, Backes K, Agarwal G, Goldstein JL, Anzia J. Mental health during residency training: assessing the barriers to seeking care. *Acad Psychiatry.* 2018;42(4):469–472. doi:10.1007/s40596-017-0881-3

33. ACGME. ACGME Common Program Requirements, VI. The learning and working environment. Published online 2017. Accessed December 21, 2022. https://www.acgme.org/globalassets/PFAssets/ProgramRequirements/CPRs_Section-VI_with-Background-and-Intent_2017-01.pdf

34. FSMB Workgroup on Physician Wellness and Burnout. Draft report and recommendations. In Federation of State Medical Boards House of Delegates Annual Business Meeting Guidebook. 2018:343–363. Accessed December 21, 2022. https://www.fsmb.org/siteassets/annual-meeting/hod/april-28-2018-fsmb-hod-book.pdf.

35. Wimsatt LA, Schwenk TL, Sen A. Predictors of depression stigma in medical students: potential targets for prevention and education. *Am J Prev Med.* 2015;49(5):703–714. doi:10.1016/j.amepre.2015.03.021

36. Hankerson SH, Suite D, Bailey RK. Treatment disparities among African American men with depression: implications for clinical practice. *J Health Care Poor Underserved.* 2015;26(1):21–34. doi:10.1353/hpu.2015.0012

37. Hall GCN. Why don't people of color use mental health services? *Psychological Science Agenda.* 2019. Accessed December 21, 2022. http://www.apa.org/science/about/psa/2019/03/people-color-mental-health

38. Moise N, Hankerson S. Addressing structural racism and inequities in depression care. *JAMA Psychiatry.* 2021;78(10):1061–1062. doi:10.1001/jamapsychiatry.2021.1810

39. Coombs A, Joshua A, Flowers M, et al. Mental health perspectives among Black Americans receiving services from a church-affiliated mental health clinic [published online ahead of print July 8, 2021]. *Psychiatr Serv.* 2021;appips202000766. doi:10.1176/appi.ps.202000766

40. Gerada C. The making of a doctor: medical self and group of belonging. In C Geralda, ed. *Beneath the White Coat: Doctors, Their Minds and Mental Health.* Routledge; 2020:3–11.

41. Hunt J, Eisenberg D. Mental health problems and help-seeking behavior among college students. *J Adolesc Health.* 2010;46(1):3–10. doi:10.1016/j.jadohealth.2009.08.008

42. Drum DJ, Brownson C, Denmark AB, et al. New data on the nature of suicidal crises in college students: shifting the paradigm. *Prof Psychol Res Pr* 2009;40(3):213–222.

43. Ketchen Lipson S, Gaddis SM, Heinze J, Beck K, Eisenberg D. Variations in student mental health and treatment utilization across US colleges and universities. *J Am Coll Health.* 2015;63(6):388–396. doi:10.1080/07448481.2015.1040411

44. Dyrbye LN, Eacker A, Durning SJ, et al. The impact of stigma and personal experiences on the help-seeking behaviors of medical students with burnout. *Acad Med.* 2015;90(7):961–969. doi:10.1097/ACM.0000000000000655

45. Elharake JA, Frank E, Kalmbach DA, Mata DA, Sen S. Racial and ethnic diversity and depression in residency programs: a prospective cohort study. *J Gen Intern Med.* 2020;35(4):1325–1327. doi:10.1007/s11606-019-05570-x

46. Lipson SK, Kern A, Eisenberg D, Breland-Noble AM. Mental health disparities among college students of color. *J Adolesc Health.* 2018;63(3):348–356. doi:10.1016/j.jadohealth.2018.04.014

47. The JED Foundation. JED's Comprehensive Approach to Mental Health Promotion and Suicide Prevention for Colleges and Universities. July 19, 2021. Accessed December 21, 2022. https://jedfoundation.org/wp-content/uploads/2021/07/JED-Comprehensive-Approach_FINAL_July19.pdf

48. Association for University and College Counseling Center Directors. Annual report. 2020. Accessed December 21, 2022. https://www.aucccd.org/assets/documents/Survey/2019-2020%20Annual%20Report%20FINAL%20March-2021.pdf

49. Center for Collegiate Mental Health. Annual report. 2020. Accessed December 21, 2022. https://ccmh.psu.edu/assets/docs/2020%20CCMH%20Annual%20Report.pdf

50. Di Carlo F, Sociali A, Picutti E, et al. Telepsychiatry and other cutting-edge technologies in COVID-19 pandemic: bridging the distance in mental health assistance. *Int J Clin Pract.* 2021;75(1):e13716. doi:10.1111/ijcp.13716

51. U.S. Equal Employment Opportunity CommissionADEA issues: Background: equal benefits. In EEOC Compliance Manual Directive 915.003 Section 3: Employee Benefits. October 3, 2000. Accessed December 21, 2022 https://www.eeoc.gov/laws/guidance/section-3-employee-benefits#II.%20Backgro und:%20Equal%20Benefits.

52. Ey S, Moffit M, Kinzie JM, Brunett PH. Feasibility of a comprehensive wellness and suicide prevention program: a decade of caring for physicians in training and practice. *J Grad Med Educ*. 2016;8(5):747–753. doi:10.4300/JGME-D-16-00034.1

53. Goldman ML, Bernstein CA, Summers RF. Potential risks and benefits of mental health screening of physicians. *JAMA*. 2018;320(24):2527–2528. doi:10.1001/jama.2018.18403

54. American Psychological Association. Stress in America: generation Z. Stress in America™ survey. 2018. Accessed December 21, 2022. https://www.apa.org/news/press/releases/stress/2018/stress-gen-z.pdf

55. Place S, Talen M. Creating a culture of wellness: conversations, curriculum, concrete resources, and control. *Int J Psychiatry Med*. 2013;45(4):333–344. doi:10.2190/PM.45.4.d

56. Boone MS, Edwards GR, Haltom M, et.al. Let's talk: getting out of the counseling center to serve hard-to-reach students. *J Multicult Couns Devel*. 2011;39(4):194–205.

57. Dyrbye LN, Massie FS Jr, Eacker A, et al. Relationship between burnout and professional conduct and attitudes among US medical students. *JAMA*. 2010;304(11):1173–1180. doi:10.1001/jama.2010.1318

58. West CP, Shanafelt TD. Physician well-being and professionalism. *Minn Med*. 2007;90(8):44–46.

59. NEJM Knowledge+ Team. Exploring the ACGME core competencies: professionalism (Part 7 of 7). Published online January 12, 2017. Accessed December 21, 2022. https://knowledgeplus.nejm.org/blog/acgme-core-competencies-professionalism/-competencies-professionalism/

60. Duaso MJ, McDermott MS, Mujika A, Pursell E, While A. Do doctors' smoking habits influence their smoking cessation practices? A systematic review and meta-analysis. *Addiction*. 2014;109(11):1811–1823. doi:10.1111/add.12680

61. Cummings KM, Giovino G, Sciandra R, Koenigsberg M, Emont SL. Physician advice to quit smoking: who gets it and who doesn't. *Am J Prev Med*. 1987;3(2):69–75.

62. Pederson LL. Compliance with physician advice to quit smoking: a review of the literature. *Prev Med*. 1982;11(1):71–84. doi:10.1016/0091-7435(82)90006-8

63. Lewis CE, Clancy C, Leake B, Schwartz JS. The counseling practices of internists. *Ann Intern Med*. 1991;114(1):54–58. doi:10.7326/0003-4819-114-1-54

64. Reed BD, Jensen JD, Gorenflo DW. Physicians and exercise promotion. *Am J Prev Med*. 1991;7(6):410–415.

65. Center C, Davis M, Detre T, et al. Confronting depression and suicide in physicians: a consensus statement. *JAMA*. 2003;289(23):3161–3166. doi:10.1001/jama.289.23.3161

66. van Heeringen K, Mann JJ. The neurobiology of suicide. *Lancet Psychiatry*. 2014;1(1):63–72. doi:10.1016/S2215-0366(14)70220-2

67. Mann JJ. A current perspective of suicide and attempted suicide. *Ann Intern Med*. 2002;136(4):302–311. doi:10.7326/0003-4819-136-4-200202190-00010

68. Luoma JB, Martin CE, Pearson JL. Contact with mental health and primary care providers before suicide: a review of the evidence. *Am J Psychiatry*. 2002;159(6):909–916. doi:10.1176/appi.ajp.159.6.909

69. Dyrbye LN, Thomas MR, Massie FS, et al. Burnout and suicidal ideation among U.S. medical students. *Ann Intern Med*. 2008;149(5):334–341. doi:10.7326/0003-4819-149-5-200809020-00008

70. Gould MS, Midle JB, Insel B, Kleinman M. Suicide reporting content analysis: abstract development and reliability. *Crisis*. 2007;28(4):165–174. doi:10.1027/0227-5910.28.4.165

71. Gould MS. Suicide and the media. *Ann N Y Acad Sci*. 2001;932:200–224. doi:10.1111/j.1749-6632.2001.tb05807.x

72. Higher Education Mental Health Alliance. Postvention: a guide for response to suicide on college campuses. 2014. Accessed December 21, 2022. https://hemha.org/wp-content/uploads/2018/06/jed-hemha-postvention-guide.pdf

73. Drybye L, Moutier C, Wolanskyj-Spinner A, Zisook S. After a Suicide: A Toolkit for Medical Schools. American Foundation for Suicide Prevention. 2018. Accessed December 21, 2022. https://www.dato cms-assets.com/12810/1578318822-13719afspmedicalschooltoolkitm1v3.pdf

74. Drybye L, Konapasek L, Moutier C. After a Suicide: A Toolkit for Residency/Fellowship Programs. American Foundation for Suicide Prevention. 2018. Accessed December 21, 2022. https://www.dato cms-assets.com/12810/1578318836-after-a-suicide-a-toolkit-for-physician-residency-fellowship-prog ram.pdf

75. Drybye L, Jin J, Moutier C, Bucks C. After a Physician Suicide: Responding as an organization toolkit. AMA STEPS Forward. 2022. Accessed December 21, 2022. https://www.ama-assn.org/practice-man agement/physician-health/after-physician-suicide-responding-organization-toolkit

76. Chew QH, Chia FL, Ng WK, et al. Perceived stress, stigma, traumatic stress levels and coping responses amongst residents in training across multiple specialties during COVID-19 pandemic-a longitudinal study. *Int J Environ Res Public Health.* 2020;17(18):6572. doi:10.3390/ijerph17186572

77. Shanafelt T, Ripp J, Trockel M. Understanding and addressing sources of anxiety among health care professionals during the COVID-19 pandemic. *JAMA.* 2020;323(21):2133–2134. doi:10.1001/jama.2020.5893

78. Maunder RG, Lancee WJ, Balderson KE, et al. Long-term psychological and occupational effects of providing hospital healthcare during SARS outbreak. *Emerg Infect Dis.* 2006;12(12):1924–1932. doi:10.3201/eid1212.060584

79. Wu P, Fang Y, Guan Z, et al. The psychological impact of the SARS epidemic on hospital employees in China: exposure, risk perception, and altruistic acceptance of risk. *Can J Psychiatry.* 2009;54(5):302–311. doi:10.1177/070674370905400504

80. Dzau VJ, Kirch D, Nasca T. Preventing a parallel pandemic—a national strategy to protect clinicians' well-being. *N Engl J Med.* 2020;383(6):513–515. doi:10.1056/NEJMp2011027

81. Lai J, Ma S, Wang Y, et al. Factors associated with mental health outcomes among health care workers exposed to coronavirus disease 2019. *JAMA Netw Open.* 2020;3(3):e203976. doi:10.1001/jamanetworkopen.2020.3976

82. Rossi R, Socci V, Pacitti F, et al. Mental health outcomes among frontline and second-line health care workers during the coronavirus disease 2019 (COVID-19) pandemic in Italy. *JAMA Netw Open.* 2020;3(5):e2010185. doi:10.1001/jamanetworkopen.2020.10185

83. Shechter A, Diaz F, Moise N, et al. Psychological distress, coping behaviors, and preferences for support among New York healthcare workers during the COVID-19 pandemic. *Gen Hosp Psychiatry.* 2020;66:1–8. doi:10.1016/j.genhosppsych.2020.06.007

84. Mellins CA, Mayer LES, Glasofer DR, et al. Supporting the well-being of health care providers during the COVID-19 pandemic: the CopeColumbia response. *Gen Hosp Psychiatry.* 2020;67:62–69. doi:10.1016/j.genhosppsych.2020.08.013

85. Bernstein CA, Bhattacharyya S, Adler S, Alpert JE. Staff emotional support at Montefiore Medical Center during the COVID-19 pandemic. *Jt Comm J Qual Patient Saf.* 2021;47(3):185–189. doi:10.1016/j.jcjq.2020.11.009

86. Ripp J, Peccoralo L, Charney D. Attending to the emotional well-being of the health care workforce in a New York City health system during the COVID-19 pandemic. *Acad Med.* 2020;95(8):1136–1139. doi:10.1097/ACM.0000000000003414

87. Ey S, Soller M, Moffit M. Protecting the well-being of medical residents and faculty physicians during the COVID-19 pandemic: making the case for accessible, comprehensive wellness resources. *Glob Adv Health Med.* 2020;9:2164956120973981. doi:10.1177/2164956120973981

88. Smith S, Woo Baidal J, Wilner PJ, Ienuso J. The heroes and heroines: supporting the front line in New York City during Covid-19. *NEJM Catalyst.* 2020. doi:10.1056/CAT.20.0285

89. Grilo SA, Catallozzi M, Desai U, et al. Columbia COVID-19 Student Service Corps: harnessing student skills and galvanizing the power of service learning [published online ahead of print November 18, 2020]. *FASEB Bioadv.* 2020;3(3):166–174. doi:10.1096/fba.2020-00105

90. Feingold JH, Peccoralo L, Chan CC, et al. Psychological impact of the COVID-19 pandemic on frontline health care workers during the pandemic surge in New York City. *Chronic Stress (Thousand Oaks).* 2021;5:2470547020977891. doi:10.1177/2470547020977891

91. Kaplan CA, Chan CC, Feingold JH, et al. Psychological consequences among residents and fellows during the COVID-19 pandemic in New York City: implications for targeted interventions

[published online ahead of print August 10, 2021]. *Acad Med.* 2021;96(12):1722–1731. doi:10.1097/ACM.0000000000004362

92. Al-Humadi SM, Cáceda R, Bronson B, Paulus M, Hong H, Muhlrad S. Orthopaedic surgeon mental health during the COVID-19 pandemic. *Geriatr Orthop Surg Rehabil.* 2021;12:21514593211035230. doi:10.1177/21514593211035230

93. Civantos AM, Byrnes Y, Chang C, et al. Mental health among otolaryngology resident and attending physicians during the COVID-19 pandemic: National study. *Head Neck.* 2020;42(7):1597–1609. doi:10.1002/hed.26292

94. Sen S. Stress, depression and suicide among training physicians: Insights from the intern health study. Presented at National Physician Suicide Awareness; Sept 15, 2021; Columbia University Irving Medical Center, NY, NY.

95. Shechter A, Chiuzan C, Shang Y, et al. Prevalence, incidence, and factors associated with posttraumatic stress at three-month follow-up among New York City healthcare workers after the first wave of the COVID-19 pandemic. *Int J Environ Res Public Health.* 2021;19(1):262. doi:10.3390/ijerph19010262

96. Ghahramani S, Lankarani KB, Yousefi M, Heydari K, Shahabi S, Azmand S. A systematic review and meta-analysis of burnout among healthcare workers during COVID-19. *Front Psychiatry.* 2021;12:758849. doi:10.3389/fpsyt.2021.758849

97. Wan W. Burned out by the pandemic, 3 in 10 health-care workers consider leaving the profession. *Washington Post.* Published online April 22, 2021. Accessed December 21, 2022. https://www.washingtonpost.com/health/2021/04/22/health-workers-covid-quit/

98. Plater R. Doctors are returing due to COVID-19: Why you might have a hard time finding one. *Healthline.* Published online November 27, 2022. Accessed December 21, 2022. https://www.healthline.com/health-news/doctors-are-retiring-due-to-covid-19-why-you-might-have-a-hard-time-finding-a-new one

99. Dzau V, Kirch D, Murthy V, Nasca T. Letter from the Co-Chairs. National Academy of Medicine Action Collaborative on Clinician Well-being and Resilience. 2022. Accessed December 21, 2022. https://nam.edu/wp-content/uploads/2022/01/Letter-from-the-Co-Chairs_We-Stand-with-Our-Nations-Healthcare-Workforce.pdf

10

Addressing and Meeting Regulatory Requirements

Tara K. Cunningham and Michael Leitman

These are the duties of a physician: first, to heal his mind and to give help to himself before giving it to anyone else.
—Epitaph of an Athenian physician, 2 AD[1]

Undergraduate Medical Education
Background

The Premedical Journey

Aspiring physicians begin preparing for a career in medicine at various stages in life; initial interest in medicine may occur during the primary school years, in college, or even after contributing first to society as a member of the working class in their adult years prior to medical school matriculation. Reasons to enter medicine vary and include such drivers as familial legacy, a desire to help others, financial stability, or the pursuit of knowledge and fascination with the human body. Regardless of the reason, the pathway to medicine requires years of planning, persistence, dedication, and resolve to become a life-long learner in the ever-evolving field of medicine.

To prepare for the rigors of medical education, medical school applicants are often encouraged to complete a well-rounded undergraduate degree in an area of personal interest while also acquiring a foundation in the core sciences and other prerequisite courses, often packaged as the premedical ("premed") curriculum. Outside of the classroom, premed students generally engage in medicine-focused extracurricular activities to gain important leadership skills and demonstrate a commitment and sense of duty to care for others' needs. They also often spend a significant amount of time observing, or "shadowing," practicing physicians to witness meaningful doctor–patient relationships. They may seek student research positions, attend scientific and organized medicine meetings and conferences, and absorb conversations about rapidly changing technologies, patient needs, therapies, and the future of medicine. In short, demonstration of sustained dedication to a career in medicine is, itself, part of the process of matriculating into medical training.

In addition to academics, research, and other activities, premedical students study for and take the standardized Medical College Admissions Test (MCAT). Revised in 2015 to broaden the content and scope of testable material, the MCAT includes questions related to social determinants of health, social inequality, and other factors that affect the wellness and well-being of self and others, in addition to assessing problem-solving, critical thinking, and fundamental basic science knowledge.[2]

The decision of who is given the opportunity to study medicine lies with medical school admissions committees, which choose applicants based on data collected over a nearly year-long selection process. The exhaustive application collects information about personal and academic accomplishments, extracurricular activities (as described above), hobbies, volunteer and paid positions, and personal reflections shared through written essays. To assess other characteristics, such as the "soft skills" of communication, compassion, empathy, and more, applicants undergo interviews with medical school faculty, students, and others.[3] The 2020–2021 US allopathic medical school admission data highlight the competitive nature of entering medicine. Of the 53,030 applicants seeking admission, 42%, or 22,239, were admitted to medical school, leaving 58% of applicants to turn to another career choice or try again for admission in a subsequent application cycle.[4]

Considering that the path to the front door of medicine demands high academic and nonacademic expectations honed to a competitive edge, it is perhaps not surprising that premed students report a high prevalence of burnout and depression even prior to matriculation into medical school, as further described in Chapter 3.[5,6] Medical schools have moved toward considering applicants through a holistic approach which credits the "distance-traveled" of a person seeking a career in medicine and provides an opportunity for students who have been historically underrepresented in medicine to demonstrate readiness through lived experiences. As a result of this holistic review in admissions paradigms, medical schools have increased the diversity of the student body.[7] Nevertheless, the process of becoming a medical student, with its emphasis on achievement, high-stakes testing, and standing out in a field of highly accomplished peers, is already fraught with many of the stressors that are known to contribute to burnout in physicians.

The Medical Student Experience

Although each of the 155 US MD degree-granting institutions has a unique curricular structure,[8] the start of medical education often includes a short transition period, or orientation, to acclimatize students to the culture of medicine, including an introduction to professional and behavioral expectations and academic requirements, as well as essential policies and processes. This time also often serves to help with socialization into the student body.[9] During this time, students are typically introduced to school support staff and services in areas such as financial aid, career and academic advisement, tutoring, and disability accommodations, along with personal and mental health resources dedicated to their well-being. Furthermore, there is often an introduction to student-led activities and organizations to encourage connection with like-minded peers, create networks with residents and faculty, explore specialties, and establish meaningful mentorship for research. Some schools also include during this period the donning of the student's first white coat, a ceremonial introduction to medicine known as the White Coat Ceremony.[10] During this ceremony, students profess their commitment to becoming compassionate healers by reciting the Hippocratic Oath or an alternative oath authored by the students themselves. An additional pledge to care for oneself or an "Oath to Self-Care and Well-Being" is also being included in some medical schools.[11] Families, friends, and the medical school community bear witness to their joy and pride as the newly minted physicians-to-be stand proud and ready to learn at the start of their journey toward becoming a physician. The beginning of medical school, with its high emphasis on community and celebration of joining the profession, is often a high point for those who have just completed the premedical pathway.

However, as described in prior chapters, well-being generally begins to decline shortly after the beginning of medical school. Earning a medical degree occurs in as few as 4 years and is an immersive on-the-job experience with a full-time course load, clinical rotations, research, co-curricular activities, and near-weekly examinations. In addition to the required curriculum, students complete 2 of the 3 parts of the US Medical Licensing Examination (USMLE) examination, a high-stakes milestone important to the career advancement of students. In all, attending medical school often requires a lifestyle that can lead many students to put personal life priorities on hold (e.g., buying a home, getting married, starting a family, etc.). Students also amass an average of $200,000 in medical education debt by graduation.[12] In contrast to other professional terminal degrees (i.e., law, business), medical students are not considered fully trained upon graduation; rather, medical school is the first phase of training that continues after graduation in hospital-based residencies which may last another 3–7 years in a hospital setting. Impressively, the US medical school 4-year graduation rate is 84%, and the 6-year rate climbs to 96%.[13]

As described above, the graduation rate suggests a high degree of resilience among medical students; however, due to the above factors and inherent challenges of the nature of the work, medical school may also be a time of psychological distress which can lead to a decline in empathy, unwillingness to care for the chronically ill, increased cynicism, academic dishonesty, alcohol and substance abuse, sleep deprivation, financial concerns, and an overall negative impact related to being surrounded by disease and death.[13] (See Chapters 3-5 for more discussion on the psychological impact on medical students.) In recognition of the prevalence of medical student distress, medical schools are now required by their accrediting body, the Liaison Committee on Medical Education (LCME), to screen, identify, and implement well-being programming and services to protect the future physician workforce from further burnout and other mental health consequences. While personal factors may contribute to distress, medical schools are responsible for monitoring the learning environment wherein students study medicine and ensure student safety and the ability to learn.

The Need for Regulatory Support for Well-Being: The Example of Mistreatment

> Our students' mental health was very good at orientation but deteriorated across their four years of medical school. The only plausible conclusion: We were harming our students.[14]
> —Stuart Slavin, MD, former curriculum dean, Saint Louis University School of Medicine

As described in Chapter 8, mistreatment is another common experience in medical school and has had a significant impact on the medical school regulatory and accreditation process. Medical student mistreatment has been reviewed and written about since the 1980s, although not always under the contemporary definition of mistreatment to which medical schools are currently held accountable. Early reports of sexual harassment[15] in some cases were met with denial of such abuse occurring when medical school deans were surveyed.[16] In a national survey representing 72% of graduating medical students, 35% reported being the recipient of one or more forms of mistreatment.[17]

In recognition of the impact of mistreatment on the learning climate and well-being and mental health, the LCME has prioritized identifying and addressing instances of mistreatment. The Association of American Medical Colleges (AAMC) surveys students across all medical schools during enrollment, upon matriculation, before starting the third year, and in the months prior to graduation. Annually, medical schools receive aggregate data from each survey and are encouraged to utilize the information to enhance program and curricular development. The Graduation Questionnaire (GQ), which includes questions about preclinical and clinical experiences, school debt, and career and academic counseling has also expanded to include questions about mistreatment. The definition of mistreatment has been revised at least five times since 1991,[18] and today's GQ defines mistreatment as "behaviors performed by faculty, nurses, residents/interns, other institutional employees or staff, and other students."[19] Patient interactions, however, are not included in the GQ. Students are asked to self-report the frequency of and person(s) engaged in the behaviors, as well as any observed behaviors directed at other students. A list of behaviors defined as reportable mistreatment experienced during medical school can be found in the GQ, available on the AAMC website https://www.aamc.org/data-reports/students-residents/report/graduation-questionnaire-gq.[20]

As we transition to a more detailed discussion of regulatory requirements and their role in well-being, consider the case study below as an illustration of mistreatment, microaggressions, and overt bias that may be experienced during medical school. Note that such experiences may be insidious and can accumulate over the course of medical education. Students who are in the position of being evaluated frequently do not feel that they can safely speak up or ask for support in addressing these instances for fear of retaliation. This case poignantly illustrates the importance of regulations and reporting systems to detect and intervene on mistreatment and bias in the clinical learning environment.

Medical student Jane Smith recalls the first moment that becoming a surgeon came to her mind at the age of 9. Her favorite stuffed animal's leg was torn and stuffing began to escape through the growing hole. She asked her mother for a needle and thread and with steady hands and detail, she performed her first surgical procedure. She grew up biracial in a single-parent household and was the first in her family to attend medical school. Starting third-year of medical school meant that she would finally get a chance to observe and learn the art of surgery first-hand, and, despite the early mornings, she was excited to begin her surgery clerkship. She started her 6 weeks on the surgery clerkship with an orientation led by the faculty and teaching residents and entered the locker room to store her belongings. As she neared her locker, she was surprised to hear the residents commenting on a fourth-year student who had recently been interviewed for a residency position. "I'm tired of Black students feeling they are owed something; he had an attitude and is not the face I would want to see before I went under the knife."

Although she knew this was not the right thing to say about someone, she remembered the advice of a mentor who told her that you cannot fight other peoples' fights. For the next 6 weeks, she needed to keep her head down and work hard to make sure she received the highest grade possible—Honors—otherwise, in her view, her future as a surgeon would never happen.

Two days later, she scrubbed in on an appendectomy case and quickly recognized the resident on service as the same person she saw in the locker room earlier in the week. During the procedure, the resident expressed frustration with the "disgusting amount of fat" on the patient and joked that instead of an appendectomy, "the patient really needed liposuction." The others in the room laughed and, nervously, she giggled as quietly as possible so as not to be seen as disinterested. After all, this resident would be the one to grade her performance for the day.

The most exciting case occurred near the end of her clerkship during the rotation with the trauma service. She knew trauma surgery would be eye-opening, fast-paced, and exhilarating given the life-threatening nature of the surgical needs. The patient was her age, a 23-year-old, who lived in the same neighborhood as her mother. The patient had been stabbed and suffered lacerations to his liver and stomach. She scrubbed in and recognized the trauma surgeon as someone considered to be a specialty advisor for students interested in surgery. She had heard him speak at a career event in her second year of medical school and enjoyed hearing about the stories told from a 35-year career in medicine. The room felt different from other surgeries: there was no music, there was no chatter about weekend plans, and it was as if others knew something that the student did not know. The only words spoken were his commands for instruments and time spent on the procedure. Knowing a bit about the patient's neighborhood and his age, she asked if a family member was in the waiting room. She wanted to make a personal outreach after the case ended if she knew the family. Frustrated by her question and for thinking about something other than the procedure, the surgeon threw his scalpel across the room and told her, "Get out of my operating room. This is not a time to care about his gang family!"

Jane is now second-guessing her place in medicine and future as a surgeon. She has sought counseling and feels overwhelmed by the burden of feeling the need to, on her own, correct the racism and bias in medicine. She entered into medicine because she wanted to heal her community, and now she is beginning to question the road ahead. Spending at least 4 more years after graduation surrounded by the people she experienced in the past 6 weeks on her surgery rotation wrecked her resolve to fulfill a childhood dream. On the final day of the clerkship, she sat next to her classmate to take the surgery final exam. He was beaming with energy and told her that he's been invited to shadow "the guys in trauma" later that day and whenever else he wants. Unaware of her career aspirations, he shares that he's been told, "The head of the surgery department told me I am guaranteed to match with him because I fit what they want: humor and I like to cut."

Current LCME Standards

Since 1942, the LCME has served as the accrediting agency for medical schools granting the MD degree in the United States and Canada. Sponsored by the American Medical Association (AMA) and the AAMC, the LCME coordinates a peer-reviewed process based on a set of accreditation standards with which schools are required to demonstrate compliance on a regular schedule. In 1957, the LCME created the *Functions and Structure of a Modern Medical School*, the accreditation standards by which medical schools would be evaluated and, in 1962, an accreditation guidebook was created to help schools prepare for the accreditation process. In February 1993, the American Medical Student Association (AMSA) first called on the LCME to address the well-being of medical students. The LCME rejected the call and believed the accreditation process adequately addressed the topic in existing standards.[21]

It took 10 years from those initial discussions for the well-being conversation to emerge in several new accreditation elements. In February 1998, a working group was formed by the LCME to address the growing awareness of medical student mistreatment and abuse. A year later, an element to address access to mental health services was approved, and, in 2003, attention to the learning environment and "hidden curriculum" was added. In all, medical schools now are required to address these broad topics in the accreditation process. Failure to demonstrate sufficient programs, policies, and processes could lead to monitoring, probation, or the removal of accreditation. In 2014, the Data Collection Instrument (DCI), the standards required to be addressed during the accreditation process, were reduced from 132 to 12. Within the 12 standards, there are

> ## BOX 10.1 2021–2022 LCME Standards
>
> Standard 1: Mission, Planning, Organization, and Integrity
> Standard 2: Leadership and Administration
> Standard 3: Academic and Learning Environments
> Standard 4: Faculty Preparation, Productivity, Participation, and Policies
> Standard 5: Educational Resources and Infrastructure
> Standard 6: Competencies, Curricular Objectives, and Curricular Design
> Standard 7: Curricular Content
> Standard 8: Curricular Management, Evaluation, and Enhancement
> Standard 9: Teaching, Supervision, Assessment, and Student and Patient Safety
> Standard 10: Medical Student Selection, Assignment, and Progress
> Standard 11: Medical Student Academic Support, Career Advising, and Educational Records
> Standard 12: Medical Student Health Services, Personal Counseling, and Financial Aid Services

93 elements that require a written response, data, tables, and other metrics, all required to be provided by medical schools within the 18- to 24-month period leading up to the accreditation and on-site review visits that occurs every 8 years.[22]

Of note, medical students provide data themselves for use during this process, and these data are considered to provide a critical perspective during the accreditation. Students participate formally in the accreditation process in three ways: by serving on the school committees preparing responses for the 12 standards (Box 10.1), by leading a peer-developed and -administered survey which functions as the basis of a comprehensive report of the student perception of the institution, and by participating in the meetings that occur during the LCME's on-site visit.[23] The LCME uses these data along with the AAMC's GQ responses from the most recent survey administration to determine compliance with accreditation standards. In the following section, we describe several standards that have particular relevance to medical student well-being. While other standards have elements within them that may also be relevant to medical student well-being, for the scope of this review, we focus on Standards 3, 8, and 12. For each of these standards, some examples of interventions that may support institutions in successfully meeting these standards are listed in Table 10.1. Full text of the LCME standards with additional description is available at the LCME website: https://lcme.org/publications/#Standards24

The Academic and Learning Environment, Professionalism, and Mistreatment

The LCME Standard 3, focusing on the Academic and Learning Environment, is defined on page 4 of the 2021 LCME *Functions and Structure of a Medical School* as follows:

TABLE 10.1 Liaison Committee on Medical Education (LCME) Standards related to well-being and example strategies to support meeting these standards

LCME Standard	Example strategies to support meeting standard
Standard 3: The Academic and Learning Environment 3.5 Learning environment/professionalism 3.6 Student Mistreatment	• Establish a Teacher-Learner Compact to create a shared responsibility of respect and professionalism. • Create a Professionalism or Ombuds Office to address violations of professional standards and provide remediation. • Include students in the remediation process when possible. • Provide a real-time reporting mechanism for students to raise issues of unprofessional comments or content. • Conduct climate surveys to identify areas of persistent and negative influence for action. • Give feedback to faculty based on student comments. • Remove faculty from the learning environment who continue to demonstrate unprofessional behavior. • Establish and widely publicize a mechanism for reporting mistreatment/professionalism concerns that can be accessed easily. • To reduce fear of retaliation or retribution, offer delayed action after an alleged report of mistreatment. • Publicly report mistreatment outcomes and findings and ensure that leadership is aware of consistent sources of mistreatment. • Inform students of confidential support services and protect the identity of a student unless required to report by law. • Ensure that well-being resources and mistreatment resources are distinct in order to encourage help-seeking by making it clear that one can both report mistreatment and access support without a connection being made.
Standard 8: Curricular Management, Evaluation, and Enhancement 8.8: Monitoring student time	• Set a standard start/end time for educational activities each week that includes protected time during the week that cannot be scheduled for learning (i.e. protected lunch hour). • Conduct a thorough curriculum review to identify redundant or inflated content. • Create uniformity in the number of hours allowed for teaching across all courses and faculty. • Ensure students have adequate rest between clinical shifts, especially when overnight or weekend clinical learning occurs. • Enforce requirements through oversight by an educational committee that holds faculty accountable. • Survey students often about hours spent in required activities, and address violations quickly.
Standard 12: Medical Student Health Services, Personal Counseling, and Financial Aid Services 12.3: Personal Counseling/Well-being Programs	• Create a dedicated role in the medical school (e.g., Student Affairs) to address student well-being. • Provide the necessary funding and resources to build sustainable programs and initiatives. • Introduce well-being programs at the start of a student's medical education in orientation. • Involve students in the conversation around mental health and counseling and stigma reduction. • Use available well-being data to preemptively plan events or activities around times of high stressors (e.g., board exams). • Build well-being, mental health and counseling resources that meet the scheduling demands of students.

A medical school ensures that its medical education program occurs in professional, respectful, and intellectually stimulating academic and clinical environments, recognizes the benefits of diversity, and promotes students' attainment of competencies required of future physicians.[24]

Within this standard are two elements that address the learning environment/professionalism (3.5) and student mistreatment (3.6). Schools are required to evaluate the learning environment to maintain professional standards and to have policies defining mistreatment and mechanisms to report and respond to any concerns about mistreatment. Importantly, the institutions must ensure that violations can be reported without fear of retaliation.[24]

Curricular Management, Evaluation, and Enhancement

The LCME Standard 8, Curricular Management, Evaluation and Enhancement, page 12 of the 2021 LCME, *Functions and Structure of a Medical School*, reads as follows:

The faculty of a medical school engage in curricular revision and program evaluation activities to ensure that medical education program quality is maintained and enhanced and that medical students achieve all medical education program objectives and participate in required clinical experiences and settings.[24]

The link to well-being here is the attention needed to ensure that students do not become overwhelmed with curricular demands. With the explosive growth in medical knowledge, there can be a tendency to add curricular components without cutting back, leading to curricular bloat and increased time demands on the student. As described in subsection 8.8 of the standard, institutions are specifically required to establish policies to monitor time, including total number of hours spent in required activities.[24]

Medical Student Health Services, Personal Counseling, and Financial Aid Services

The LCME Standard 12, Medical Student Health Services, Personal Counseling, and Financial Aid Services, page 19 of the 2021 LCME *Functions and Structure of a Medical School*, reads as follows:

A medical school provides effective student services to all medical students to assist them in achieving the program's goals for its students. All medical students have the same rights and receive comparable services.[24]

In addition to physical health supports, as described in subsection 12.3 of the standard, medical schools are required to have systems in place for counseling and programming to support student well-being.[24]

Challenges of Compliance with the LCME Standards

Creating a culture of student well-being in the medical school is complex, multifaceted, and requires buy-in among and between faculty, staff, administrators, and clinical environments. An increasingly diverse group of medical school applicants and matriculants have questioned centuries-old traditional mindsets and assumptions that medicine requires one to forego life plans until training is complete, sometimes leading to tensions between faculty and students. Residents and practicing physicians themselves are overworked and often burned out, leaving little time to teach and mentor the next generation of physicians. Furthermore, factors beyond the medical school's control, such as global pandemics, political unrest, systemic racism and bias in society, and more, have a direct impact on the well-being of our students. While these complex challenges may have impacts that influence responses to annual student surveys, none can be easily solved with simple actions or quick fixes.

Future Directions

In all, meeting the complex needs of our students is the responsibility of the medical education community, and current regulatory requirements provide a formal mechanism to assess how well a school is meeting these needs. Just as other accreditation standards have evolved to meet training needs of the future physician workforce, future emphasis on well-being may harness the concept of the growth mindset and continuous self-improvement along with addressing systems to support the well-being and mental health of learners. To meet the standards of the LCME, a school must pass the scrutiny of students and peers at every cycle and in between and ensure adequate attention to continuous quality improvement, including for well-being and mistreatment.

Graduate Medical Education

Background

Residency Training and Work Hours

Physicians spend 3 to 10 years in graduate medical education (GME) developing their skills and mastering the knowledge necessary for independent practice. This time is a period of great intensity that impacts sleep, exercise, emotional and physical health, and family and personal relationships, but is required to enter the practice of medicine in the United States.

Residency and fellowship programs have evolved a great deal over the years in terms of their support for well-being. Many will recall the former "boot camp-like" attitude toward GME trainees. In prior generations, training programs did not provide well-being resources. And, in the past, for many programs, attrition during training was not necessarily seen as a negative since there was a need to eliminate residents from the pyramid of programs that, by design, accommodated fewer trainees per postgraduate year as training progressed. The emphasis on clinical service supporting hospital and departmental staffing needs (residents and fellows having a primary role as members of the hospital workforce) made it challenging for most GME trainees to have a strong educational experience. Well-being was certainly not a focus in those years.

Attention to work-hour limitations arguably was the first focus on graduate medical trainee well-being. The primary intent in initial work-hour reforms, however, was not to foster optimal learning conditions for residents, but rather to protect patients from fatigued residents who were too exhausted from working excessive hours to focus on the details necessary to deliver safe patient care.

Prior to the unfortunate death of Libby Zion in a New York City academic teaching hospital in 1984, there were few regulations that governed resident duty hours. Although it remains unclear what led to Zion's death, it appears that a missed diagnosis of iatrogenic serotonin syndrome due to medication administration was a significant factor in the fatal outcome. Two years later, a grand jury concluded that the factors contributing to her death included inadequate faculty supervision of the residents caring for her both in the emergency room and on the hospital floor and fatigue related to the 36-hour duty shifts of some of those residents. These findings led the New York State Health Commission to form what became known as the Bell Commission, which subsequently recommended a maximum 80-hour work week and no more than 24 hours of consecutive work for resident physicians. These recommendations were then incorporated into New York State's health code.[25] New York remains the only state that *legislated* the limitation of GME trainee work hours into its health codes. The focus of early work-hour rules and policies was on developing strategies to recognize and mitigate fatigue, rather than on enhancing the well-being of residents and fellows or optimize sleep health.[26,27]

The Role of the ACGME

The majority of GME in the United States is overseen by the Accreditation Council for Graduate Medical Education (ACGME), which accredits training programs and monitors compliance with requirements. In 1989, the Review Committee for Internal Medicine, the largest accredited specialty, instituted an 80-hour weekly limit, averaged over 4 weeks, to become effective in July 1989; by the early 1990s, six specialties had established a weekly duty-hour limit. Residency programs of some specialties were initially reluctant to implement work-hour restrictions based on concerns that continuity of patient care might be disrupted and, for some surgical specialties, concerns about a negative impact on the surgical training experience and potential for reduced operative case numbers. In actuality, the negative impact on experiential learning was quite minimal with these reforms.[28-31]

In September 2001, the ACGME authorized the formation of a working group on resident duty hours and the GME learning environment. This group was charged with the development of standards for resident work hours and with providing recommendations in a number of related areas. The resulting work-hour requirements were implemented in 2003, under the threat of federal legislation, to place a limit on resident hours.

National work-hour limitations were further refined in 2011.[28] Reports on the impact of work-hour reductions on patient outcomes, such as complications and mortality, were mixed.[32,33] While residents were more rested and less fatigued[34] and in turn may have made fewer patient care errors,[35] it became clear that some vital information passed between residents during work-hour shift transitions was lost during those "handoffs." The findings from cluster randomized trials related to the 2011 work-hour changes are described in additional detail in Chapters 4 and 8. The reduction in the number of hours that residents and fellows could work also markedly increased costs to hospitals, which needed to hire nonresident staffing to fill in gaps left by the reduction in GME trainee work hours.[36] Recognizing the implicit pressures residents may face to demonstrate compliance with work hours, whether residents accurately report their work hours is also a subject of debate.[37,38]

With studies on the impact of work-hour limitations showing mixed impacts on well-being, subsequently, there has been a growing recognition that GME trainee well-being is more complicated than simply the number of hours worked. It is the *work intensity* (inclusive of the total number of hours, the acuity and number of patients, the complexity of the work, and the amount of nonphysician work required) that likely has the greatest effect on well-being outcomes. As a new resident, Colleen M. Farrell used the metaphor of the beating heart to describe the emotional impact of residency training.

> During my first month on the wards as an intern, I held steady against the torrent of admissions, pages, progress notes, rapid responses, and discharge paperwork. My mind darted incessantly from one urgent issue to the next. After that month, I was given a reprieve: two weeks of primary care clinic. Weekends off. Evenings at home. Patients who were, on balance, much healthier. One of the cardiology attendings calls this primary care time our diastole. I had to remind myself that diastole is not a passive process. It takes work for the heart to relax. Energy must be expended. It is not enough to simply be away from the inpatient wards for two weeks. To seize diastole, I must continue doing the hard work of processing my fear, frustration, and grief.[39]

Over the past decade, the increased awareness of burnout, depression, and physician suicide contributed to the increased prominence of a national discussion on GME trainee well-being, with increased urgency related to the concern that 300–400 physicians were dying by suicide every year.[40]

In 2017, the ACGME revised its Common Program Requirements (CPRs) to address well-being more directly and comprehensively. These requirements emphasized that psychological, emotional, and physical well-being are critical to the development of the competent, caring, and resilient physician. Section VI of the CPRs for accredited residency and fellowship programs addressed more comprehensively the issue of resident and fellow well-being. Changes included requiring access to appropriate tools for self-screening and for programs to provide support to individual residents through 24/7 access to urgent and emergent mental health care, as well as confidential mental health assessment, counseling, and treatment. Institutions were charged with the identification of burnout, depression, and substance abuse among trainees.[41]

These program requirements went into effect in July 2018 and have been updated and refined multiple times since then. Separate requirements for residency and fellowship now exist, but the requirements that focus on well-being are the same. There is also new recognition that GME training occurs in clinical settings that establish the foundation for practice-based and life-long learning. The professional development of the physician includes modeling faculty who demonstrate the effacement of self-interest in a humanistic environment emphasizing a joy in curiosity, problem-solving, academic rigor, and discovery. This transformation is often physically, emotionally, and intellectually demanding and occurs in a variety of learning environments that are committed to the well-being of patients, residents, fellows, faculty members, students, and all members of the health care team. The ACGME well-being requirements acknowledge this complex milieu and the importance of supporting well-being as part of professional development. Discussion about ensuring compliance with these requirements in GME follows.

Current ACGME Common Program Requirements

The transformation of the learning environment from one that focused primarily on work and service to one that also includes a focus on well-being was a revolution brought about by public recognition that GME training resulted in high rates of burnout and depression. The concept of well-being is woven into the entirety of the most recent version of the ACGME CPRs, with the intent to provide flexibility within an established framework, allowing programs and GME trainees more discretion in structuring clinical education in a way that best supports the principles of personal and professional development. Examples of ways to meet CPRs relevant to well-being are summarized at the end of this chapter in table 10.2.

Institutional and Program Resources (Section 1.D)

The sponsoring institution and the training program are required to ensure that the following basic elements are present in the training environment:

- access to food while on duty
- safe, quiet, clean, and private sleep/rest facilities available and accessible for residents, with proximity appropriate for safe patient care
- clean and private facilities for lactation that have refrigeration capabilities, with proximity appropriate for safe patient care
- security and safety measures appropriate to the participating site
- accommodations for residents with disabilities consistent with the Sponsoring Institution's policy.[41]

The Learning and Working Environment: Professionalism (Section VI.B)

With increased flexibility comes the responsibility for programs and residents to continue to adhere to an 80-hour maximum weekly limit and to utilize flexibility in a manner that optimizes patient safety, GME trainee education, and well-being. These requirements are intended to support the development of a sense of professionalism by encouraging GME trainees to make decisions based on patient needs *and* their own well-being, without the fear of jeopardizing their program's accreditation status. This change is a modernization of the traditional professionalism focus (which involved self-effacement of one's own needs) in which an individual physician's well-being needs are now considered *along with* the patient's needs. Clinical and educational work hours represent only one part of the larger issue of learning and working environment conditions. With flexibility also comes a responsibility for residents, fellows, and faculty members to recognize the need to hand off responsibility to another provider when a GME trainee is too fatigued to provide safe, high-quality care and for the training programs to ensure that GME trainees remain within the 80-hour maximum weekly limit.[41] Self-care and responsibility to support other members of the health care team are now important components of professionalism; they are also skills that must be modeled, learned, and nurtured in the context of other aspects of GME training, as described in detail in Chapter 7. A positive culture in a clinical learning environment models constructive behaviors and prepares GME trainees with the skills and attitudes needed to thrive throughout their careers. For example, a culture which encourages the coverage of colleagues who are out during an illness without the expectation of reciprocity (i.e., having to pay back time taken off when ill) can help support ideals of professionalism.

Well-Being (Section VI.C)

Psychological, emotional, and physical well-being are critical to the development of the competent, caring, and resilient physician and require proactive attention to life both inside and outside of medicine. Well-being requires that physicians retain the joy and fulfillment found in the medical profession while managing their own real-life stresses. Residents, fellows, and faculty members are all at risk for burnout and depression. As such, programs, in partnership with their sponsoring institutions, have the same responsibility to address well-being as other aspects of GME trainee competence. Physicians and all members of the health care team share responsibility for the well-being of each other.

Goldman and colleagues provide one framework of suggested interventions for programs to meet the new requirements that address GME trainee well-being.[42] Interventions in this framework focus on educating physicians about the negative physical and emotional impacts of GME training, developing dedicated faculty (in addition to their program leadership) to regularly focus departmental efforts toward wellness (e.g. wellness champions), implementing well-being activities such as providing a time and space for reflection, teaching mindfulness and other self-care skills, building a community to support well-being, ensuring access to care, improving the workplace environment, and transforming the institutional culture.

Residency program teaching faculty are required not only to foster the well-being of GME trainees, but also attend to their own well-being. The basis of the ACGME focus on the clinician's well-being to improve patient care and reduce burnout among residents, fellows, and practicing physicians is considered an organizing principle in the provision of high-quality patient care.[43] Training programs and institutions are required to meet specific responsibilities to address well-being as outlined in Section VI.C.1 of the CPRs. The requirements align with published frameworks to support well-being and include:

- Undertaking efforts to enhance meaning and connection to patients and reducing administrative or nonphysician work that does not contribute to meaningful patient care (VI.C.1.a)
- Paying attention to scheduling, work intensity, and work compression (VI.C.1.b)
- Evaluating and addressing resident and faculty workplace safety (VI.C.1.c)
- Acknowledging that well-being includes time to attend to nonwork interests and personal needs (VI.C.1.d), which includes policies to support resident and faculty member well-being and allowing time for GME trainees to attend physical and mental health appointments
- Giving attention to resident and faculty burnout, depression, and substance use (VI.C.1.e):
  a. Educating faculty members and GME trainees about signs of burnout, mental health conditions, and substance abuse, including means to personally seek care as well as assist those who experience these conditions
  b. Encouraging GME trainees and faculty members to notify program leadership if they are concerned about a GME trainee's well-being, mental health, or substance use
  c. Providing access to tools for self-screening and access to mental health counseling, including 24-hour access to urgent and emergent care.

Programs are also required to understand that external personal influences might impact a resident's well-being, including but not limited to fatigue, illness, family emergencies, and parental leave. Programs are required to support GME trainees to be absent from patient care responsibilities for an appropriate length of time without fear of negative consequences while ensuring that systems for continuous patient coverage exist (Section VI.C.2).[41]

Fatigue Mitigation (Section VI.D)

Fatigue mitigation is also essential to the physical and emotional health of residents and the patients for whom they are responsible to provide care. GME training programs are required to educate all faculty members and GME trainees to recognize the signs of fatigue and sleep deprivation, practice alertness management, and use fatigue mitigation strategies. Furthermore, they are required to encourage GME trainees to avail themselves of fatigue mitigation processes that enable them to manage the potential negative effects of fatigue on patient care and learning.[44] Programs are required to have clear contingencies in the event that a resident may be unable to perform their patient care responsibilities due to excessive fatigue. Each clinical teaching site is required to have adequate sleep facilities and safe transportation options for residents who might be too fatigued to safely return home.[41]

Clinical Responsibilities, Teamwork, and Transition of Care (Section VI.E)

Understanding the work-hour limitation in the context of providing continuous high-quality patient care has necessitated attention to the concern that important information not be lost during transitions of care. Training programs are therefore required to design clinical assignments that optimize transitions in patient care, including their safety, frequency, and structure. As such they must ensure and monitor effective, structured hand-over processes to facilitate both continuity of care and patient safety. To attend to these concerns, GME trainees must develop competency in communicating with team members during the hand-over process. This must be achieved under the framework that clinical sites maintain and communicate the schedules of attending physicians and GME trainees who are actively responsible for patient care. Programs are required to have policies in place in the event that a resident may be unable to perform their patient care responsibilities due to excessive fatigue, illness, or family emergency.[41]

Clinical Experience, Education, and Work Hours (Section VI.F)

Work-hour limitations continue to be a central focus within the ACGME program requirements. These requirements limit hours per week to 80, averaged over 4 weeks and set requirements for 1 day in 7 (averaged over 4 weeks) free from required work, call frequency, and time off between scheduled shifts. There is also a recognition that the time spent at home on patient-related activities impacts a GME trainee's well-being. Therefore, the time spent on patient care activities by residents on at-home call needs to be counted toward the 80-hour maximum weekly limit. Additionally, related to well-being, the requirements also provide more specific guidelines for structuring clinical work. Specifically, programs must ensure that workload is manageable during scheduled hours and must support time for education within the work week. Programs are required to pay attention to needed time off for rest and well-being, including full 24-hour periods during which residents are free from all assigned clinical and nonclinical responsibilities. The full requirements can be accessed under Section VI.F of the CPRs: https://www.acgme.org/what-we-do/accreditation/common-program-requirements/.[41]

One strategy to allow for complying with duty-hour limitation requirements while providing continuous patient care is the use of an in-house "night float" resident assignment. Understanding that switching from daytime to nighttime work also has impacts on well-being, policies regarding night float have also been developed.[45] The ACGME requires supervision and education during a night-float rotation. Night-float must also occur within the context of the 80-hour work week and 1-day-off-in-7 requirements. The maximum number of consecutive weeks of night float and maximum number of months of night float per year may be specified by the specific specialty review committee (Section VI.F.6).[41]

Challenges of Compliance with the ACGME Common Program Requirements

Implementing cultural change at teaching hospitals has resulted in operational challenges. The change in perception of residents and fellows as learners rather than simply as laborers has created tension within their departments by misaligning hospital incentives.[46] And it remains unclear what the impact of these requirements has been on measurable well-being outcome metrics. Much more work still needs to be done in this area. From a GME trainee perspective, work-hour reduction resulted in more clinical efficiency, enhanced responsiveness to problems, and a collegial environment that has contributed to an ability to meet clinical and learning goals. However, GME trainees did not associate work-hour compliance with patient safety, which may be more related to the presence or absence of supervision.[47] The cost of full compliance with the new well-being requirements is also hefty. Additional costs to each program may be as much as $247,000 per year for an average training program.[48]

As described in prior chapters, a diverse array of GME interventions exist to enhance the well-being of residents and fellows through both individual and systems interventions, which often are most effective when integrated into educational programs. In some surgery programs, for example, opportunities for well-being activities, dedicated faculty and GME wellness champions, and assistance to decrease clerical burden were all associated with lower rates of burnout and depression compared to programs without such resources,[49] though it remains difficult to attribute reduction in trainee burnout directly to specific interventions.[50] Programs are encouraged to innovate and develop well-being initiatives for their constituents in collaboration with those who are experienced in creating meaningful resources.[51,52] With the continued recognition that residents and fellows remain at significant risk for burnout, depression, and suicide without clear evidence on the optimal approach for mitigating these outcomes, programs need to continue to explore and investigate novel methods that further enhance GME trainee well-being.[53]

Future Directions

New GME trainee well-being resources are under development. Smart device applications are available that introduce users to common cognitive routines which can contribute to their stress and burnout.[54] Future efforts will further focus on enhancing work–life integration for residents and fellows to foster a healthy balance between training and life outside of the GME space. Parental leave continues to challenge residents and fellows during their reproductive years, especially now that women comprise about half of all GME trainees.[55] Due to current challenges with parental leave and parenting during training, many opt to delay starting families, possibly increasing career dissatisfaction and burnout. Attention to enabling GME trainees to start a family during training will also no doubt become an increasing focus of many programs and specialty boards.[56]

Conclusion

Despite a lack of scientific evidence on outcomes from the implementation of well-being initiatives in requirements that govern medical student and GME training, public and professional recognition of the stress of residency and fellowship has resulted in a seismic shift toward a more trainee-focused learning environment. Even with changes such as restrictions on work hours, the complexity of patient care and acuity of illness in our health care system continues to place significant demands on our medical students, residents and fellows. Additional work is required to further optimize learning and professional development in the context of the demands of patient care.

Summary Points

- Responding to the needs of medical students, residents and fellows is complex and accreditation standards are not always responsive to these needs.
- The struggles between the traditions of medical education and responsibilities to provide the optimal learning environment require that we constantly measure the well-being of our learners and strike an ever-shifting balance.
- Accreditation is one of several frameworks that structure our work but internal and external forces must be constantly considered in preparing the next generation of physicians for practice of medicine in a dynamic global health care system.

Putting It into Practice

- Strategies for meeting LCME standards related to well-being include structures, policies, and curricula to support medical students: examples are listed in Table 10.1.
- Strategies for meeting ACGME requirements related to GME trainee well-being include policies, clinical and nonclinical supports, and curricular interventions. Examples are listed in Table 10.2.

TABLE 10.2 Accreditation Council for Graduate Medical Education (ACGME) requirements related to well-being and example strategies to support compliance

ACGME requirement	Example strategies to support compliance
VI.B Professionalism	■ Develop a culture that encourages handing off patient care when fatigued or sick. ■ Role model that professionalism values patient care and provider well-being simultaneously.
VI.C Well-being ■ Enhancing meaning ■ Workplace safety ■ Time for personal interests/ needs ■ Attention to resident/faculty burnout and mental health	■ Schedule routine community-building activities such as retreats and social events. ■ Create systems supports to reduce work that takes residents away from direct patient care. ■ Educate about the causes and incidence of needlestick injuries or exposure to infectious agents. ■ Create a hospital committee to review and develop policies to support workload and time off for all members of health care team. ■ Allow flexibility in scheduling vacation. ■ Take into account the need for time to attend appointments in scheduling and staffing models, and consider scheduled or preplanned wellness days. ■ Develop transparent emergency coverage systems to allow residents time off for personal emergencies or illness without fear of negative consequences. ■ Provide access to mobile apps or well-based screening platforms (e.g., American Foundation for Suicide Prevention, Well-Being Index). ■ Provide an on-call phone system for after-hours support. ■ Establish a wellness champion within the program and/or GME to oversee approach to initiatives that meet section VI.C requirements. ■ Establish/link to institutional wellness and mental health resources.
VI.D Fatigue mitigation	■ Promote strategic napping and use of caffeine on longer shifts. ■ Minimize external distractions at end of long shifts to prioritize sleep. ■ Institute formal fatigue mitigation training.
VI.E Clinical responsibilities, Teamwork, and Transitions of Care	■ Create policies for handing off patient care. ■ Ensure easily available access to attending physician contact information for support and back-up.
VI.F Clinical Experience, Education, and Work Hours	■ Set a culture of work hours limitations during orientation. ■ Designate protected conference time (consider academic half days). ■ Incorporate educational time and work from home into anticipated weekly work hours. ■ Enhance nonresident clinical staffing and nonclinical staffing to support long-term needs to adhere to work hours and well-being requirements.

References

1. Maas PL, Oliver JH. An ancient poem on the duties of a physician. *Bull Hist Med.* 1939;7:315–323.
2. AAMC. Taking the MCAT® exam. 2022. Accessed May 12, 2022. https://students-residents.aamc.org/taking-mcat-exam/taking-mcat-exam
3. AAMC. Applying to medical school. 2022. Accessed May 12, 2022. https://students-residents.aamc.org/applying-medical-school/applying-medical-school

4. AAMC. Table 1: Applicants, matriculants, enrollment, and graduates of U.S. MD-granting medical schools, 2012–2013 through 2021–2022. 2021. Accessed May 12, 2022. https://www.aamc.org/data-reports/students-residents/interactive-data/2021-facts-applicants-and-matriculants-data.

5. Fang DZ, Young CB, Golshan S, Moutier C, Zisook S. Burnout in premedical undergraduate students. *Acad Psychiatry*. 2012;36(1):11–16. doi:10.1176/appi.ap.10080125

6. Grace MK. Depressive symptoms, burnout, and declining medical career interest among undergraduate pre-medical students. *Int J Med Educ*. 2018;9:302–308. doi:10.5116/ijme.5be5.8131

7. AAMC.Aspiring docs. 2022. Accessed May 12, 2022. https://students-residents.aamc.org/aspiring-docs/aspiring-docs.

8. LCME.Accredited U.S. programs. 2022. Accessed May 12, 2022. https://lcme.org/directory/accredited-u-s-programs/

9. Ellaway RH, Cooper G, Al-Idrissi T, Dubé T, Graves L. Discourses of student orientation to medical education programs. *Med Educ Online*. 2014;19:23714. doi:10.3402/meo.v19.23714

10. The Arnold P. Gold Foundation. White coat ceremony. Accessed May 12, 2022. https://www.gold-foundation.org/programs/white-coat-ceremony/

11. Panda M, O'Brien KE, Lo MC. Oath to self-care and well-being. *Am J Med*. 2020;133(2):249–252.e1. doi:10.1016/j.amjmed.2019.10.001

12. Education Data Initiative. Average medical school debt. Updated December 9, 2021. Accessed May 12, 2022. https://educationdata.org/average-medical-school-debt

13. Dyrbye LN, Thomas MR, Shanafelt TD. Systematic review of depression, anxiety, and other indicators of psychological distress among U.S. and Canadian medical students. *Acad Med*. 2006;81(4):354–373. doi:10.1097/00001888-200604000-00009

14. Paturel A. Healing the very youngest healers. AAMC. 2020. Accessed May 12, 2022. https://www.aamc.org/news-insights/healing-very-youngest-healers

15. Silver HK. Medical students and medical school. *JAMA*. 1982;247(3):309–310. doi:10.1001/jama.1982.03320280029024

16. Mavis B, Sousa A, Lipscomb W, Rappley MD. Learning about medical student mistreatment from responses to the medical school graduation questionnaire. *Acad Med*. 2014;89(5):705–711. doi:10.1097/ACM.0000000000000199

17. Hill KA, Samuels EA, Gross CP, et al. Assessment of the prevalence of medical student mistreatment by sex, race/ethnicity, and sexual orientation. *JAMA Intern Med*. 2020;180(5):653–665. doi:10.1001/jamainternmed.2020.0030

18. Mavis B. Measuring mistreatment: honing questions about abuse on the Association of American Medical Colleges graduation questionnaire. *AMA J Ethics*. 2014;16(3):196–199. doi:10.1001/virtualmentor.2014.16.3.stas1-1403

19. AAMC. 2022 AAMC medical school graduation questionnaire. 2022. Accessed May 12, 2022 https://www.aamc.org/media/59071/download?attachment.

20. AAMC. Graduation questionnaire (GQ). 2022. Accessed May 12, 2022. https://www.aamc.org/data-reports/students-residents/report/graduation-questionnaire-gq.

21. AAMC. Academic quality and public accountability in medical education: the 75-year history of the LCME. 2017. Accessed May 12, 2022. http://www.lcme.org/wp-content/uploads/filebase/articles/October-2017-The-75-Year-History-of-the-LCME_COLOR.pdf

22. LCME. Overview of accreditation process. 2022. Accessed May 12, 2022. https://lcme.org/accreditation-preparation/students/#Overview-of-Accreditation-Process

23. LCME. Student participation in accreditation. 2022. Accessed May 12, 2022. https://lcme.org/accreditation-preparation/students/#Student-Participation-in-Accreditation

24. LCME. Functions and structure of a medical school: standards for accreditation of medical education programs leading to the MD degree. AAMC and AMA. 2021. Accessed May 12, 2022. https://lcme.org/publications/#Standards.

25. Greenberg WE, Borus JF. The impact of resident duty hour and supervision changes: a review. *Harv Rev Psychiatry*. 2016;24(1):69–76.

26. Papp KK, Stoller EP, Sage P, et al. The effects of sleep loss and fatigue on resident-physicians: a multi-institutional, mixed-method study. *Acad Med*. 2004 May;79(5):394–406.

27. Raj KS. Well-being in residency: a systematic review. *J Grad Med Educ.* 2016 Dec;8(5):674–684.

28. Simien C, Holt KD, Richter TH. The impact of ACGME work-hour reforms on the operative experience of fellows in surgical subspecialty programs. *J Grad Med Educ.* 2011;3(1):111–117.

29. Vaporciyan AA, Yang SC, Baker CJ, Fann JI, Verrier ED. Cardiothoracic surgery residency training: past, present, and future. *J Thorac Cardiovasc Surg.* 2013;146(4):759–767.

30. Mirmehdi I, O'Neal CM, Moon D, MacNew H, Senkowski C. The interventional arm of the flexibility in duty-hour requirements for surgical trainees trial: first-year data show superior quality in-training initiative outcomes. *J Surg Educ.* 2016;73(6):e131–e135.

31. Lieberman JD, Olenwine JA, Finley W, Nicholas GG. Residency reform: anticipated effects of ACGME guidelines on general surgery and internal medicine residency programs. *Curr Surg.* 2005;62(2):231–236. doi:10.1016/j.cursur.2004.06.015. PMID: 15796946.

32. Fletcher KE, Reed DA, Arora VM. Patient safety, resident education and resident well-being following implementation of the 2003 ACGME duty hour rules. *J Gen Intern Med.* 2011;26(8):907–919.

33. Roses RE, Foley PJ, Paulson EC, Pray L, Kelz RR, Williams NN, Morris JB. Revisiting the rotating call schedule in less than 80 hours per week. *J Surg Educ.* 2009;66(6):357–360. doi:10.1016/j.jsurg.2009.07.005. Erratum in: J Surg Educ. 2010 Jan-Feb;67(1):59. PMID: 20142135.

34. Reiter ER, Wong DR. Impact of duty hour limits on resident training in otolaryngology. *Laryngoscope.* 2005 May;115(5):773–779. doi:10.1097/01.MLG.0000157696.03159.24. PMID: 15867638.

35. Landrigan CP, Rothschild JM, Cronin JW, et al. Effect of reducing interns' work hours on serious medical errors in intensive care units. *N Engl J Med.* 2004; 351(18):1838–1848.

36. Parthasarathy S. Sleep and the medical profession. *Curr Opin Pulm Med.* 2005;11(6):507–512.

37. Blitz JB, Rogers AE, Polmear MM, Owings AJ. Duty hour compliance: a survey of U.S. military medical interns and residents. *Mil Med.* 2017;182(11):e1997–e2004. doi:10.7205/MILMED-D-17-00105. PMID: 29087871.

38. Sticca RP, Macgregor JM, Szlabick RE. Is the Accreditation Council for Graduate Medical Education (ACGME) Resident/Fellow survey, a valid tool to assess general surgery residency programs compliance with work hours regulations? *J Surg Educ.* 2010;67(6):406–411. doi:10.1016/j.jsurg.2010.09.007. Epub 2010 Nov 7. PMID: 21156299.

39. Farrell CM. Systole and diastole, strength and openness. *JAMA.* 2019;321(19):1871–1872.

40. American Foundation for Suicide Prevention. Physician and medical student depression and suicide prevention. 2017. Accessed October 21, 2016. https://afsp.org/ our-work/education/physician-medical-student-depression- suicide-prevention/.

41. ACGME. Common program requirements. ACGME. February 3, 2020. Accessed May 12, 2022. https://www.acgme.org/globalassets/PFAssets/ProgramRequirements/cprresidency2020.pdf

42. Goldman ML, Bernstein CA, Konopasek L, Arbuckle M, Mayer LES. An intervention framework for institutions to meet new ACGME common program requirements for physician well-being. *Acad Psychiatry.* 2018;42(4):542–547.

43. Berwick DM, Nolan TW, Whittington J. The triple aim: care, health, and cost. *Health Aff (Millwood).* 2008;27(3):759–769. doi:10.1377/hlthaff.27.3.759

44. Puddester D. Managing and mitigating fatigue in the era of changing resident duty hours. *BMC Med Educ.* 2014;14(Suppl 1):S3. doi:10.1186/1472-6920-14-S1-S3

45. Cavallo A, Jaskiewicz J, Ris MD. Impact of night-float rotation on sleep, mood, and alertness: the resident's perception. *Chronobiol Int.* 2002;19(5):893–902. doi:10.1081/cbi-120014106. PMID: 12405552.

46. Wolpaw JT. It is time to prioritize education and well-being over workforce needs in residency training. *Acad Med.* 2019;94(11):1640–1642. doi:10.1097/ACM.0000000000002949. PMID: 31425182.

47. Philibert I. Resident perspectives on duty hour limits and attributes of their learning environment. *BMC Med Educ.* 2014;14 Suppl 1(Suppl 1):S7.

48. Kempenich JW, Willis RE, Campi HD, Schenarts PJ. The cost of compliance: the financial burden of fulfilling Accreditation Council for Graduate Medical Education and American Board of Surgery requirements. *J Surg Educ.* 2018 Nov;75(6):e47–e53. doi:10.1016/j.jsurg.2018.07.006. PMID: 30122641.

49. Bui AH, Ripp JA, Oh KY, Basloe F, Hassan D, Akhtar S, Leitman IM. The impact of program-driven wellness initiatives on burnout and depression among surgical trainees. *Am J Surg.* 2020;219(2):316–321. doi:10.1016/j.amjsurg.2019.10.027. PMID: 31668706.

50. Chung A, Mott S, Rebillot K, Li-Sauerwine S, Shah S, Coates WC, Yarris LM. Wellness interventions in emergency medicine residency programs: review of the literature since 2017. *West J Emerg Med.* 2020;22(1):7–14. doi:10.5811/westjem.2020.11.48884. PMID: 33439796; PMCID: PMC7806318.

51. Jordan SG, Robbins JB, Sarkany D, et al. The Association of Program Directors in Radiology well-being 2019 survey: identifying residency gaps and offering solutions. *J Am Coll Radiol.* 2019;16(12):1702–1706. doi:10.1016/j.jacr.2019.06.017. Epub 2019 Jul 11. PMID: 31302059.

52. Oliveira A, Slanetz PJ, Catanzano TM, Sarkany D, Siddall K, Johnson K, Jordan SG. Strengthening the clinical learning environment by mandate-implementing the ACGME common program requirements. *Acad Radiol.* 2020:S1076-6332(20) 30671–30671. doi:10.1016/j.acra.2020.11.019. PMID: 33303348.

53. Zaver F, Battaglioli N, Denq W, Messman A, Chung A, Lin M, Liu EL. Identifying gaps and launching resident wellness initiatives: the 2017 resident wellness consensus summit. *West J Emerg Med.* 2018;19(2):342–345. doi:10.5811/westjem.2017.11.36240. PMID: 29560064; PMCID: PMC5851509.

54. Sullivan AG, Hoffman A, Slavin S. Becoming AWARE: ACGME's new suite of well-being resources. *J Grad Med Educ.* 2020;12(1):122–124. doi:10.4300/JGME-D-19-00967.1. PMID: 32064068; PMCID: PMC7012532.

55. Vassallo P, Jeremiah J, Forman L, et al. Parental leave in graduate medical education: recommendations for reform. *Am J Med.* 2019;132(3):385–389. doi:10.1016/j.amjmed.2018.11.006. PMID: 30503884.

56. Spruce MW, Gingrich AA, Phares A, Beyer CA, Salcedo ES, Guralnick S, Rea MM. Child-rearing during postgraduate medical training and its relation to stress and burnout: results from a single-institution multispecialty survey. *Mil Med.* 2021:usab029. doi:10.1093/milmed/usab029. Epub ahead of print. PMID: 33580698.

Bringing It Home and Making the Case

Diagnosing Your Institution's Readiness to Address Trainee Well-Being

Larissa R. Thomas, Irina Kryzhanovskaya, and Saadia Akhtar

Introduction

Change is unavoidable in the health care industry. The decision to pursue well-being as an institutional priority involves a significant evolution in strategic thinking for organizations. A number of theories regarding change management exist that can help leaders ready their institutions to thrive amid change by using practical strategies to solve common problems related to clinician well-being. In this chapter, we share some theories of change management commonly used in organizational science and discuss some concepts specific to change for organizational well-being in a health care setting. We then describe a practical approach for assessing your organization's readiness for change that includes considerations for successful change management, such as identifying stakeholders, building alliances, anticipating roadblocks, and reflecting on progress. Finally, we provide practical suggestions for "quick wins" that can build momentum in the early stages of change management and tips for getting started in your institution.

Theories of Change Management

Change is inevitable in every industry, and health care is no exception. Health care organizations therefore need to be strategic in anticipating and reacting to change using nimble approaches that adapt to evolving circumstances. Institutions that handle change in a successful manner provide a healthy environment not only for their patients, but also for their learners and employees. All theories of change management have in common an emphasis on preparing for the change, implementing the change, and studying the change to identify expected and unexpected effects and reactions in the organization. Some examples of frequently referenced theories of change management are described in more detail below

Lewin's Model: "Unfreeze-Change-Refreeze"

In the 1940s, Kurt Lewin, a physicist and social scientist, developed the Theory of Planned Change. His model incorporates a three-stage process: unfreeze, change, and refreeze.[1] It uses the analogy of changing the shape of a block of ice. In relation to organizational change, the first stage in Lewin's model is for the organization to understand that change is needed and prepare to accept that change is necessary (Unfreezing Stage). This stage comprises breaking down the status quo before a new process of functioning can exist within an institution. During the change stage, individuals within the institution initiate new ways to do things (Change Stage). They let go of uncertainty and decide to move forward by accepting the change. Two key resources that institutions can utilize to make the transition from the unfreezing stage to the change stage successful are time and communication. Employees need time to understand the changes, and leaders need to communicate about the forthcoming change on a consistent basis with transparency and clarity. The institution is ready for the third stage when employees have accepted the changes and when the changes are forming (Refreeze Stage). This stage allows the changes to be institutionalized and implemented on a daily basis. Through this process, employees are more likely to feel confident about the changes and the overall organization.[1,2]

Kotter's Eight-Step Change Model

In 1995, John Kotter developed the Eight-Step Change Model.[3] These steps help move organizations from planning and "setting the stage," to stakeholder buy-in and plans for implementation, to actual implementation, feedback, and, ultimately, making the changes stick. The first step is to create a sense of urgency for change. Institutional leadership can identify potential threats and examine opportunities, ultimately convincing employees about the need for change. The second step is forming a powerful coalition team that consists of influential individuals with a diverse background in their experience and job title. Once this change coalition is created, it is important to create a vision and plan for change, which involves the third step of Kotter's Change Model. In the fourth step, leadership should communicate the change vision and plan with stakeholders. All aspects of institutional operations should be tied to the change vision. Leadership should also address employee concerns in an open and honest manner. The fifth step deals with removing obstacles. By removing change obstacles, individuals can feel more empowered and be more supportive of the change plans. Creating short-term wins is part of the sixth

TABLE 11.1 Applying Lewin's Change Management Model to well-being interventions

Stage	Considerations
Unfreeze	Timing Stakeholders Identify measures of success Identify quick wins Avoid zero-sum traps
Change	Communication Involve students or GME trainees Pilot and scale Expect pitfalls Gather data
Refreeze	Pause new interventions Review data Reflect on unanticipated challenges or interim events Communicate results Identify next steps

step. The change coalition can play a key role in identifying short-term targets that are set up for success. Accomplishing these wins will motivate the entire staff. The next step is to build on these short-term wins. The quick wins are the beginning of what ultimately needs to be accomplished within the institution on a long-term basis. The last step of Kotter's Change Model is to anchor the changes in corporate culture. The change should become part of the foundation of the institution, with continued support from leadership.[3]

In this chapter, we integrate strategies from Kotter's model with Lewin's Theory of Planned Change to outline ways to apply these theories to organizational change for well-being (Table 11.1).

Change Management for Organizational Well-Being

General Principles

Change management strategies apply to organizational well-being in two important ways. First, impacts on well-being can and should be anticipated from any major organizational change. The role of well-being leaders in this context can be to help other institutional leaders anticipate effects on well-being and mitigate negative impacts. Second, since large changes to an organization are inherently complex, implementing changes to improve well-being will often have impacts (both anticipated and unanticipated) on other domains of the organization. This type of system, in which the effects of an input are complex and often cannot be fully anticipated, are known as *complex adaptive systems*. As described in Chapter 1, for these types of complex systems, such as health care, a fundamental component of change management is knowing that, even with careful

TABLE 11.2 Well-being as an organizational competency

Novice	Competent	Expert
Aware of the problem and desire to act	Understand potential causes and solutions	Integrate well-being into organizational strategy

Adapted from Shanafelt, *JAMA IM* 2017; 77(12): 1827

planning, there will be unintended effects of the change. Frequent feedback and monitoring for these impacts can help to mitigate negative effects and even detect unanticipated benefits that may not have been immediately apparent.[4] Proactive communication and ensuring stakeholder buy-in at the early stages of any major change can help set the stage for a smoother implementation. Follow-up throughout implementation can help to support integration and adoption.

Shanafelt and colleagues have described a competency framework for organizational well-being.[5] With its aspiration for integrating well-being into the core fabric of organizational strategy and operations as part of the Quadruple Aim,[6] this continuum illustrates common steps organizations can take to progress toward this goal. Because viewing well-being as a pillar of the health care system is itself a change in strategic thinking on the part of an organization, few organizations to date have achieved expert status. Yet many organizations have begun to progress along the early stages of competency. Awareness that well-being is important and taking actions such as establishing a well-being committee and opportunities for individually focused well-being activities are common first steps along this continuum. Assessing well-being and identifying unit- or program-level hot spots are common next steps, followed by interventions at the program or system level and, finally, progressive integration of well-being into key decision-making within the program/organization.[5]

We encourage you to examine Table 11.2 and consider where your organization or program is along this continuum. You may note that different parts of your organization may be at different stages or that your program or school may be at a different level than the institution as a whole. This chapter will provide tools and strategies to help you take your organization to the next level and specifically highlight important considerations for organizational change to promote well-being in medical education.

As you examine where your own institution is along the continuum, consider the following case example of a change to enhance organizational well-being.

Case

An institution's C-suite meets with undergraduate (UME) and graduate medical education (GME) leadership to consider the current state of organizational well-being. Specifically, the GME Well-Being Director, Chief Wellness Officer, Chief Financial Officer, and Dean of the School of Medicine meet after a recent survey administered by a group of internal medicine residents indicated that 30% of the residents felt that they would have benefitted from mental health screening and treatment since the start of their training, but only 25% actually received treatment. The Dean is concerned with this finding but suggests that since the residents all have health insurance, they should be able to access mental health services when needed and thus wants to know what her role should be. The Chief Wellness Officer is concerned about the documented increase in depression and suicidal ideation among resident physicians. The Chief Financial Officer notes that the institution has just spent a considerable amount on administrative resource support (to help with nonphysician work) and is bound by budgetary constraints in a difficult fiscal year for the institution. The GME Well-Being Director is concerned about an upcoming Clinical Learning Environment Review visit where there will be questions about how residencies provide access to mental health screening and treatment.

Setting the Stage for Success: Planning to "Unfreeze"

The first phase of change management can often make or break a major change. The timing of a change within the institutional landscape can either benefit or hinder progress. Before considering a change, identifying the stakeholders and how the change might affect them and working to build alliances will increase the likelihood of successes. Since many changes for well-being do not result in immediately apparent effects, identifying a possible "quick win" can help to build momentum for forthcoming larger-scale changes.

Timing Is (Sometimes) Everything

The timing of a major change to improve well-being can be one of the most important factors to consider. As will be further discussed in Chapter 12, similarly to other institutional needs, the feasibility of enacting a major change often depends on a combination of motivation to enact change and the business case for investing resources. Additionally, as described in Chapter 10, regulatory requirements (Liaison Committee on Medical Education [LCME] and the Accreditation Council for Graduate Medical Education [ACGME]) can also compel leaders to invest resources in trainee well-being. However, because the impetus for organizational change to support well-being may differ from that of other institutional priorities, a recent tragic event (such as a suicide) or the moral imperative (such as the COVID pandemic) can help spur significant organizational investment in changes to promote well-being even during years of fiscal constraint. When proposing change to enhance well-being, the well-being leaders should consider what impetus is most compelling for health care leadership, along with contextual factors within the institution that can affect the timing of a proposed change.[7] Similarly, it is important not to be discouraged if a proposal or request to fund an initiative is not initially successful. It may be necessary to revisit the proposal again in the future when circumstances might better favor receptiveness and feasibility.

Identifying Stakeholders and Building Alliances

The first step in considering a major change to improve well-being (e.g., increased funding for leadership or mental health resources, or a major systems intervention to enhance clinical support) is to identify all stakeholders who would be affected and what impact a change would have. While some changes are perceived as a "win-win," even changes that everyone agrees are important for well-being often have significant financial implications and may have unintended impacts on other groups if work is shifted.

Considering what each stakeholder has to gain or lose with the change can help to identify points of leverage, areas of possible negotiation, and metrics to gauge success from each vantage point. Additionally, anticipating each stakeholder's readiness for change (from inertia to readiness for action) will help to identify the optimal timing of the change, or, if timing is not negotiable, to anticipate and mitigate potential barriers to implementation. Finally, it is important to consider which parties hold power (for financial resource or policy change), which parties will do the work, and which parties are the "end users" for whom the intervention is designed.

Figure 11.1 lists some of the common stakeholders who should be considered when considering changes to improve well-being in undergraduate and graduate medical education. At the center of this figure are those who are in the clinical learning environment. While this audience centers learner well-being, in a holistic model considering stakeholders, it is helpful to consider that students and GME trainees have needs for well-being that are interrelated to all members of the health care team. Additionally, and as previously discussed, centering patient care also includes attending to the well-being of all members of the health care team. Maintaining these groups at the center as the "end

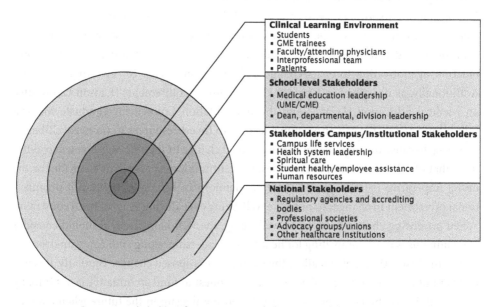

FIGURE 11.1 Common stakeholders for organizational change in well-being.

users" of an intervention helps to focus priorities on "lifting all boats" rather than pitting one group against another. The concentric circles illustrate stakeholders who are often involved in major organizational changes to support well-being at the medical school/departmental level, at the institutional level, and at the national/policy level. For smaller-scale changes, a subset of such stakeholders may be involved in planning, communication, or implementation.

Importantly, it is easiest to lay the groundwork for change before a change is imminent. Significant changes in a complex environment are generally realized over years of consensus-building, rather than as overnight successes. Establishing relationships and collaborations locally and externally will position the well-being leader both to implement large changes over the long term, and to be able to act with agility when an opportunity for rapid innovation arises (e.g., a donor who wishes to fund an initiative to support frontline workers during the pandemic) or a mandate for immediate change occurs (due to an ACGME citation or CLER visit, for example). Holding regular meetings among well-being leaders with different stakeholder groups is one way to build these alliances. A retreat can also be a way to galvanize support across stakeholder groups. Successful retreats are predicated on a defined scope and leadership's endorsement of moving a vision forward afterward. Building collaborations with other institutions can also help the well-being leader to provide benchmarks for their own health system about where their organization is on the continuum compared to peer institutions.

Considering How to Measure Success

In initial planning, leaders should consider how they will demonstrate success or impact and what qualitative and quantitative data are needed (or available) to measure that impact. It is important to consider "survey fatigue" and balance desire for gathering data for each intervention with the additional impact of more surveys on well-being. Leaders may choose to align interventions with the timeframe of larger ongoing surveys such as the ACGME or LCME survey, or institutional well-being or climate surveys. Additionally, they may consider process metrics that are already available and tracked, such as work hours or amount of time spent on the electronic health record.

One general challenge with implementing systems interventions in a complex adaptive system is that randomized trials are rarely feasible because of the complexity of the real-world environment. As a result, well-being outcomes are often not directly attributable to one specific intervention because the environment is constantly evolving and one intervention may have anticipated or unintended impacts on the culture, which can either amplify or diminish well-being impacts.[4] For this reason, structural metrics that demonstrate capacity, or process metrics that demonstrate access to or education about well-being efforts, are often easier to gather than outcome measures (impacts on well-being scores such as burnout) in the short term.[8] For example, access and utilization metrics, such as number of mental health providers and percentage accessing care, are often helpful when implementing a mental health screening tool or new mental health service.

Outcome measures (such as decreased prevalence of depression or burnout) may take much longer to measure and are often affected by other events happening independently of the intervention itself. Qualitative feedback can help to identify examples of success and opportunities to improve. Planning which metrics to track and how to obtain qualitative feedback in addition to measuring well-being outcomes can help to demonstrate success and guide next steps for further change.

Creating Quick Wins

In the consensus-building and planning stages of change, creating quick wins can consolidate support and build momentum for larger, more complex changes. During needs assessments and feedback sessions, it is necessary to keep an eye out for a process that could easily be changed, an oversight that could be easily corrected, or misunderstandings that can be addressed with improved communication. Although quick wins are not usually "game-changers" in terms of systems impact, such efforts can still be impactful and indicate commitment to investing in well-being and listening to feedback, and thus can help to build trust among stakeholders while the groundwork for larger-scale changes is established. When considering quick wins, an *effort-impact analysis* is often helpful. Known as a "Pick" chart, an effort-impact matrix is a 2 × 2 table that can help to prioritize interventions (Figure 11.2).[9] Anything that is low effort but high impact should be considered first, but low effort, lower impact interventions can also have a larger impact if several of these "nice-to-haves" are coupled together and packaged as a collective win. It is important to recognize that a focus *only* on low effort, low impact interventions, however, can lead to cynicism if these appear to be the only interventions that leadership is considering, so communicating plans for longer-term, higher effort (major initiative) interventions at the same time is key to maintaining momentum.

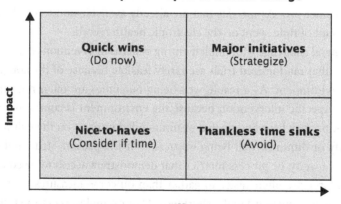

FIGURE 11.2 Effort–impact matrix of potential well-being interventions. Adapted from Impact Effort Matrix | ASQ. Accessed May 18, 2022. https://asq.org/quality-resources/impact-effort-matrix.

Avoiding the "Zero-Sum" Well-Being Trap

One common challenge that institutions face in addressing well-being is the "zero-sum" well-being trap: if one side wins, another side must lose. When resources are finite, improving well-being for one group can, in fact, worsen well-being for another group by shifting resources toward the beneficiary of the initiative, with a concurrent shifting of work or reduced support for another group. In this scenario, being the "squeaky wheel" can seem advantageous, but, in the long run, improving well-being for one group at the expense of others has negative effects on the entire health care team. For example, as Figure 11.3 illustrates, resident work compression (having to do more work in a defined period of time without other responsibilities removed) negatively affects well-being and can lead to work-hours violations. The risk of an ACGME work-hours citation with resulting threat to accreditation could compel institutions to limit or "cap" the number of patients a resident team cares for in an effort to reduce work hours and address the citation. While this intervention could have a positive impact on resident well-being if it reduces work compression, without sufficient resources added to the health system, the work merely becomes shifted to other members of the health care team. As a result of this work compression, faculty who take up the slack may then be at higher risk for burnout themselves. Faculty who are burned out may be less able to contribute to a supportive workplace culture, and therefore, resident well-being may ultimately further diminish as a result. Some stakeholders in the health system may also see well-being as a zero-sum between clinicians and patients: in this mindset, prioritizing clinician well-being can be falsely conflated with deprioritizing investment in patient care.

How can the "zero-sum" trap be avoided? First, collaborations among stakeholders for all affected groups can ensure an environment of co-advocacy. In scenarios in which immediate action to benefit one group is needed (e.g., to address a citation or grievance),

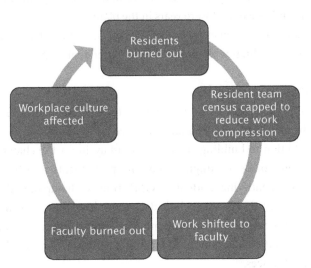

FIGURE 11.3 Example of a "zero-sum" well-being trap.

proactive communication among stakeholders could still provide the opportunity for leaders of other groups to make a business case for simultaneous interventions/plans to avoid downstream effects of work-shifting.[5] Additionally, well-being leaders can draw on literature showing the impact of clinician well-being on patient care, as described in Chapter 5, or use examples from the business world to illustrate how investment in employee well-being can improve client (patient) satisfaction.[10,11]

Implementing the Change

Communication

Nearly all leaders have had the experience of extensively planning an important change and then realizing in retrospect that the change had not been clearly communicated in advance to everyone who would be affected. For changes that have been discussed for months or years, it is common to think that everyone is aware of the change when it finally is implemented. Consider adding communication strategy as a specific element of a strategic plan, including timing, content, platform/method, and who will be sending communications during each stage of an intervention. Inevitably, however, any change will appear to catch a segment of the target audience off guard.

While Chapter 18 will discuss specific strategies related to crisis or disaster communication, principles of communication are just as important for slow-moving, gradual changes. In fact, in the medical education environment in which institutional memory is short due to short training times, a gradual or years-long change is often implemented after the original stakeholders who gave input into planning have graduated. In this situation, the students and GME trainees may feel that a carefully considered change that checked all the boxes and involved the target community in planning was a rash or sudden change done without their input. For the medical student or GME audience, frequent communication about past efforts and ongoing quick wins can help to bridge institutional memory gaps. For very large initiatives that were years in the planning, a pause to examine the scale of the necessary communication effort before the launch of the initiative can be helpful in mitigating misunderstandings with groups that have frequent turnover.

Participatory Leadership

When implementing changes, using leadership strategies that include engagement of those who will be affected by the change may have an independent positive impact on well-being[12] in addition to building consensus and buy-in for the change. Participatory leadership strategies can be as simple as inviting participants to a listening or brainstorming session or identifying student or GME trainee champions. Formal strategies for engaging participants in change include design thinking (human-centered design) to involve end-users in the development of an intervention. Such strategies not only provide real-time feedback on the intervention to improve its implementation,[13] but may also enhance trust among trainees.[14]

Pilot and Scale

Since most organizational well-being challenges are complex problems, identifying a small pilot or "test-of-change" project serves as a proof of concept to further the case for investment of resources, builds trust among end-users for implementation of larger-scale changes, and helps to build momentum for initiatives that may take a long time to demonstrate changes in well-being outcomes. Using a strategy of pilots or small tests of change also ensures that well-being leaders can remain nimble and pivot to a different strategy if initial pilots are not successful. A common reason that well-being initiatives lose steam is that they become "too big to fail," meaning that so much time and so many resources are invested that it becomes difficult to change strategy once plans are set in motion. While major systems changes ultimately require extensive planning, strategic initiatives building on prior successes and collaborations are more likely to succeed and be sustained if initial pilots have demonstrated success.[15]

Expect Pitfalls and Roadblocks

As we have described, although changes to improve well-being intuitively would seem easier to implement than other changes (such as, e.g., billing practices), well-being is a complex problem that is no easier to solve than the most vexing problems of our time. At the same time, because clinician address well-being is deeply personal, the stakes for not meeting expectations can feel particularly high. For all of these reasons, it is important that leaders anticipate that there will be pitfalls, unintended consequences, and barriers to implementation of any major change to address well-being. It can be helpful to recognize that resistance to change is an *expected* stage of change. Changes in support of trainee well-being, in particular, can frequently be met with skepticism from those who trained under different circumstances, concerns about prioritization of clinicians over patients, and financial concerns. Anticipating these concerns can help well-being leaders prepare a proactive communication strategy to address them.

Additionally, a sentinel event (such as medical error that requires immediate changes) or institutional crises (such as the COVID-19 pandemic) can upend the most thoughtful of plans and require pivoting resources. It is helpful for leaders to consider the priority of their intervention, the urgency of need, and what the consequences of delaying the intervention will be so that they are ready to advocate for prioritizing the intervention, as appropriate, or putting it on hold if an emergency need arises.

Gathering Data

Including a plan to track key metrics is critical to enabling successful change. Although changes in well-being outcomes (such as burnout or depression) are generally the desired impact of interventions to improve well-being, as described above, it is rarely possible (and sometimes not ethical) to implement randomized interventions in a complex system. Therefore, outcomes can be influenced by many circumstances other than the change itself. Additionally, several iterations of change may be necessary before quantitative impacts on well-being outcomes can be assessed. Additionally, while quantitative measures (scales or surveys) will assess the "who, what, and when," qualitative data will capture the "how and why" of an intervention. Focus groups, end-user interviews, and on-the-ground qualitative feedback are particularly useful during pilot stages to help quickly assess success and pivot interventions to meet end-user needs. This type of interim data can continue to justify ongoing investment in or scaling up of initiatives that may not deliver outcomes over the short term.

Pause ("Refreeze"), Reflect, and Make It Stick

An essential but often-overlooked element of change management is pausing (or "refreezing") after a change is implemented to assess the impact, review progress, and plan for the next stage. In addition to helping leaders to ensure that they are reviewing the success of the intervention, pausing is essential to establish stability. Humans crave order and stability; even when there is a desire to rapidly implement changes to support well-being, too many changes at once can lead to a sense of chaos and undermine the desired well-being impacts. During the stage of pausing and reflecting, leaders should review feedback, communicate progress, and decide and communicate next steps. During this stage, new priorities and needs may emerge, and previous "burning platforms" may no longer be of highest concern. Setting an intention to pause and reflect also helps to scope expectations for what can be accomplished in a given time frame and encourages leaders to also remain open to new ideas and course correction.

During this pause period, leaders may review planned project-specific metrics as well as ongoing institutional survey data to examine to what extent changes to metrics may be attributed to the intervention. Pausing to reflect on whether the organization/unit has shifted along the continuum of organizational competency in well-being (Table 11.1) as a result of this change may also inform the extent to which an intervention was successful in contributing to long-term institutional strategy. It is important to also consider unanticipated challenges or new external forces that arose within the timeframe of intervention implementation (e.g., the COVID pandemic was an unanticipated influence that could have eroded any positive effects from systems interventions evaluated over that time period). In such cases, reviewing process metrics, feedback on acceptability of the intervention, and qualitative feedback can still help to demonstrate whether an intervention was successful at face value and guide next steps for further change.

Conclusion

While change management is a daunting part of any well-being leader's job, using a strategic approach to plan, implement, and reflect on change can help to ensure success. Key components include stakeholder involvement, communication, anticipating resistance, ability to change course, and taking time to pause and reflect before implementing further changes. In complex adaptive systems, controlled interventions are rarely feasible, and the dynamic environment means that unintended impacts should be expected and examined. Remembering that the well-being of all members of the health care team is intertwined and supports patient care can help to avoid zero-sum traps that enhance well-being of one group at the expense of another.

Summary Points

- Using change management theory can help well-being leaders move an organization along a continuum in addressing well-being as a systems issue.
- Planning a change should include determining the right timing, involving stakeholders, defining measures of success, identifying quick wins and avoiding zero-sum traps.
- When implementing a change, it is important to engage those who will be affected by the planned change, use a comprehensive communication strategy, and gather data from pilots before scaling.
- A critical component of change management is pausing after the change has been implemented in order to reflect on and communicate successes and identify opportunities to improve.

Putting It into Practice

Reflect back on the case presented at the start of this chapter or an example at your own institution:

- Identify the stakeholders who would be affected by any change to screening and referral to treatment and the impact of that change.
- Consider which groups may experience work being shifted to them with the implementation of a new screening and referral mechanism. What communications and resources may be helpful to mitigate negative impacts on these groups?
- Look for quick wins that can consolidate support and build momentum for larger, more complex changes.
- Choose some process measures that might help you to demonstrate early success. How will you measure if your change produced the desired outcome?

References

1. Shirey MR. Lewin's Theory of Planned Change as a strategic resource. *J Nurs Adm*. 2013;43(2):69–72. doi:10.1097/NNA.0b013e31827f20a9

2. Cummings S, Bridgman T, Brown KG. Unfreezing change as three steps: rethinking Kurt Lewin's legacy for change management. *Hum Relat*. 2016;69(1):33–60. doi:10.1177/0018726715577707

3. Harrison R, Fischer S, Walpola RL, et al. Where do models for change management, improvement and implementation meet? A systematic review of the applications of change management models in healthcare. *J Healthc Leadersh*. 2021;13:85–108. doi:10.2147/JHL.S289176

4. Sterman JD. Learning from evidence in a complex world. *Am J Public Health*. 2006;96(3):505–514. doi:10.2105/AJPH.2005.066043

5. Shanafelt T, Goh J, Sinsky C. The business case for investing in physician well-being. *JAMA Intern Med*. 2017;177(12):1826–1832. doi:10.1001/jamainternmed.2017.4340

6. Bodenheimer T, Sinsky C. From triple to quadruple aim: care of the patient requires care of the provider. *Ann Fam Med*. 2014;12(6):573–576. doi:10.1370/afm.1713

7. Shanafelt T, Trockel M, Ripp J, Murphy ML, Sandborg C, Bohman B. Building a program on well-being: key design considerations to meet the unique needs of each organization. *Acad Med*. Published online August 2018:1. doi:10.1097/ACM.0000000000002415

8. Donabedian A. The quality of care: how can it be assessed? *JAMA*. 1988;260(12):1743–1748. doi:10.1001/jama.1988.03410120089033

9. ASQ. Impact effort matrix. 2022. Accessed May 18, 2022. https://asq.org/quality-resources/impact-effort-matrix.

10. Friedman R. How to support employee health instead of sapping it. *Harv Bus Rev*. Published online November 30, 2015. Accessed May 18, 2022. https://hbr.org/2015/11/how-to-support-employee-health-instead-of-sapping-it

11. Beard A, Hornik R, Heather Wang ME, Presnal S. It's hard to be good. *Harv Bus Rev*. Published online November 1, 2011. Accessed May 18, 2022. https://hbr.org/2011/11/its-hard-to-be-good.

12. Shanafelt TD, Gorringe G, Mcnaker R, et al. Impact of organizational leadership on physician burnout and satisfaction. *Mayo Clin Proc*. 2015;90(4):432–440. doi:10.1016/j.mayocp.2015.01.012

13. Brown T. Design thinking. *Harv Bus Rev*. 2008;86(6):84–92.

14. Thomas LR, Nguyen R, Teherani A, Lucey CR, Harleman E. Designing well-being: using design thinking to engage residents in developing well-being interventions. *Acad Med J Assoc Am Med Coll*. 2020;95(7):1038–1042. doi:10.1097/ACM.0000000000003243

15. Brown T, Martin R. Design for action. *Harv Bus Rev*. 2015;93(9):56–64.

Making the Case
for Institutional
Commitment to Well-Being

Elizabeth Harry, Katherine Morrison, and
Elizabeth Lawrence

Introduction

Health care institutions have changed dramatically in recent years to meet the so-called
triple aim of improving the patient health care experience, enhancing population health,
and reducing health care costs.[1] These innovations include new payment and reimbursement models, electronic health record requirements, quality metrics, patient portals, patient satisfaction surveys, and productivity benchmarks. This rapid evolution in health
care has resulted in an increased physician and trainee workload, with a concurrent decrease in physician autonomy and face-to-face time with patients, together contributing
to an epidemic of physician and trainee burnout.[2,3] As described in Chapter 1, health care
professional burnout and distress have led physician thought leaders to call for an expansion of the triple aim to include the fourth aim of improving the work life of health care
providers.[4]

In this chapter, we examine the rationale for health care institutions incorporating
this fourth aim of clinician well-being into their organizational strategic plans, and we
explore five common reasons why institutions choose to invest in physician well-being.
The supporting literature is reviewed in each of these five domains. In addition, we argue
that addressing clinician well-being at a systems level additionally includes addressing
institutional responsibilities around gender equity, social justice, and diversity. We also

include discussion around a model for institutional change with detailed practice boxes to help the reader make their own case for institutional support of well-being.

Why Institutions and Leaders Choose to Invest in Well-Being

Executive leadership endorsement is essential to incorporate well-being into institutional strategic plans, budgets, and policies. The most common catalysts of leadership support for well-being, as described by Shanafelt and colleagues, include the *moral imperative* to focus on professional well-being, the *tragedy* of physician suicide, the *regulatory* requirements to invest in learner well-being, the identified association between physician and trainee well-being and *high-quality health care*, and the *financial benefits* or "business case" of investing in well-being (Table 12.1).[5] Leaders who recognize these forces will be more likely to support well-being initiatives. Additionally, a given impetus may be compelling for one leader to decide to support well-being as a strategic priority, while a different factor may motivate another leader. Therefore, well-being leaders and advocates can leverage a specific rationale for supporting well-being needs based on their knowledge of which approach may best strike a chord with the executive leadership at their institution.

The Moral Imperative

Medical students enter medical school with a higher quality of life, lower rates of depression, and lower rates of burnout than their age-matched peers.[6] As they progress through their training and learn how to become competent physicians, they develop higher rates of depression and burnout than their peers, a finding that continues throughout their medical training. Twenty-seven percent of medical students endorse depressive symptoms,[7] 11% have suicidal ideation, and 45–56% have symptoms indicating burnout.[8] Shortly before starting internship, 49% of responding medical students had burnout, 38% endorsed depressive symptoms, and 34% had low mental quality of life. Similar

TABLE 12.1 Reasons for leadership to support well-being initiatives

Moral imperative	Tragedy	Regulatory requirements	Quality and safety	Cost
Learner distress	Motor vehicle Accidents	LCME	Medical error	Unnecessary orders
Wellness-centered leadership	Substance use		Communication skills	Remediation/ unprofessional behavior
Oath of Geneva	Divorce or breakups	ACGME	Patient outcomes	Medical malpractice
Equity and diversity	Suicide		Patient experience	Recruitment and retention

rates of distress persist in residency training.[9,10] Chapter 3 describes these findings in greater detail. The suggestion from these observed data that bright, hard-working, and empathic young people matriculating into medical school must sacrifice their own well-being to join the medical profession is unacceptable. Leaders of health care institutions should not countenance this sacrifice but instead practice "wellness-centered leadership" by adhering to the foundational imperative to "care about people always."[11] By respecting our learners, we can cultivate community, engender trust, foster institutional loyalty, and contribute to a culture of compassion oriented to minimize learner distress.[12] Respect for medical student and graduate medical education (GME) trainees includes acknowledging their hard work, assisting them to recognize that burnout is a systemic issue,[13] and validating their needs for personal safety, mental health, and support resources.

The Oath of Geneva is the modern version of the Hippocratic Oath and includes the statement, "I will attend to my own health, well-being, and abilities in order to provide care of the highest standard."[14] The inclusion of this declaration in an oath that is taken by our students, residents, and fellows reflects a moral commitment of the profession to which academic medical center leaders should respond by prioritizing physician, GME trainee, and medical student well-being.

The moral imperative to address physician well-being is also informed by the interdependence of well-being and inclusion, as described in Chapter 8. Medical students and GME trainees must learn and practice in an environment in which all feel included and valued and in which people from diverse backgrounds can share their perspectives.[15] Working to eliminate bias and racism not only is the right thing to do on moral grounds; it also advances the well-being of learners. Learner mistreatment is associated with burnout,[16] and resident burnout is associated with greater explicit and implicit bias.[17] Discrimination should be confronted in all of its forms, including race- and gender-based mistreatment and microaggressions.[18,19] A true culture of well-being will address systemic racism in admissions and recruitment processes, mentoring programs, salaries, and job expectations.

Tragedy as Imperative for Change

Burnout, anxiety, and depression in our medical students, residents, and fellows can lead to tragedy. As described in Chapter 5, burnout is associated with myriad consequences, including motor vehicle accidents, divorce or broken relationships, an increased risk for substance use, and leaving the profession of medicine.[20-23] Although there is some uncertainty and controversy about the incidence of medical student suicide,[24] as described in Chapter 2, suicide remains the first leading cause of death for male residents and the second leading cause of death for female residents.[25] It has been reported that 300-400 physicians kill themselves each year,[26] and the fact that suicide is considered by some to be a known occupational hazard of becoming a physician speaks to the magnitude of the problem.[27]

Convincing health care institutional leadership to recognize and address physician well-being and to change institutional culture to prevent tragedy can be a daunting challenge. To make the case for such a change, the model of cultural transformation proposed by Shanafelt in 2019 is useful (Figure 12.1).[28] In this model, the authors propose that institutions exist in an equilibrium created by survival anxiety ("If we don't change, something bad will happen") and learning anxiety ("Making the needed changes may be impossible"). Tragedy is an event that may disrupt equilibrium and precipitate institutional change.[28] Providing the tools and skills needed for change and the motivation to prevent tragedy can shift the equilibrium toward positive change. While the timing of such conversations needs to be carefully considered depending on circumstances, a recent institutional experience of tragedy can sometimes unite people with a clear focus and sense of purpose that can result in removal of prior logistic or financial obstacles to implementing change.

Regulatory Requirements

In addition to the moral imperative and desire to avert tragedy, health care organizations are obliged to meet regulatory requirements set by their accrediting bodies. As discussed in Chapter 10, the Liaison Committee for Medical Education (LCME) and the Accreditation Council for Graduate Medical Education (ACGME) have both enacted mandatory requirements for well-being programs to support learners. The LCME states clearly that "A medical school has in place an effective system of personal counseling for its medical students that includes programs to promote their well-being and to facilitate their adjustment to the physical and emotional demands of medical education."[29] The ACGME Common Program Requirements Section VI.C states, "Self-care and responsibility to support other members of the health care team are important components of professionalism; they are also skills that must be modeled, learned, and nurtured in the context of other aspects of residency training."[30] The ACGME further specifies that both faculty and house staff need to engage in well-being education and initiatives.

Health care institutions with medical students and GME trainees must meet LCME and ACGME regulatory standards in order to maintain accreditation. These standards, therefore, drive changes that *affect* medical student and GME trainee well-being although it is not always clear that they *improve* medical student and GME trainee well-being. For example, the limits on resident work hours have not consistently shown benefit for resident well-being.[31] The ACGME nonetheless reaffirmed its commitment to resident and fellow well-being by making work-hour restrictions one of its "inviolate principles" in the face of the COVID-19 pandemic.[32] And, because funding remains limited across the health care system, this regulatory lever can be a powerful mechanism to advocate for allocation of necessary resources to support compliance with regulatory requirements. The downside of this approach is that making changes only in response to the risk of losing accreditation tends to be more reactive than proactive and forward-thinking.

Factors driving survival anxiety

- Physician suicide
- Decreased quality/medical errors due to distress
- Turnover
- Productivity issues
- Decreased patient satisfaction
- Fear we may not achieve our organizational goals

Concerns contributing to learning anxiety

- Can we change?
- I do not know what to do
- What will I give up/lose?
- It will be too hard (will it work?)
- Fear loss of power or prestige
- Fear temporary incompetence

Steps to create psychologic safety and reduce learning anxiety

- Involvement in the implementation of change
- Education and formal training
- Positive role models
- Advisors and coaches
- Opportunities to practice
- Bidirectional communication between leaders and those affected
- Supportive structures, processes, rewards, and controls

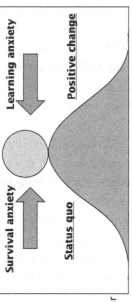

A

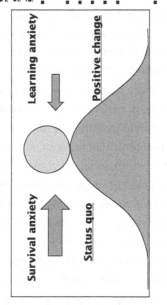

B

FIGURE. Balance of forces. A. Survival anxiety driving change in medicine offset by learning anxiety. B. Reducing learning anxiety to tip the balance in favor of change.

FIGURE 12.1 Reducing learning anxiety to promote change. Reproduced with permission from Shanafelt TD, Schein E, Minor LB, Trockel M, Schein P, Kirch D. Healing the professional culture of medicine. Mayo Clin Proc. 2019;94(8):1556–1566.

Providing Quality Health Care

Burnout reduces the ability of medical students and GME trainees to provide high-quality, patient-centered, evidence-based care.[2] Medical students who are distressed or burned out show a decline in empathy[33] and are more likely to engage in dishonest behavior, such as stating that a test had been ordered when it had not and engaging in relationships with industry that are inconsistent with professional guidelines.[34] These students are also less likely to want to provide care to the medically underserved.[34]

As described in Chapter 5, resident burnout has been associated with suboptimal patient care[35-37] and self-reported medical errors,[38] including medication errors.[39] Cognitive impairment in the form of lower standardized test scores and difficulty in skill acquisition has been seen in burned out residents.[40] The need to provide safe, high-quality care to all patients is another reason that health care institutions should address physician, medical student, and GME trainee burnout and distress.

Many additional studies have demonstrated the potential institutional impact of burnout on patient experience, patient safety, and quality outcomes. In a 2016 systematic review of publications of patient outcomes and health care worker well-being and burnout, the authors concluded that addressing the mental health and professional well-being of health care workers should be considered when designing any patient safety initiative. In fact, a decline in patient safety, quality of care, and patient satisfaction potentially jeopardizes long-term institutional survival.[41]

One study found that physician burnout, fatigue, and work unit safety grades were independently associated with self-reported major medical errors.[42] It is worth noting that the evidence to date does not support an association between well-being metrics and medical errors measured *objectively* through chart audits, official error reports, and direct observation.[43,44] This discrepancy may reflect a difference between actual care and individual perception of low performance and low self-valuation, an independent predictor of burnout.[45] In what may be a vicious cycle, self-perceived medical errors have also been found to substantially increase personal distress among trainees as well as decrease empathy, a key characteristic for optimal patient experience.[46]

Physician burnout also has a negative impact on patient-reported experience of patient–provider communication with a 0.43-point decrease in adjusted patient–provider communication (as measured by the Clinician and Group Consumer Assessment of Health care Providers and Systems [CG-CAHPS] survey) scores for every 1 point increase in provider burnout.[47] Furthermore, patient satisfaction scores decline in patients cared for by more burned-out clinicians[48,49] and are higher for those physicians who are more satisfied with their job.[50]

In addition, physicians who are burnt out are more likely to order unnecessary lab tests and consultations[51,52] and less likely to be cost-conscious.[46] Furthermore, physicians who have burnout also often role-model these behaviors to the medical students and GME trainees with whom they work, potentially contributing to the perpetuation of these clinical practice patterns. The quality imperative can be a compelling motivating force for change because it centers excellence in patient care (the purported primary role of health care organizations) as inextricably linked with clinician well-being, rather than framing clinician well-being in isolation.

Business Case

Recognition of the impact that burnout has on clinical productivity and physician turnover is essential to understanding the financial implications of burnout for a health care institution. The impact of a burned out clinician on their team members,[53-55] the additional cost associated with the remediation of clinicians demonstrating increased unprofessional behavior potentially resulting from burnout,[56] and a possible increased risk of malpractice[49] all potentially contribute to the financial impact of burnout. One study estimates that in a 400-bed hospital, "the combined costs for disruptive physician behaviors (due to staff turnover, medication errors and procedural errors) exceeds $1 million."[56]

Burnout is one of the major reasons physicians plan to reduce the amount of time they spend in direct patient care.[23,57,58] Distressed physicians are less productive[59,60] and more likely to leave their institution.[23,61] Researchers at Stanford University used their own institution as a case study and, after adjusting for multiple confounding variables in a logistic regression model, concluded that physicians who were burned out were almost twice as likely to leave their institution in the subsequent 2 years than physicians who were not burned out.[62] In the same study, researchers estimated that the 2-year cost due to the estimated loss of 60 physicians from burnout was between $15,544,000 and $55,506,000.[62]

The full cost of replacing an existing attending physician includes the costs of recruitment, travel, interviewing, lost billings, and onboarding expenses and is currently estimated at between $500,000 and $1,000,000 per physician. The American Medical Association (AMA) has developed a calculator that can be used to assess the cost incurred by an institution from physician turnover due to burnout.[63] An example using this calculator is shown in Table 12.2. A recent cost-consequence analysis, using the best available input parameters, including current rates of physician burnout, estimated that the national cost of burnout in physician turnover and lost productivity in the United States is $4.6 billion per year.[64]

While institutions might not immediately recognize a local business case for supporting medical student and GME trainee well-being, the costs to society and schools are more apparent. A 1997 review estimated total educational resource costs at approximately $72,000 to $93,000 per student per year. Using this estimate, if approximately 400 physicians per year continue to die by suicide, this is a potential loss to society of $148,800,000 dollars per year. This estimate was made almost 25 years ago and the authors predicted that the social cost would increase over time as the medical knowledge base increases and curricular innovations become more time-intensive.[65]

TABLE 12.2 Example projection of operational costs of physician burnout

Data needed	Example
# physicians in your group	800
Rate of physician burnout	54%
Current Turnover Rate/Year	7%
Cost of physician Turnover*	$400,000–1,000,000
Calculations	
1. Calculate rate of Turnover of those w/o burnout Formula (Turnover/1 + Burnout)	.07/1 + .54 = .045 or 4.5% turnover w/o burnout
2. Calculate % physicians turning over due to burnout Formula (%turnover – % turnover w/o burnout	.07 – .045 = .025 or 2.5% of physician turnover/yr due to burnout
3. Calculate # physicians turning over due to burnout/year	.025 × 800 = 20 physicians leaving per year due to burnout
4. Projected cost of physician turnover/yr due to burnout	20 × $400,000 = $8,000,000/year

*estimated to be 2x cost of salary (recruitment, relocation and replacement costs)

Source: American Medical Association. Steps Forward. Accessed December 2021: https://edhub.ama-assn.org/steps-forward/interactive/16830405

A challenge with identifying costs attributable to burnout is that funding streams and budgets are frequently focused only on a fiscal year, while the costs attributed to burnout may manifest (and accrue) over a longer period of time. The above calculator can therefore be a helpful way for an institution to recognize the costs it may not have previously attributed to burnout. An important caveat is that these calculations and models do not take into account that physicians bring different strengths to their work. One physician may be able to bill more relative value units (RVUs), another produce more academic papers, and a third mentor a large number of junior colleagues and learners. There is also the incalculable cost of burnout on the ability of faculty to teach and create a positive learning environment for medical students and GME trainees, a cost for which literature is just now emerging.[66] Ultimately, making a business case will require using available survey data on well-being (or initiating such a survey if existing data do not meet the need); identifying appropriate stakeholders, as described in Chapter 11; and calculating the costs that may be attributable not only to turnover, but also to malpractice risk, patient experience/attrition, and remediation of unprofessional behavior.

As described in the prior four imperatives for change, even if there were not a business case to be made, there are compelling reasons to support well-being. The fact that

---

BOX 12.1 Presenting Your Business Case

Improvement is possible.

Investment is justified.

ROI is measurable.

Build a picture of a road to success.

---

leaders can indeed also expect a long-term return on investment is a powerful "bonus" argument but may in itself be enough motivation for some health care institutions to invest in well-being. Suggestions for framing a business case are outlined in Box 12.1.

Conclusion

Medical training and our current health care system often lead to burnout for both medical students and GME trainees. This has costly outcomes for health care organizations, patients, and communities, in addition to the learners themselves. While the moral imperative to prevent the suffering of our health care workforce must be kept at the forefront, a strong business case can and should be made to health care organizations for investment in the well-being of our medical students and GME trainees. The medical and business scholarly literature demonstrates the impact of clinician burnout on patient safety and quality outcomes, clinician turnover, medical errors, and total team care. By elevating the importance of and attention to the well-being of medical students, trainees, and clinicians, we are likely to achieve a more efficacious, equitable, and affordable health care system.

Summary Points

- There is a moral imperative to reduce distress, mental illness, and suicide in physicians and those training to be physicians.
- Physician and trainee distress negatively impacts the cost and quality of patient care.
- The Liaison Committee for Medical Education (LCME) and the Accreditation Council for Graduate Medical Education (ACGME) have both enacted mandatory requirements for well-being programs to support learners.
- Physician turnover, physician reduction in clinical time, increased malpractice litigation and remediation of unprofessional behavior are just some of the contributing factors to the high cost of burnout for individual institutions and society as a whole.

Putting It into Practice

- Survey your institution to gather data on well-being outcomes or identify existing sources of data.
- Identify your stakeholders and which imperative may be most compelling to respective stakeholders and leaders.
- Use tools and institutional data to calculate potential financial costs of burnout at your institution.
- Create a sense of optimism that change is possible by reducing learning anxiety and building a picture of a road to success.

References

1. Donald M. Berwick, Thomas W. Nolan, and John Whittington. The triple aim: care, health, and cost. *Health Aff* 2008;27(3):759–769.
2. Dyrbye L, Shanafelt T. A narrative review on burnout experienced by medical students and residents. *Med Educ.* 2016;50(1):132–149.
3. Dyrbye LN, Shanafelt TD, Sinsky CA, et al. Burnout among health care professionals: a call to explore and address this underrecognized threat to safe, high-quality care. *NAM Perspect.* Published online July 5, 2017. doi:10.31478/201707b
4. Bodenheimer T, Sinsky C. From triple to quadruple aim: care of the patient requires care of the provider. *Ann Fam Med.* 2014;12(6):573–576. doi:10.1370/afm.1713
5. Swensen SJ, Shanafelt TD. *Mayo Clinic Strategies to Reduce Burnout: 12 Actions to Create the Ideal Workplace.* Oxford University Press; 2020.
6. Brazeau CMLR, Shanafelt T, Durning SJ, et al. Distress among matriculating medical students relative to the general population. *Acad Med J Assoc Am Med Coll.* 2014;89(11):1520–1525. doi:10.1097/ACM.0000000000000482
7. Rotenstein LS, Ramos MA, Torre M, et al. Prevalence of depression, depressive symptoms, and suicidal ideation among medical students: a systematic review and meta-analysis. *JAMA.* 2016;316(21):2214–2236. doi:10.1001/jama.2016.17324
8. Dyrbye LN, Thomas MR, Massie FS, et al. Burnout and suicidal ideation among U.S. medical students. *Ann Intern Med.* 2008;149(5):334–341. doi:10.7326/0003-4819-149-5-200809020-00008
9. Dyrbye LN, Moutier C, Durning SJ, et al. The problems program directors inherit: medical student distress at the time of graduation. *Med Teach.* 2011;33(9):756–758. doi:10.3109/0142159x.2011.577468
10. Mata DA, Ramos MA, Bansal N, et al. Prevalence of depression and depressive symptoms among resident physicians: a systematic review and meta-analysis. *JAMA.* 2015;314(22):2373–2383. doi:10.1001/jama.2015.15845
11. Shanafelt T, Trockel M, Rodriguez A, Logan D. Wellness-centered leadership: equipping health care leaders to cultivate physician well-being and professional fulfillment. *Acad Med.* 2021;96(5):641–651. doi:10.1097/ACM.0000000000003907
12. Berry LL, Awdish RLA. Health care organizations should be as generous as their workers. *Ann Intern Med.* 2021;174(1):103–104. doi:10.7326/M20-5172
13. Bohman B, Dyrbye LN, Sinsky CA, et al. Physician well-being: the reciprocity of practice efficiency, culture of wellness, and personal resilience. *NEJM Catal.* Published online January 23, 2018. Accessed December 12, 2021. https://catalyst.nejm.org/doi/full/10.1056/CAT.17.0429
14. Parsa-Parsi RW. The revised declaration of geneva: a modern-day physician's pledge. *JAMA.* 2017;318(20):1971. doi:10.1001/jama.2017.16230

15. Barrett E, Salas NM, Dewey C, Ripp J, Hingle T. A call to action: align well-being and antiracism strategies. *ACP Internist* Published online March 2021. Accessed December 12, 2021. https://acpinternist. org/archives/2021/03/a-call-to-action-align-well-being-and-antiracism-strategies.htm

16. Hill KA, Samuels EA, Gross CP, et al. Assessment of the prevalence of medical student mistreatment by sex, race/ethnicity, and sexual orientation. *JAMA Intern Med.* 2020;180(5):653. doi:10.1001/jamainternmed.2020.0030

17. Dyrbye L, Herrin J, West CP, et al. Association of racial bias with burnout among resident physicians. *JAMA Netw Open.* 2019;2(7):e197457. doi:10.1001/jamanetworkopen.2019.7457

18. Fassiotto M, Valantine H, Shanafelt T, Maldonado Y. Everyday heroism: maintaining organizational cultures of wellness and inclusive excellence amid simultaneous pandemics. *Acad Med.* 2020. doi:10.1097/ACM.0000000000003905

19. Sotto-Santiago S, Ansari-Winn D, Neal C, Ober M. Equity + wellness: a call for more inclusive physician wellness efforts [version 1]. *MedEdPublish.* 2021; 10:99. doi:10.15694/mep.2021.000099.1

20. Oreskovich MR, Shanafelt T, Dyrbye LN, et al. The prevalence of substance use disorders in American physicians: the prevalence of substance use disorders in American. *Am J Addict.* 2015;24(1):30–38. doi:10.1111/ajad.12173

21. Shanafelt TD, Noseworthy JH. Executive leadership and physician well-being: nine organizational strategies to promote engagement and reduce burnout. *Mayo Clin Proc.* Published online November 18, 2016. doi:10.1016/j.mayocp.2016.10.004

22. West CP, Tan AD, Shanafelt TD. Association of resident fatigue and distress with occupational blood and body fluid exposures and motor vehicle incidents. *Mayo Clin Proc.* 2012;87(12):1138–1144. doi:10.1016/j.mayocp.2012.07.021

23. Sinsky CA, Dyrbye LN, West CP, Satele D, Tutty M, Shanafelt TD. Professional satisfaction and the career plans of US physicians. *Mayo Clin Proc.* 2017;92(11):1625–1635. doi:10.1016/j.mayocp.2017.08.017

24. Laitman BM, Muller D. Medical student deaths by suicide: the importance of transparency. *Acad Med.* 2019;94(4):466–468. doi:10.1097/ACM.0000000000002507

25. Yaghmour NA, Brigham TP, Richter T, et al. Causes of death of residents in ACGME-accredited programs 2000 through 2014: implications for the learning environment. *Acad Med.* 2017;92(7):976–983. doi:10.1097/ACM.0000000000001736

26. Center C, Davis M, Detre T, et al. Confronting depression and suicide in physicians: a consensus statement. *JAMA.* 2003;289(23):3161–3166. doi:10.1001/jama.289.23.3161

27. Vogel L. Has suicide become an occupational hazard of practising medicine? *CMAJ.* 2018;190(24):E752–E753. doi:10.1503/cmaj.109-5614

28. Shanafelt TD, Schein E, Minor LB, Trockel M, Schein P, Kirch D. Healing the professional culture of medicine. *Mayo Clin Proc.* 2019;94(8):1556–1566. doi:10.1016/j.mayocp.2019.03.026

29. Kassebaum DG. LCME accreditation standards for management of the medical school curriculum: a clarification. Liaison Committee on Medical Education. *Acad Med.* 1994;69(1):37–38. doi:10.1097/00001888-199401000-00009

30. ACGME. Common program requirements. February 3, 2020. Accessed December 12, 2021. https://www.acgme.org/globalassets/PFAssets/ProgramRequirements/cprresidency2020.pdf

31. Ahmed N, Devitt KS, Keshet I, et al. A systematic review of the effects of resident duty hour restrictions in surgery: impact on resident wellness, training, and patient outcomes. *Ann Surg.* 2014;259(6):1041–1053. doi:10.1097/SLA.0000000000000595

32. Nasca TJ. ACGME's early adaptation to the COVID-19 pandemic: principles and lessons learned. *J Grad Med Educ.* 2020;12(3):375–378. doi:10.4300/JGME-D-20-00302.1

33. Thomas MR, Dyrbye LN, Huntington JL, et al. How do distress and well-being relate to medical student empathy? A multicenter study. *J Gen Intern Med.* 2007;22(2):177–183. doi:10.1007/s11606-006-0039-6

34. Dyrbye LN, Jr FSM, Eacker A, et al. Relationship between burnout and professional conduct and attitudes among US medical students. *JAMA* 2010;304(11):1173–1180. doi:10.1001/jama/2010/1318.

35. Shanafelt TD, Bradley KA, Wipf JE, Back AL. Burnout and self-reported patient care in an internal medicine residency program. *Ann Intern Med.* 2002;136(5):358. doi:10.7326/0003-4819-136-5-200203050-00008

36. Dewa CS, Loong D, Bonato S, Trojanowski L, Rea M. The relationship between resident burnout and safety-related and acceptability-related quality of healthcare: a systematic literature review. *BMC Med Educ.* 2017;17(1):195. doi:10.1186/s12909-017-1040-y

37. Baer TE, Feraco AM, Tuysuzoglu Sagalowsky S, Williams D, Litman HJ, Vinci RJ. Pediatric resident burnout and attitudes toward patients. *Pediatrics.* 2017;139(3):e20162163. doi:10.1542/peds.2016-2163

38. West CP, Tan AD, Habermann TM, Sloan JA, Shanafelt TD. Association of resident fatigue and distress with perceived medical errors. *Obstet Anesth Dig.* 2010;30(4):217. doi:10.1097/01.aoa.0000389590.11106.13

39. Fahrenkopf, Amy M., et al. Rates of medication errors among depressed and burnt out residents: prospective cohort study. *BMJ.* 2008;336(7642): 488–491.

40. West CP, Shanafelt TD, Kolars JC. Quality of life, burnout, educational debt, and medical knowledge among internal medicine residents. *JAMA.* 2011;306(9):952–960. doi:10.1001/jama.2011.1247

41. Hall LH, Johnson J, Watt I, Tsipa A, O'Connor DB. Healthcare staff wellbeing, burnout, and patient safety: a systematic review. *PLoS One.* 2016;11(7):e0159015. doi:10.1371/journal.pone.0159015

42. Tawfik DS, Profit J, Morgenthaler TI, et al. Physician burnout, well-being, and work unit safety grades in relationship to reported medical errors. *Mayo Clin Proc.* 2018;93(11):1571–1580. doi:10.1016/j.mayocp.2018.05.014

43. Mangory KY, Ali LY, Rø KI, Tyssen R. Effect of burnout among physicians on observed adverse patient outcomes: a literature review. *BMC Health Serv Res.* 2021;21(1):369. doi:10.1186/s12913-021-06371-x

44. Kwah J, Weintraub J, Fallar R, Ripp J. The Effect of burnout on medical errors and professionalism in first-year internal medicine residents. *J Grad Med Educ.* 2016;8(4):597–600. doi:10.4300/jgme-d-15-00457.1

45. Trockel M, Sinsky C, West CP, et al. Self-valuation challenges in the culture and practice of medicine and physician well-being. *Mayo Clin Proc.* 2021;96(8):2123–2132. doi:10.1016/j.mayocp.2020.12.032

46. Dyrbye LN, West CP, Hunderfund AL, et al. Relationship between burnout, professional behaviors, and cost-conscious attitudes among US physicians. *J Gen Intern Med.* 2020;35(5):1465–1476. doi:10.1007/s11606-019-05376-x

47. Chung S, Dillon EC, Meehan AE, Nordgren R, Frosch DL. The relationship between primary care physician burnout and patient-reported care experiences: a cross-sectional study. *J Gen Intern Med.* 2020;35(8):2357–2364. doi:10.1007/s11606-020-05770-w

48. Windover AK, Martinez K, Mercer MB, Neuendorf K, Boissy A, Rothberg MB. Correlates and outcomes of physician burnout within a large academic medical center. *JAMA Intern Med.* 2018;178(6):856–858. doi:10.1001/jamainternmed.2018.0019

49. Welle D, Trockel MT, Hamidi MS, et al. Association of occupational distress and sleep-related impairment in physicians with unsolicited patient complaints. *Mayo Clin Proc.* 2020 Apr;95(4):719–726. doi:10.1016/j.mayocp.2019.09.025

50. Haas JS, Cook EF, Puopolo AL, Burstin HR, Cleary PD, Brennan TA. Is the professional satisfaction of general internists associated with patient satisfaction? *J Gen Intern Med.* 2000;15(2):122–128.

51. Bachman KH, Freeborn DK. HMO physicians' use of referrals. *Soc Sci Med.* 1999;48(4):547–57.

52. Kushnir T, Greenberg D, Madjar N, Hadari I, Yermiahu Y, Bachner YG. Is burnout associated with referral rates among primary care physicians in community clinics? *Fam Pract.* 2014;31(1):44–50. doi:10.1093/fampra/cmt060

53. Bakker AB, Le Blanc PM, Schaufeli WB. Burnout contagion among intensive care nurses. *J Adv Nurs.* 2005;51(3):276–287. doi:10.1111/j.1365-2648.2005.03494.x

54. Helfrich CD, Simonetti JA, Clinton WL, et al. The association of team-specific workload and staffing with odds of burnout among va primary care team members. *J Gen Intern Med.* 2017;32(7):760–766. doi:10.1007/s11606-017-4011-4

55. Baron AN, Hemler JR, Sweeney SM, et al. Effects of practice turnover on primary care quality improvement implementation. *Am J Med Qual.* 2020;35(1):16–22. doi:10.1177/1062860619844001

56. Rawson JV, Thompson N, Sostre G, Deitte L. The cost of disruptive and unprofessional behaviors in health care. *Acad Radiol.* 2013;20(9):1074–1076. doi:10.1016/j.acra.2013.05.009

57. Shanafelt TD, Raymond M, Kosty M, et al. Satisfaction with work-life balance and the career and retirement plans of US oncologists. *J Clin Oncol.* 2014;32(11):1127–1135. doi:10.1200/JCO.2013.53.4560

58. Shanafelt TD, Balch CM, Bechamps GJ, et al. Burnout and career satisfaction among American surgeons. *Ann Surg.* 2009;250(3):463–471. doi:10.1097/SLA.0b013e3181ac4dfd

59. Dewa CS, Loong D, Bonato S, Thanh NX, Jacobs P. How does burnout affect physician productivity? A systematic literature review. *BMC Health Serv Res.* 2014;14:325. doi:10.1186/1472-6963-14-325

60. Turner TB, Dilley SE, Smith HJ, et al. The impact of physician burnout on clinical and academic productivity of gynecologic oncologists: a decision analysis. *Gynecol Oncol.* Published online June 24, 2017. doi:10.1016/j.ygyno.2017.06.026

61. Degen C, Li J, Angerer P. Physicians' intention to leave direct patient care: an integrative review. *Hum Resour Health.* 2015;13:74. doi:10.1186/s12960-015-0068-5

62. Hamidi MS, Bohman B, Sandborg C, et al. Estimating institutional physician turnover attributable to self-reported burnout and associated financial burden: a case study. *BMC Health Serv Res.* 2018;18(1):851. doi:10.1186/s12913-018-3663-z

63. American Medical Association. Steps forward. Published online September 12, 2018. Accessed December 2021. https://edhub.ama-assn.org/steps-forward/interactive/16830405

64. Han S, Shanafelt TD, Sinsky CA, et al. Estimating the attributable cost of physician burnout in the United States. *Ann Intern Med.* 2019;170(11):784. doi:10.7326/M18-1422

65. Jones RF, Korn D. On the cost of educating a medical student: *Acad Med.* 1997;72(3):200–210. doi:10.1097/00001888-199703000-00015

66. Dyrbye LN, Leep Hunderfund AN, Moeschler S, et al. Residents' perceptions of faculty behaviors and resident burnout: a cross-sectional survey study across a large health care organization. *J Gen Intern Med.* 2021;36(7):1906–1913. doi:10.1007/s11606-020-06452-3

Preparing Your Pitch

Communications and Organizational Approaches

Paul Chelminski and Mukta Panda

Introduction

Preparing organizations for change is a complex task that requires multiple skills including sophisticated communication, systematic planning, and implementation expertise. In the caring health professions, such skills for achieving change are often based on relationships rather than transactions. This chapter outlines the communication skills and organizational approaches needed to prepare an institution for positive change in an environment where health care professionals are the leaders in fulfilling missions of patient care, education, and research. We describe a creative approach to fostering institutional change based on literature that defines how change occurs in the caring professions. We present tools such as the "elevator speech" (or pitch) and the Logic Model which, respectively, create institutional awareness and a systematic framework for implementing change. We also review developments in communications and psychological sciences from the past 50 years that catalyze the respectful, inclusive, and productive conversations that motivate teams and drive change by honing an affirmative communications mindset and skillset.

The "Elevator Speech": Creating Your "Melody" and Capturing Organizational Attention

When trying to convince institutional leaders to pay attention and listen to a new proposal, concern, or innovative idea, it is helpful to have a prepared "elevator speech" (or pitch), so-named because it is meant to convey your idea in the time it takes to complete

---

BOX 13.1 The Elevator Pitch

- Introduce yourself (first and last name).
- Highlight your idea and why it is important.
- End with a plan for ongoing conversation.
- Arrange follow-up.

---

an elevator ride (Box 13.1).[1-3] This short synopsis of your issue or proposal is often an effective way to gain the attention and spark the curiosity of institutional leaders who might then desire more information. It is the melody of your mission, the prelude to your symphony. The elevator speech gives just enough information without playing the entire musical piece. There are several basic strategies that one can use in preparing an elevator speech, which should indeed be prepared and even practiced before use.

1. *Keep it brief.* Usually, one hopes to be in an elevator for no more than a minute or so; an elevator pitch is usually 30–60 seconds in length.
2. *Introduce yourself, using your first and last names, and give a brief synopsis of your idea or goal.* Plan on articulating one issue, not the entire symphony. Remember, this is brief. Do not assume that your listener knows you or your idea, and make sure you know enough about your idea or project to describe it in 1–2 sentences. (Before the elevator reaches the next floor and the doors open!) It is important to also briefly describe how you will be contributing to the idea you are mentioning.
3. *Make a connection.* Highlight what you want and why it is important, not only to you but also to the listener and the institution. Make sure to align with the institutional mission and vision and describe why this idea is unique and important.
4. *End with a plan for follow-up.* It is important to definitively "continue the symphony" by arranging for the next meeting with your listener or alternative appropriate colleague.

When addressing the need for well-being activities for students and graduate medical education (GME) trainees, the elevator speech can be a remarkable conduit for highlighting an issue that needs further discussion. Its objective—the concise and engaging transfer of important information—is not likely to be completely foreign to the health professional leader. More than likely, such a leader is used to hearing such pitches on a routine basis.

Writing the elevator speech—especially on an issue or topic that your institution may find controversial, expensive, or unique—may be challenging.

- Consider what the end goal of the pitch may be.
- Briefly explain the situation. Explain how you want to solve, evaluate, and discuss the goal you initially outlined. There is no substitute for practice when planning an elevator speech.

- Practice with a colleague, in front of a mirror, or tape (and time) the pitch. It is also important to update the pitch when you have made changes or progress on the issue.

The elevator speech is the *prelude* to the more in-depth conversation that will later offer your listener details and process information about your idea. Preparing a confident, concise elevator speech will help you connect with your listener.

Case Example (Part 1)

Dr. Melton is the program director in internal medicine. She is leaving a Graduate Medical Education Committee (GMEC) meeting in which the quantity and quality of ambulatory training of residents across specialties were described as educational and accreditation vulnerabilities. She runs into the institutional director of ambulatory operations, a senior faculty member, who sighs and says, "Haven't we been trying to make progress on this issue for the past 20 years?"

Dr. Melton says, "I'm Dr. Jane Melton. I am the program director of the endocrinology fellowship. I want to share an idea with you. I need to address the cultural concerns raised in our divisional survey, especially as it relates to the conversation we had at today's meeting about the ambulatory experience of our trainees. I have an idea for a well-being initiative that is interprofessional and may help address this issue, particularly in our clinics. Faculty, clinicians, and fellows feel that inefficiencies are hurting education and creating patient safety issues. They are not just complaining. They have some really good ideas. May I schedule a time with your assistant to discuss this further with you? Thank you so much for your interest and I look forward to our future conversation."

Creating a Mindset and Skill Set in Persons and Teams: Building and "Harmonizing the Orchestra"

The elevator pitch is the glossy and concisely reasoned invitation to a deeper, more substantive conversation. It is an anchoring melody. This conversation is not an end in itself: the long-term goal is a self-sustaining and mutually beneficial professional arrangement founded on respectful relationships. It is the starting point for the symphony itself, the creative process that requires translating ideas and information into action and outcomes.

Moving from Transactional to Learning Conversations: Bloom's Taxonomy

It might seem self-evident that all conversations are learning conversations, but this is frequently not the case, even in educational institutions. Established hierarchies and their policies and procedures often ensure that some communications are unidirectional and transactional. They are neither conversations nor invitations to a conversation, simply a transfer of information that is expected to be acted upon. For example, a program director or medical student clerkship director may learn that a new well-being survey has been developed and that it will be administered to all students and residents on a certain date (another time imposition) or that meal allowances for students and residents have been decreased. Such directive communications make the program director or clerkship director just a conduit for information, although she will certainly have to be skillful in how she communicates this information to her learners. These types of communications do not solicit input and do not fundamentally build the educational culture for faculty, students, residents, or fellows. In effect, directive communications say, "We are performing the same tune—with these alterations—but our creative state has not been elevated."

At this point, it is helpful to introduce Bloom's Taxonomy,[4] which is a common conceptual framework depicting stages of educational development starting with a rudimentary understanding and moving toward the application of knowledge and the achievement of a creative, validated process. Moving forward, communication strategies can employ this taxonomy and take us to the application, analysis, and evaluation of our actions that lead to creation. Implicit in Bloom's Taxonomy is the notion that our communications are inherently learning conversations, not transactions. While Bloom's Taxonomy provides a mental model for a speech or pitch, it does not provide an operational roadmap for achieving goals. Later in the chapter we describe a commonly used tool, the Logic Model, (Figure 13.1)[5] that allows us to fuse our aspirations for improving medical student or graduate medical education (GME)

The Logic Model

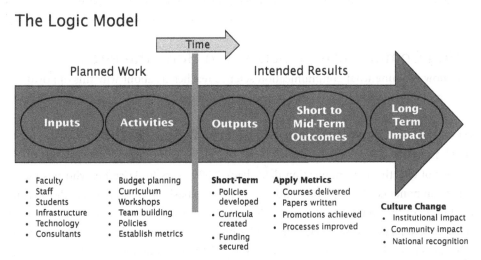

FIGURE 13.1 The Logic Model for program implementation and evaluation. Adapted from CDC Division for Heart Disease and Stroke Prevention. Evaluation Guide: Developing and Using a Logic Model. Department of Health and Human Services. Accessed February 6, 2022. https://www.cdc.gov/dhdsp/docs/logic_model.pdf

trainee well-being with a process that ensures accountability and progress over time. Metaphorically, Bloom's Taxonomy is the melody of work, the higher purpose. The Logic Model accounts for the complexity of our endeavor and allows us to harmonize the many different pieces.

Learning conversations have a much more fundamental and transformative goal. Such communications strive to change culture. They can be conceptualized as a journey that drives us vertically up Bloom's Taxonomy. Learning conversations aim to change the tune itself—even if it requires retooling and augmenting the orchestra. Such conversations require patience, reciprocity, persistence, curiosity, and humility. Leading learning conversations requires cultivating a skill set and a readiness to engage in the long game. medical student and GME educators work in frantic, time-compressed environments where the long game is eclipsed by imminently pressing clinical and educational priorities. In this setting, patience, curiosity, and humility can seem like luxuries that may undermine the mandates of efficiency, productivity, and constant decision-making. These are tools we all have, but they need to be practiced, refined, developed.

Before we consider the tools and skills that will take us beyond pass-through, informational conversations, let's return to our example of the elevator conversation.

The Case Part 2: A Relationship Begins

Dr. Melton's elevator pitch has resulted in a meeting with Dr. Powell, the institution's director of ambulatory operations, along with her chief administrative lead. Two days after the GMEC meeting, Dr. Powell sent her an email saying, "Let's meet regarding the good ideas you mentioned about improving resident ambulatory training. I am getting a lot of complaints and was thinking about our conversation. Let's meet for half an hour." Dr. Melton is surprised to have such an unexpected opportunity.

Using Communication Science to Hone the Pitch

Let's now examine what communication science teaches us about why this opportunity arose and how to make the most of it. It was not by chance.

History of Communication Theory: Ethos, Pathos, and Logos

Theory of effective communication dates back 2,500 years to Aristotle, who postulated three components: ethos, pathos, and logos.[6] *Ethos* is basically the stature, authority, and credibility of the communicator; it is who you are as a well-trained physician. *Pathos* is the ability to relate and show empathy, something that has been rebranded as "emotional intelligence" in the past 30 years. *Logos* is the ability to reason and logically discuss and argue; it is your rigorous problem-solving capacity. A developing health professional will have to do all of these things in their careers. However, as leaders and catalysts of change, we may not always accomplish our intended goals if one of these three components has not been adequately cultivated to address environmental change. We are so used to (and often very good at) "fixing" the patient or educating a student in the moment, that we do not know how to approach the more complex challenge of transforming our workplaces or environments.

The communication skill that might lag for physicians generally is not *ethos* or *logos*. Physicians often retain an ability to reason, even when presented with new information and areas of expertise to master. In our observation, generally, it is *pathos* that has not been formally trained for the challenges of organizational change.[7] Medical training prepares people superbly for empathizing and problem-solving in time-pressured environments, for communicating effectively in the short term. This same training, though, does not prepare one's communication *pathos* for the long game of creating more vibrant and harmonized professional environments that promote culture change and well-being in groups. In these scenarios, *pathos* is more than just empathizing and addressing problems in the moment with a single person. It is a respectful demeanor and relationship to be cultivated over time in a larger group rather than in the more circumscribed clinical encounter. It is team-building, which has traditionally not figured prominently in medical education.[8]

Going back to our case, developments in the sciences of communication and human growth over the past 50 years offer insight into why this conversation was solicited by the institutional leader and what it will take for it to become a learning conversation. We describe these approaches below, but let's first dissect the case further.

First, the program director opened the conversation in a spirit of generosity and reciprocity. That is, she offered to *share* information. There was no premature ask in her approach (e.g., "My fellows have too much on their plates balancing clinic with consults. You can see it in their well-being surveys. The institution has to hire more scribes." Problem solved!). Such asks generally do not come across as invitations to richer conversation, regardless of whether they are based on data, and can lead to defensiveness. Imagine for a moment how many similar asks this director of ambulatory operations is inundated with each week by people she hardly knows and without greater context. Thus, cultivating *pathos* (an empathic approach) for the long game involves not only communicating empathetically, but also refraining from ill-timed or threatening complaints. Second, the program director communicated in a positive (optimistic) and constructive(problem-solving) tone. That is, she did not pile on with more complaints about what was not working. She was using the language of possibility and exploration. What can this example tell us going forward?

Modern Frameworks for Spurring Change Through Communications

In the late 1970s and early 1980s, two powerful new communication modalities were developed that can be particularly helpful in professional and clinical learning environments.

One was the Harvard Negotiation Project (HNP). The other was the skill of motivational interviewing (MI).[9,10] These two developments had very different intended audiences. For HNP, the audience was the professional work environment. For MI, the audience was persons struggling with addiction. Despite the different audiences, the tactics and strategies are remarkably similar. Both approaches recognize that even in hierarchical work and clinical environments, fundamental change is not premised on individual influence or authority (*ethos*) alone. Both modalities put a premium on high-quality listening without rushing to judgment based on incomplete information. For the HNP, this approach involves avoiding attribution error or bias; that is, precipitously attributing bad intent, bad faith, or incompetence without a robust accounting of facts and different perspectives. The MI approach includes exploring the complex circumstances, inputs, and ambiguities of human addiction. Both approaches are premised on increasing understanding (*pathos*)—rather than the exertion of authority—as a precondition for fostering change. Both counsel against explicit, reflexive, and premature admonitions to change, something called the *righting reflex* in MI.

In addition, HNP and MI advise against rushing to solve problems reflexively. These conversations require time and perseverance. In fact, more listening and deeper discussions may reveal that there is no problem to solve immediately (once attributions and intent are sorted out) or that the nature of the problem is substantially different from what was first assumed. Premature judgments and solutions are analogous to the great diagnostic nemesis of "premature closure"; that is, settling for and anchoring on a clinical diagnosis to explain signs and symptoms without a full accounting of clinical data and perspectives. Premature closure in clinical and organizational contexts can unleash negative downstream consequences, including unnecessary, costly, and potentially harmful approaches with missed opportunities to identify and treat the right problem. Such blind alleys can be unconsciously abetted by the professional pride that health care professionals embrace as being problem-solvers (consistent with a reliance on *ethos* and *logos*). A similar cascade of harms can ensue when we pursue organizational change without a robust accounting of interests and perspectives. This tendency to "rush to judgment," and its attendant counterproductive consequences, has received widespread treatment in the behavioral economics literature.[11]

Semantic Framing to Craft a Message

As illustrated above, nonjudgmental communication and listening are critical for building a solid foundation for collaboration and pathos. So what is the next step for Dr. Melton when she has her meeting with Dr. Powell? Dr. Melton might first respond to the invitation with a brief email framing the purpose of the meeting. The email in Box 13.2 provides a simple, three-paragraph format that one of the authors has found useful when inviting colleagues on collaborative endeavors.

When using this format, it is important to borrow some of the typical language used by the stakeholder with whom one is communicating. We can call this process *semantic*

BOX 13.2 Sample Email Invitation to Collaborate

Salutation: Dear/Hi/Hello Dr. Powell,

Paragraph 1 (Purpose: Acknowledge the recipients' status and importance to the institution, their Ethos):
Thank you for the opportunity to meet and for your commitment to improving the educational experience and well-being of our residents and fellows. I know that education can be one of several competing priorities.

Paragraph 2 (Purpose: Frame the issue, their Logos):
A survey of our division confirms that the well-being of our fellows is compromised by competing demands of the hospital and the clinic. Fortunately, the results also show how to engage APPs in a way that will benefit clinical care in both environments and improve the well-being and professional identity of the fellows.

Paragraph 3 (Purpose: An invitation to collaborate, joint Pathos):
I hope that our meeting can lead to a conversation that will involve an interdisciplinary team with representatives from the hospital and other programs whose fellows may be experiencing similar stresses. I plan on bringing the results of our division survey. Please let me know if you would like me to prepare anything else.

framing, using the common language or professional dialect of the stakeholder. The language to use when speaking with someone from administration, the so-called *C-suite*, will depend on the role that person has in leadership. If the person is invested with authority over quality and safety, the elevator pitch and subsequent communication should be couched in the language of quality. If that person has financial oversight responsibilities, then the language of fiscal accountability may be appropriate as a framing device. This language will likely be different from a conversation with a clinical, educational, or research colleague who shares a common professional training. The purpose of semantic framing is to indicate respect for that other professional's role. Using their dialect also promotes the efficiency of communication in time-limited situations. Less time is lost in translating when we "pre-translate" and adapt idioms.

The Case Part 3: Meeting Day

The meeting day has arrived. Dr. Melton has her survey results in hand. After a greeting, Dr. Powell asks what the division of endocrinology has learned from its survey regarding fellow workload and well-being. Dr. Melton shares a summary of the data on one page and then explains that the fellows value their clinic experience but habitually are cutting their clinics short to attend to consult duties. They then find themselves without enough time to follow-up on issues relating to their clinic patients after finishing their hospital or on-call duties. She mentions also that the physician assistants and nurse practitioners in the practice feel as if they are not working to their highest clinical potential and find themselves doing clerical tasks for the fellows when they would prefer to be working more collaboratively with them. Dr. Melton then asks Dr. Powell about her thoughts and perspective. Dr. Powell shares that fellows across specialties are not meeting productivity targets in ambulatory settings. Dr. Melton then mentions that the surveys also show that well-being is being affected as a result of these perceived inefficiencies, overlapping responsibilities, and personal values conflict. She adds that there is an opportunity to creatively address both the concerns of fellows and advanced practice providers (APPs) and the unmet productivity with an initiative that could foster higher-level interprofessional practice.

Dr. Melton then asks Dr. Powell what she has seen that works and does not work over the years. Dr. Powell remarks that discontinuities in communication that occur as trainees move back and forth between clinical settings have been a big problem and that new forms of real-time communication occasioned by the COVID-19 pandemic might contribute to solutions. A realm of possibilities opens. The conversation flows. They agree to form a working group and consider a pilot in the endocrine clinic once they have invited other stakeholders.

This successful, albeit stylized conversation followed the script for a learning conversation. There was mutual exchange of information, and the collaborative spirit was one of mutual guiding, not direction based on hierarchy. Both sides showed humility in that they were curious to learn from each other. Neither indulged in what MI refers to as the *expert trap* or *righting reflex*, those efforts to solve problems based on expertise alone or just the customary reflex to solve a problem because it's there. Importantly, Dr. Melton continued to maintain a positive note throughout the conversations. This positivity is not a naïve or frivolous "toxic positivity." Rather, this choice displayed an optimism grounded in the possibilities of the data that she had at her disposal, reinforced by her role as an educator and her commitments to her trainees. Instead of adopting a disease model of her environment (i.e., what's wrong), she was focusing on the potential of the people and institution where she works.

Pragmatic positivity is diverse, not monolithic. It encompasses a range of redeeming emotions and states such as gratitude, pride, joy, and love. The HNP puts a particular emphasis on the positive state of curiosity and advises the development of a curiosity stance. The positive psychology movement and other strands of research support that such grounded positivity is a powerful catalyst for change and success.[12]

Maintaining a Growth Mindset in Communications

Last, it is important to note that both parties invested time in the conversation. In her book, *Mindset: The New Psychology of Success*, Dr. Carol Dweck emphasizes that growth cannot occur in the absence of the grant of time necessary for mutual understanding. "Speed and perfection are the enemy of difficulty learning," she writes. In the concept of the growth mindset there is also an admonition to avoid perfectionism as we strive to improve, *not perfect*, our environments.[13] This concept can also be embodied in the common adage that "the perfect should not be the enemy of the good." The HNP also cautions against striving for entirely satisfactory resolutions of issues because this inevitably leads to cycles of misattribution of intent, conflict, and blame that can prevent progress.

The Case Part 4: A Plan and First Steps

Another meeting is scheduled between Dr. Melton and Dr. Powell which includes the faculty lead of the consult service, two senior endocrinology fellows, the endocrine clinic nurse manager, and the lead APP, a nurse practitioner. In preparation, the endocrine clinic team has drafted a proposal with two principal goals: to mitigate the competing clinical demands on the fellows and to enhance the autonomy of the nursing staff and the APPs. The broad outlines of the proposal call for shortening the clinic schedules for fellows on days when they are doing hospital consults. Each fellow will be assigned a nurse and an APP teammate who will follow-up on patient-related tasks. The APP will also see some of the fellow's established patients for the remainder of the day. The next morning, the fellow, the APP, and the nurse will have a video huddle to address outstanding clinical issues. APPs will be relieved of some time-consuming clerical duties, such as medication and device prior authorizations, and nursing will be charged with facilitating communication among all parties. In addition, fellows will be assigned to a single attending preceptor to serve as a first-resort consultant and advisor on care and educational issues that arise. Dr. Melton describes to Dr. Powell how, in balance, the endocrine clinic will be able to see more patients and have a better system of continuity. Dr. Powell is pleased and asks Dr. Melton to present her with a model of the proposal.

We are almost ready for the final step in initiating collaborative change: the creation of a Logic Model. Before we tackle this, though, it is useful to review the progress we have made so far using the common educational framework of Bloom's Taxonomy introduced earlier. In our sample case, we moved from the understanding phase of the endeavor to early team formation. We launched a learning conversation that has created mutual understanding. This mutual understanding is based on data and shared aims to improve education and clinical care. We have now achieved the initial steps of applying our learning.

We have formed a diverse team and agreed to goals with the end in mind. How do we now keep the momentum going? The Logic Model is an excellent tool for translating intended work and inputs into outputs and outcomes. It does not, though, provide the tool to motivate the team so that it can function at its highest potential.

Achieving Mastery

The literature on human growth and excellence provides guidance for what it takes for individuals to achieve high performance. We have already discussed the emotional and affective catalysts to learning and progress that the individual can cultivate and learn: active listening, positivity, curiosity. These create a common understanding and shared purpose. We now address elements of the task that propel team members to higher levels of application in Bloom's Taxonomy. We have already identified one: "common purpose." In work by Malcolm Gladwell and Daniel Pink, autonomy is another crucial predictor of high performance.[14,15] It is this basic ability to work freely toward a goal that promotes mastery and work satisfaction. The work of these authors also highlights the importance that such work be complex and coupled closely in time with some kind of reward or benefit—the "small wins."

What are the rewards that propel individuals and teams toward progress and satisfaction? In the late 1960s, researchers at the *Harvard Business Review* identified two important catalysts. These were work progress and recognition for achievement. This may seem obvious to the point of irrelevance. More recent research has built on what this means. Authors Amabile and Kramer took a closer look at potential motivators in the workplace. In addition to work progress and recognition for good work, they looked at incentives, clear goals, and interpersonal support. Of these five factors, work progress—every "small win"—emerged as the most powerful driver of fulfillment.[16] There findings align with the work of Mihaly Csikszentmihalyi who studied peak performance in many occupations, from farming to sports to industrial workers. Peak performance was consistently associated with a feeling of "flow" in which workers experienced unimpeded progress in their work.[17] Theoretically, promotion of everyday mastery makes flow. Psychologically, it moves people from the basic levels up Maslow's Hierarchy of Needs to belonging and esteem.[18] Operationally, mastery situates the worker in the application zone of Bloom's Taxonomy.

The Case Part 5: The Help of a Mentor

After the last meeting with Dr. Powell, Dr. Melton contacted one of her mentors. She was a little intimidated about the scope of the project and the expertise it would require. Dr. Melton had heard of the Logic Model but had never created one. Her mentor oriented her to the large amount of readily available resources on the subject. She also pointed out to her how the Logic Model is an ideal tool to create the operational and psychological conditions for success just discussed.

The Logic Model: Moving from the Elevator Pitch to the Orchestra Pit

Dr. Melton has many ideas, and the Logic Model (Figure 13.1) can help her to get started inputting the ideas in a systematic way that allows her to articulate them to all stakeholders. The Logic Model provides a framework for the process and defines the goals and vision. It is a very clear and linear way of being able to define the input and resources present, the activities to be planned, and the outputs and the outcomes intended. This model is analogous to a road map or a compass to graphically display the "What" and the "How." Logic models also help in thinking with intentionality about the context of the program. It starts with the end in sight. Eventually, the Logic Model allows for the measurement of the impact of our outcomes on the environment. As described in Box 13.3, it helps reframe the guiding questions "What is being done?" to "What needs to be done?" A Logic Model also allows for reflection and consideration around the beliefs of the program, the external factors associated with the program, and those whom the program is intended to influence—the "what" that is to be accomplished. The Logic Model may be influenced by available stakeholder resources, community partnerships, and accreditation mandates which can help with program implementation.[19]

Graphically, the model is the sheet music, where the members of the team are the members of the orchestra. Whereas the *elevator speech* is about creating a melody and "striking the right notes," the Logic Model is the orchestration and harmonization that transcends the "one-on-one" starting point for the initiative and includes multiple organizational stakeholders. The visual representation provides focus, with clear and stepwise goals, about what change is expected to be seen, by whom, and over what period of time (Figure 13.1). All the interventions and actions are tied to outcomes that are measurable over time. The model follows the "If-Then hypothesis" (i.e., if we implement this program, then this outcome can occur, and can be measured) which enables program evaluation, can provide an inventory to stay on target, and allows for adjustments as needed to avoid untoward effects. Thus, the Logic Model facilitates change and growth by embedding a framework for evaluation (and re-evaluation) within the creative process itself.

BOX 13.3 Considerations in Building a Logic Model

- What is the current situation that we intend to impact?
- What will it look like when we achieve the desired situation or outcome?
- What behaviors need to change for that outcome to be achieved?
- What knowledge or skills do people need before the behavior will change?
- What activities need to be performed to cause the necessary learning?
- What resources will be required to achieve the desired outcome?

The Logic Model capitalizes on the communication techniques reviewed above. It is quite literally the *logos*. Just as communication from a learning stance prepares us for the "long game of change," the Logic Model graphically depicts this long game in a fashion that illustrates the important human relationships that drive the processes—the configuration of the orchestra. There is also an affinity with the "small wins" approach to progress, discussed previously, because the Logic Model allows for ready targeting and identification of areas ripe for progress—the small, concrete steps that have large and beneficial psychological impact. It portrays a systematic supply line to the future. Most importantly, this configuration of processes and relationships within a timeline stimulates creativity, innovation, and accountability. It can help Dr. Melton advocate and justify, step-by-step, how the program can work across other programs in the institution. Conceptually, the process moves to higher levels on Bloom's Taxonomy, to the level of creation. It is a way of putting communication *logos* into action.

How does such a model enhance the likelihood of success for an idea such as a wellness program and demonstrate its impact? The Logic Model organizes the ideas of the various stakeholders into outcomes and impact by identifying what inputs and outputs will complete the symphony. The Logic Model identifies the aspirations and needs of the stakeholders at the outset of planning and then outlines what efforts would be needed (inputs) to achieve a direct product (output) and what will be the impact of such an outcome now and in the future. Graphically, it does so systematically and "logically." It depicts a landscape of "small wins" leading to greater outcomes and impacts.

The Case Conclusion: Dr. Melton Populates the Logic Model

Dr. Melton has made substantial progress already in creating her Logic Model without realizing it. Her mentor points out to her that in a short amount of time she has built two diverse teams: one is her leadership team; the other is the clinical and educational team. These are considered inputs in a Logic Model. In addition, there are already specified clinical outputs (new work flows) for the clinical and educational team. Other outputs might include existing measures of clinical productivity (e.g., outpatient visits and inpatient consults) that can be trended. She also decides that utilization of telehealth will be a new output to be tracked. Dr. Melton reminds herself that the long-term goals (or impact) of the project are to improve the wellness of educators and trainees and also patient care. On the road to impact, she will need to specify outcomes on the Logic Model. Understanding GME trainee satisfaction will be important. Dr. Melton will measure fellow satisfaction more broadly with regard to clinical and educational endpoints. In addition, Dr. Melton will develop metrics related to the important interprofessional practice and education elements of the initiative to judge how they are affecting outcomes.

She realizes that within a year she will have usable data on most of her outputs but that measuring and trending outcomes will require several years. She also realizes that this endeavor will require a substantial data collection and analytic burden. At their next meeting, she presents her Logic Model to Dr. Powell, and she adds another input with an "ask" to the leadership: institutional data analytic support for the project at 0.3 FTE. Dr. Powell is impressed with the Logic Model and offers 0.2 FTE data analysis and quality improvement support from the institution.

Conclusion

Those seeking to propose and operationalize changes to improve well-being in medicine can benefit from communication and operations strategies used in the business world and public health. Translating the elevator speech into concrete action leading to change requires intentional cultivation of core communication and organizational skills. The elevator pitch is analogous to a concise patient presentation given to a colleague. It ignites a sense of common *higher* purpose and is the prelude to communication strategies that build teams and a *common* practical purpose. Hallmarks of this communication include respect, gratitude, and curiosity. Small wins are essential to maintain the momentum of the endeavor. The Logic Model can ensure that all elements are systematically accounted for and rationally depicted as change progresses from inputs and outputs to outcomes and impact.

Summary Points

- The elevator speech is a concise invitation to start a conversation about change.
- Change conversations in academic medicine are premised on a cultivated ability to listen, affirm, and show respect while a common agenda is created.
- The Logic Model offers a tool to creatively operationalize change and evaluate it.
- Using these techniques successfully for any project enhances the possibility of impact and sustainability.

Putting It into Practice

Consider a well-being intervention you would like to propose to your leadership.

- *Are you trying to start the conversation?* Craft an "elevator pitch" to concisely introduce and explain your idea. Practice this pitch with a trusted colleague.
- *Do you already have initial interest, and seek to deepen the conversation?* Consider the type of semantic framing that may resonate with a leader from whom you are

hoping to gain support. How might you tailor your approach to shift to a learning conversation?

- *Do you already have a commitment of initial support?* Consider using the Logic Model framework to flesh out how you might operationalize and evaluate your idea.

References

1. Dzara K, Kesselheim J. Going up? Tips for the medical educator's "elevator pitch." *Acad Med.* 2018;93:1884.
2. Goedereis EA, Gray-Graves A. Make your pitch: a flexible assignment for engaging students in aging. *Int J Aging Hum Dev.* 2020;91(4):435–442.
3. Taylor E. 7 steps to deliver your best elevator pitch. 2014. Accessed March 4, 2021. http://money.usn ews.com/money/careers/articles/2014/01/17/7-steps-to-deliver-your-best-elevator-pitch.
4. Bloom BS, ed. *Taxonomy of Educational Objectives Book 1. Cognitive Domain.* McKay; 1956.
5. Renger R. A three-step approach to teaching logic models. *Am J Eval.* 2002;23(4):493–503.
6. Edinger S. The three elements of great communication according to Aristotle. *Harv Bus Rev.* 2013. Accessed February 6, 2022. https://hbr.org/2013/01/three-elements-of-great-communication-according.
7. Perry J, Mobley F, Brubaker M. Most doctors have little or no management training, and that's a problem. *Harv Bus Rev.* 2017. Accessed February 6, 2022. https://hbr.org/2017/12/most-doctors-have-little-or-no-management-training-and-thats-a-problem.
8. Lee TH. Turning doctors into leaders. *Harv Bus Rev.* 2010. Accessed February 6, 2022. https://hbr.org/2010/04/turning-doctors-into-leaders.
9. Stone D, Patton B, Heen S. *Difficult Conversations: How to Discuss What Matters Most.* Penguin Books; 2000.
10. Miller WR, Rollnick S. *Motivational Interviewing: Preparing People for Change.* Guilford Press, 2002.
11. Kahneman D. *Thinking Fast and Slow.* Farrar, Straus, and Giroux; 2011.
12. Fredrickson B. *Positivity: Groundbreaking Research Reveals How to Embrace the Hidden Strength of Positive Emotions, Overcome Negativity, and Thrive.* Crown Publishers/Random House; 2009.
13. Dweck CS. *Mindset: The New Psychology of Growth.* Random House; 2006.
14. Gladwell M. *Outliers: The Story of Success.* Little, Brown, and Co.; 2008.
15. Pink D. *Drive.* Canongate Books; 2011.
16. Amabile T, Kramer S. The power of small wins. *Harv Bus Rev.* 2011. Accessed February 6, 2022. https://hbr.org/2011/05/the-power-of-small-wins.
17. Csikszentmihalyi M. *Flow and the Foundations of Positive Psychology: The Collected Works of Mihaly Csikszentmihalyi.* Springer; 2014.
18. Maslow AH. *Motivation and Personality.* Harper and Row; 1962.
19. CDC Division for Heart Disease and Stroke Prevention. Evaluation guide: developing and using a logic model. Department of Health and Human Services. Updated May 22, 2017. Accessed February 6, 2022. https://cdc.gov/dhdsp/docs/logic_model.pdf

Initial Steps
in Program Development

Saadia Akhtar, Sakshi Dua, Paul Rosenfield, and
Jonathan A. Ripp

Introduction

In establishing a comprehensive well-being program, engaging in a methodological and stepwise approach will facilitate the development of a successful effort. Creating an organized development strategy is necessary to ensure the direction, coordination, organization, and leadership required to operationalize complex and multiple well-being program elements. Ultimately, keeping in mind such organizational considerations can be instrumental in securing the level of program support needed for a broad scope of offerings that can result in organizational change.[1] Once stakeholders of an institution are ready to take action in addressing medical student or graduate medical education (GME) trainee well-being, a number of important steps and structural elements will aid the formation of an advanced program that spans silos of the institution (Box 14.1). This chapter provides guidance on building support from stakeholders, developing and clarifying a program mission and model, setting up a broad organizational structure, and instituting policies that advance the overall goals of the program. This chapter provides concrete examples from the authors' experience in designing and implementing a comprehensive well-being program at their institution.

Establishing Support
Initial Planning

The motivating forces for creating a comprehensive undergraduate medical education (UME) or GME well-being program may vary across an institution, as described in

Chapter 12. The initial support for change often comes from stakeholders most closely connected to those forces. Each motivational factor typically aligns with potential stakeholders who may be invested in well-being initiatives. Frontline clinicians, for example, may demand change. Faculty and GME trainees may step up to make the case that burnout is a major problem and engage hospital and GME administration to help drive a supportive effort. Supervisors, undergraduate medical education (UME) educational leaders, GME training program directors, and other mid-level leaders who are concerned about depression and burnout in their constituents may be strong advocates for providing support. Such leaders may not only wish to improve the learning experience of their students and trainees, but also feel the need to comply with regulations that mandate attention to well-being. Hospital leaders and administrators may be convinced that the business case to invest in the work environment speaks for itself.[2,3] Other stakeholders may emerge in the process, including patients, nurses, ancillary staff, and more. And it goes without saying that all stakeholders are affected by tragic events which at times have been the catalyst for the initiation of well-being programs. A student or GME trainee suicide rocks a community, challenges an institution to examine its culture, and galvanizes action. The circle of colleagues closest to the loss are often most deeply impacted and may be motivated to agitate for change, while more distantly connected colleagues often wonder if there is a broader problem that needs addressing. Furthermore, an institution may suffer reputational damage in the wake of tragedy, when inevitably there is a desire to seek the underlying cause. At such moments, leaders may be more inclined to examine the learning environment and appropriately commit resources where needed.[4] As described in Chapter 12, there are numerous other major motivations for institutions to develop well-being programs. Establishing the support of stakeholders to help translate these motivating factors into action is a critical initial step.

Engaging Stakeholders

The leaders of any nascent well-being initiative need to engage stakeholders from both the "bottom up" (e.g., frontline clinicians and trainees) and "top down" (e.g., hospital, medical school and GME leaders) in an effort to enlist broad interest, support, and participation in a well-being planning committee. Such committees can seek representation from trainees, faculty, and leadership, with the inclusion of individuals from underrepresented backgrounds and across genders to ensure diversity of perspectives. Committee leads may consider seeking out members from among the various stakeholders who have been previously invested in well-being efforts and specifically invite them to join. A town hall meeting (or set of meetings) introducing a plan to address well-being can be a helpful step to initiate and invite broad participation.

> **Case Example**
>
> The program director in pediatrics has established innovative projects and has become a local leader in well-being efforts over the past 2 years since one of her residents attempted suicide, and she has been sought out by other program directors to help address areas of concern in their own programs. Together they have enlisted GME leadership to advocate for expanding efforts to attend to GME trainee mental health and the workplace environment and enable the administration of a broad well-being survey which demonstrates high levels of burnout and depression. The results of the survey help make the case to hospital leadership for the need to take steps in creating a comprehensive well-being program across their institution.

Data Gathering and Needs Assessment

An essential early task to establish support and determine direction is conducting a needs assessment. Surveys of medical students and GME trainees can provide important data about the local prevalence of burnout, depression, suicidal ideation, and, perhaps more importantly, the drivers and potential areas for intervention. These survey data can in turn inform and prioritize the roll-out and composition of initial well-being program components. Additionally, focus groups and feedback solicited from stakeholders themselves can further inform a planning committee in its identification of areas for attention and intervention. Sometimes the data may already exist in the form of Accreditation Council for Graduate Medical Education (ACGME) program or well-being survey results, or Clinical Learning Environment Review (CLER) visit reports. The offices of the deans for undergraduate and graduate medical education may additionally have important data regarding areas of concern, such as mistreatment complaints, work-hour violations, service-over-education misalignment, and more. Gathering these forms of data can provide a strong case for establishing or expanding well-being efforts when speaking with school or hospital leadership and the broader community.

Prioritizing Efforts

Those involved in planning will want to consider where to focus and prioritize efforts. There will almost certainly be more areas of focus than can be prioritized at once. To aid with prioritization, it is not only important to assess needs, but also to take an inventory of existing resources. By determining what efforts are already in place and how effective they are, those in charge of coordinating well-being efforts can ascertain the extent to which existing resources match existing needs. For example, leaders may explore whether access to mental health care for medical students and GME trainees matches the need for treatment or screening, or to what extent existing support staff offload noneducational clerical burden from students or GME trainees. The well-being committee or planning leads should also attempt to ascertain whether an institution is willing to support incremental or more comprehensive/transformational change. If the need for a particular well-being priority is great and the impact may be significant, but the cost is prohibitive, then it may be infeasible to prioritize it in the immediate term. The planning team will also need to consider the extent to which it balances advocating for the development of evidence-based individual self-care programs, such as mindfulness training, compared with prioritizing more systemic interventions for medical students and GME trainees. As described in Chapter 8, systemic interventions, such as providing personnel resources to reduce work intensity and compression, limiting clerical task burden, and enforcing duty-hour limitations are likely to have a greater impact than individual-level interventions, but also are likely to require greater resource investment.

Closely tied to well-being are the impacts of bias, discrimination, mistreatment, and harassment based on sex, race, or other aspects of identity, as described in Chapter 8. The planning committee may seek input from those involved in the school's or hospital's diversity, equity, and inclusion efforts to understand whether these issues are being adequately identified, addressed, and rooted out. Another consideration is whether or not adequate and effective well-being policies and procedures exist or are in need of revision. Effective policies and procedures can ensure an impactful commitment to well-being. Ultimately, even if the policies exist, the planning committee must consider the possibility that the institutional or leadership practices are not consistent with its espoused values. All of these considerations must be kept in mind as the well-being leaders plan out their program development.

Deciding on a Home for Oversight

Decisions must be made about the home for oversight of a well-being program, with options ranging from being embedded within a local training program or specialty department, to being situated in the medical school or GME office, or located at the hospital or system administrative level. Although those tasked with well-being work may not hold authority for determining the organizational and reporting chart, the reporting structure will ultimately impact who runs the well-being initiatives as well as the size, breadth, and scope of a comprehensive program. Locally-based programs have been successful in promoting well-being, as has been seen in the case of training program–specific initiatives, by improving the on-call experience, increasing social activities, supporting preventative care, and promoting wellness education.[5] Clinical departments may decide to take action and implement a well-being program targeted to their specialty. These local initiatives can be quite helpful in directing efforts to particular needs, but will be less effective in changing larger system-level issues and may be potentially limited in funding, thus restricting scope and sustainability. Programs located within the medical school dean's office or GME office may be able to garner additional leverage to address medical student and GME trainee well-being needs more broadly and apply resources directed to their concerns. These offices tend to be already highly motivated to address well-being and can provide strong leadership. Finally, hospital system leadership can promote a powerful message of well-being through acknowledgment of the challenges, provision of resources to improve the work environment, and reinforcement of policies that promote safety, equity, and quality.[2]

Generating a Proposal to Establish a Well-being Program

A broad effort across a medical system has the potential advantages of greater visibility, universality, and sustainability. When data have been collected and initial planning has been completed, the well-being leads or committee can begin to think about generating a proposal to present to the appropriate leadership that details the needs assessment and specific recommendations, as well as the potential positive impact of implementing a comprehensive program. Establishing tangible support and a source of funding are essential to the success of any comprehensive well-being program. Lofty goals without financial resources and leadership commitment may end in disappointment, disillusionment, and frustration. Potential sources of financial support include departments, medical schools and GME offices, hospital systems, philanthropy, and even malpractice carriers. As described earlier, many arguments make a powerful case for attending to well-being, including decreased sick days, regulatory compliance, improved quality and efficiency of patient care, enhanced student and GME trainee engagement, institutional reputation, and more. The committee's ability to make its case, address doubts or reservations, and explain the well-being return on investment will likely affect the level of funding available to implement its recommendations. When support and funding are established, the next steps are to formulate a mission, decide on a budget, hire staff as part of putting together a team, establish priorities and policies, and oversee implementation.

Developing a Mission and Model

Once there is considerable stakeholder support for establishing a comprehensive well-being program at the GME or UME level, it is important to consider developing a mission, vision, and model of well-being. At this phase in program development, most institutional bodies with administrative oversight for UME and GME will likely have established a core group tasked with developing and running a systematic approach to addressing well-being. This group may overlap with the planning committee or be distinct, and may in fact ultimately evolve into the membership of the governance structure overseeing GME or UME well-being, as discussed in the next section. To be effective, such a group should be aligned around a common mission and therefore can benefit from developing a mission statement.

Mission, Vision, and Purpose

When beginning to craft a mission statement, it is important to distinguish mission from vision and purpose.[6,7] These terms are sometimes used interchangeably, but their distinction is important as they do represent different constructs.

At a minimum, a *mission statement* is necessary for a well-being initiative. A mission statement is really what an organization (or an organized well-being effort) wants to accomplish now and in the future. If well-constructed, pithy, and to the point, it will be inspiring and convey the meaning behind the work. There is also a temporal component—it is where the organization wants to be *now* and going forward, as illustrated by examples in Box 14.2.

A *vision statement* is really about where the effort would like to be some years down the road and how it will look like to have a broad impact. A vision statement is often grander and more aspirational than a mission statement and provides a long-term direction for employees or group members to look toward. It may incorporate meaning behind the work but is more of a future state to provide a path forward for the current effort.

Purpose can overlap somewhat with mission and vision but probably can best be distinguished by considering who is the target audience. The mission statement speaks to both the employees (or well-being team group members) and the intended beneficiary of the product of the work. Purpose is really all about the intended beneficiaries of the product of the work. It is tightly linked to the meaning derived by the producers of that product, which may in fact be what leads to some of the interchangeability of the two terms. One other means by which to distinguish mission from purpose is parsing out the "what" from the "why." The mission is what we do; the purpose is why we do it. But, with that said, the purpose (or the "why") should be implied from the mission (or the "what") in order for the mission to be imbued with the meaning of the work.

Establishing a mission and vision has numerous important advantages. To start, developing these concepts within an organization can elucidate a level of meaning that

---

BOX 14.1 Steps to Implement a Well-Being Plan

Initial Planning by Leaders of Well-Being Effort

Formation of planning committee with diverse representation

Data gathering and needs assessment

Prioritization of efforts and decision on local versus system-wide level for plan

Writing and presentation of report on findings and recommendations

Establishment of funding, governance, and organizational structure

Appointment of leadership and team

Formulation of mission and model

Implementation of plan

will help drive forward and unlock the passions of the group engaged in the work. Since well-being and meaning are so closely tied, the mission of an organized well-being initiative can complement or enhance the mission of the parent organization. In many cases, the mission of the core well-being group will correlate with the larger mission statements of its parent institution since most organizations have established workforce well-being as a priority. And the corollary is likely true: when employees feel that their work has worth, they are more likely to be engaged in what they do because of a connection they feel with the organization and the part they play within it. Mission and vision statements can effectively communicate and convey the message of how the individual is linked to the meaning of their work. As such, one important consideration might be to explicitly link the mission statement of the well-being initiative to that of the institution as a whole.[8] One critical consideration is to be sure that the well-being group's mission statement is actually carried out. As such, it is important to establish a mission that is likely to be feasible. If the mission statement is all talk and not reflected through action, it could potentially backfire by leading employees to feel that the words spoken are not reflective of what they see in their actual work.

One process for developing a mission statement is outlined here. The process of developing mission and vision statements should not be underestimated. Though the product is often a handful of words or a couple of sentences, creating these statements requires considerable thought, energy, and time to do it right. To begin with, organizational (or well-being program) leaders ideally would convene and commit a dedicated session or sessions of uninterrupted and focused time to develop the statement. For many large organizations that are matrixed and complex, there will be a long history of other internal groups that have gone through similar endeavors. Such organizations may in fact have a team of facilitators, perhaps through marketing or human resources, who are skilled in guiding groups through the mission and vision statement development process. Such institutional experts can often be quite helpful in assisting groups to navigate the drafting sessions. There also must be commitment from those who participate in statement-drafting to take the process seriously because it often requires considerable contributory discussion. At times, a group may spend hours trying to get just a few words right to best capture the mission and vision. This labor-intensive process is critical since these statements will likely become part of the well-being group's brand and connected with well-being efforts, thereby contributing to the way the community perceives the well-being program. Example mission and vision statements are included in Box 14.2.

Adopting a Model

Once the mission and vision have been crafted, an organized well-being effort should strongly consider adopting a model of well-being.[4] Whereas it is quite common for organizations and corporations to craft mission and vision statements, developing or adopting a model may be less common. Chapter 1 describes considerations for choosing a model and several of the commonly used models of well-being in medicine. The rationale for

---

BOX 14.2 Example Organizational Mission and Vision Statements

Organization 1:

Mission:

To educate, serve, and advocate for best practices to support resilience and well-being for school of medicine faculty and learners.

Vision:

Create a medical culture in which health care workers and learners do not have to sacrifice their own well-being to serve others.

Organization 2:

Mission:

The mission of the Office of Clinician Experience is to design and shape a uniquely positive, supportive, and productive operational environment and workplace experience for all clinicians. This will be achieved through organizational interventions that remove barriers in order to highlight and develop the innate talent, skills, knowledge, and collaborative nature of our clinical teams. This will create a close community of clinicians who are highly valued by the organization and committed to the highest possible caliber of performance and productivity, as well as to each other's success and the success of the organization. The end result will be optimal well-being and professional satisfaction for clinicians.

Vision:

The vision of the Office of Clinician Experience is to be an exemplar in manifesting an inspiring model of the ideal clinician experience.

---

placing a priority on committing to a model as an organization is three-fold: (1) to help categorize drivers that promote or erode well-being, (2) to organize the interventions that address these identified drivers, and (3) to help manage the message when communicating what the program is trying to accomplish.

Having a model is particularly helpful to address the scope of a well-being leader's work. It is not uncommon for new well-being program leads to quickly become overwhelmed with all of the requests or identified contributors to well-being. In part, this sense that well-being touches so many domains of work life may stem from the diverse and sometimes unclear definition(s) of well-being. In a group discussion about well-being, there are frequently wide-ranging opinions about what well-being means. Furthermore, and perhaps to be expected, individual constituents or employees may reach out to the new well-being group upon recognizing that well-being can be used as a lever for change. Various stakeholders from every direction may lobby for the well-being program to see to their needs. For example, here are some paraphrased examples based on the authors' experience:

> I feel that my well-being is being affected by the limited size of my retirement package (or salary, or moonlighting rate, or other monetary benefit). Your office should work to increase my take-home compensation.
>
> It is very annoying for me to get so many email messages from the health system. It is affecting my well-being. Can you get them to decrease the e-mail messages?
>
> The lack of access to the hospital gym after 10 PM makes it hard for me to get my workout. It is affecting my well-being.

Without a model, it can be unclear whether these examples are under the purview of the well-being leader or group. A model can therefore help to outline which priorities the well-being leader is responsible for addressing, categorize concerns that arise, and identify the workflow or partners needed to address them. Typically, once an issue is categorized, the decision to intervene will depend on the well-being burden (e.g., association with burnout), feasibility, cost, and support from school or institutional leadership.

Finally, a model helps convey a consistent message to the community. It shows to the constituents of an organized well-being effort how the well-being program is organized in its efforts to meet their needs. Over time this messaging can build support and alignment around priority issues and help allow the well-being group to focus on those issues likely to be most impactful.

As described in Chapter 1, many existing models already nicely capture the components of well-being, and it is not necessary for each new program to develop its own model. In fact, creating a de novo model is not recommended since extensive work and research have gone into the development of existing models. Well-being program leadership and team members should commit significant time and thought energy to identifying which model will best address organizational needs. Again, partnering with marketing and branding colleagues may be helpful here, and approval by school or system leadership will also be necessary if the model will be used in communications.

Governance and Organizational Structure

After developing a mission, vision, and model of well-being, actually implementing comprehensive well-being programs at the UME and GME levels often requires building infrastructure to ensure appropriate allocation of resources, development of policies and processes, and adoption of mechanisms for accountability. An organizational chart can be useful to illustrate a clear reporting structure and oversight that specifies designated roles and supervisory responsibilities (Figure 14.1).

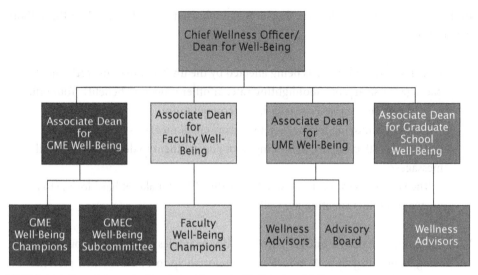

FIGURE 14.1 Sample organizational chart for an institutional well-being program.

Institution-Wide Well-Being Reporting Structures

While not all institutions house all members of their well-being teams within one organizational chart or reporting structure, some institutions may choose to organize
their UME and GME well-being programs across a larger system-wide structure. One
example of this type of institution-wide well-being reporting structure is overseen by
a Chief Wellness Officer (CWO). As a member of senior leadership, the CWO can engage members of the organization, provide relevant and actionable data to other leaders,
and develop an organization-wide action plan for improving clinician well-being.[9] To
be effective, the CWO should ideally directly report to a Dean, CEO, or similarly positioned leader within an institution. The roles and responsibilities of CWOs are described
in more detail in Chapter 16.

If given the oversight over multiple constituent groups, a CWO can be successful
by developing a leadership team organized according to constituent group (e.g., Director
of Well-being for Graduate Medical Education, Undergraduate Medical Education,
Faculty, etc.) all of whom report up to the CWO. Such constituent-based well-being
leaders generally will have numerous responsibilities that contribute to the institution's
efforts in meeting constituent-specific well-being goals. Goals can include efforts to address burnout, physical and mental health needs, clinical work intensity, educational/
curricular demands, mistreatment, and the development and integration of well-being
curricular activities. The GME or UME constituent-based well-being leader might hold
various roles within their own constituency, such as chairing a dedicated GME or UME
Well-Being Committee, while concurrently participating as a member of the larger institutional well-being team organized under the CWO.

Independent Constituent Group Reporting Structures

In institutions without a designated CWO, constituent-based well-being leaders may be charged with overseeing certain institutional efforts for well-being within their constituency groups, such as efforts to ensure effective mental health resources. While in this model the different constituent leaders may network and collaborate, the constituent-based well-being leader is generally positioned to report directly to the institutional leader overseeing GME (e.g., DIO) or UME (Dean for Medical Education). As a well-being leader, the constituent-specific well-being leader may also function in developing and overseeing the administration of survey instruments used to measure well-being and/or the effectiveness of interventions utilized to combat burnout and clerical burden. By providing mentorship and consultation, the constituent-specific well-being leader might also encourage project development and scholarly activities related to the domains of medical student or GME trainee well-being. The downside of this structure which does not involve reporting directly to a CWO is that there may be duplication of efforts or lack of communication about important initiatives that are occurring in one constituent group.

Work Within Constituencies

Constituent-based well-being leaders may work independently but ideally will work to meet the aforementioned responsibilities with their own team, which could be comprised of clinicians, administrators, psychosocial support personnel, and others. Furthermore, some institutions may support or encourage the development of additional well-being champions or directors, with the goal of increasing structure and developing programming and engagement at a more local level, such as at the level of a GME training program or medical student year/cohort.

GME Well-Being Champions

At the level of the GME trainee, the GME champion/director is often a faculty member in the same discipline as the residency or fellowship program which they represent. This champion may or may not be part of the existing leadership of the training program depending on program structure and available resources. There are certain advantages for the champion/director to be a member of the program leadership team, such as having a greater knowledge about the training program and being able to leverage resources and buy-in more easily. However, there may also be disadvantages of the champion/director being a member of the program leadership. For example, trainees may feel that they cannot raise concerns in a confidential manner if the champion/director is also a member of the training program's leadership team.

The GME champion/director can work closely with training program leadership to promote a culture of well-being within a given residency/fellowship program. The ultimate goal of this structure is to incorporate well-being into the daily function of the learning environment, in both the curricular and extracurricular domains. Ideally, the GME champion/director should be supported either financially and/or with protected time to conduct these activities. If no incentive is provided to take on this role, the individual cannot be expected to effectively dedicate a large portion of effort toward this position, thereby limiting the impact on a program. Finally, the GME champion/director should serve as a role model and resource for physician well-being for both faculty and trainees, help to educate them about the importance of self-care and seeking mental health treatment when needed, and encourage participation in institutional well-being programs that are available.

UME Well-Being Champions

At the medical student level, the UME constituent-based well-being leader has roles and responsibilities that are both similar and distinct from those of the GME well-being champion/director. In this role, the UME well-being leader is a faculty member who can oversee the creation, implementation, and assessment of evidence-based programming that focuses on medical student well-being. The UME constituent-based leader also might oversee the implementation of a well-being curriculum across all 4 years of medical school and help develop interventions that address the system-level drivers that undermine medical student well-being. In addition, the UME well-being leader can enable regular monitoring of well-being measures. Similarly to the GME champion, a UME constituent-based well-being leader or champion needs adequate time and resources in order to have an impact within their constituency.

The UME constituent-based well-being leader might also oversee a group of UME well-being champions/directors who work with smaller cohorts within the larger medical school. Such UME champions/directors can also serve in a capacity to help address concerns and identify and advocate for resources that enhance medical student well-being, and they may have one of several professional backgrounds, including within psychosocial support disciplines. Such UME champions/directors typically meet with medical students on a regular basis and might conduct one-on-one support sessions or self-care or resilience-building activities to address their needs. The UME champions/directors may also serve as supportive resources to a specific cohort of students during identified high-stress points throughout the year.

Well-Being Committees

In addition to these leadership roles, committee structures within constituent groups can be instrumental in advancing the well-being initiatives of an institution. These well-being committees ideally should include constituent representatives (medical students and resident/fellows) to provide an opportunity to share perspectives and solutions for well-being matters. Well-being committees can also be formed at the department and training program levels so that well-being issues related specifically to each specialty can be addressed by the relevant stakeholders. Once roles and committees have been established, developing policies related to well-being is often a next step.

Instituting Policies and Guidelines

Every institution should aim to develop a policy (or set of policies) or guideline that embodies a specific approach to promoting a culture and learning environment that supports the psychological, emotional, and physical well-being of all students and trainees at the institution. Policies or guidelines can be developed using several approaches. One such example process is described in Figure 14.2

1. *Identify initial need and focus.* Well-being needs can be identified through a number of means, including through town halls or focus groups with trainees or medical students; by getting input from established house staff or medical student well-being committees, planning committees, councils, or advisory boards; or by implementing structured well-being needs assessment surveys. All these sources can provide vital information about the well-being themes to address as priorities for policy development.
2. *Create policy draft.* After leveraging thematic data, a working group within the well-being planning committee can create an initial policy draft, which can then be shared with other well-being planning committee group members for suggestions, edits, and ultimate approval.
3. *Share working draft.* Once a working draft has been approved by the planning committee, it can be shared with training program and institutional leaders to "socialize" the document and solicit comments through a "feedback period" to further refine the policy.
4. *Approve final draft.* Once finalized, depending on the institutional organizational structure, the policy may need to be submitted to institutional or school leadership, the DIO, the GME Committee, possibly board members, and ultimately the dean's office for approval. Execution of well-being policies requires a structured approach

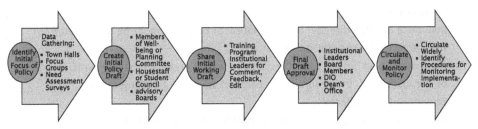

FIGURE 14.2 Pathway for instituting well-being policies.

whereby the sponsoring institution provides both oversight and well-being resources to students and individual training programs.

5. *Circulate and monitor policy.* Once approved, the policy should ideally be widely circulated as a "mandate" or established institutional best practice, recognizing that the policy will only be as effective as the extent to which it is adhered to. Some flexibility can then be built in for tailoring to specific needs, but with a high level of accountability. Procedures to identify nonadherence via anonymous reporting or program dashboards are helpful to monitor the implementation of the policy.

Since a policy is a deliberate system of principles to guide decisions and achieve rational outcomes, it must be noted that while there can be overarching well-being–related regulations (ACGME- or LCME-mandated) that may influence policy components, specific institutional policies account for and address precise institutional well-being needs. The resultant policy should be of sufficient scope to meet both regulatory and local needs, which often overlap. A policy on provision of resident wellness days, for example, is in keeping with the section on Well-Being found in the ACGME's Common Program Requirements Section VI, which requires residents/fellows to be given the opportunity to attend medical, dental, and mental health appointments during working hours. See Boxes 14.3 and 14.4 for example policies.

BOX 14.3 Sample Policy: Access to Mental Health Resources Free of Charge

- All students (medical and graduate) and GME trainees (residents, clinical fellows, and postdoctoral fellows) have access to confidential services through a mental health program.
- A wide range of mental health services are offered, including initial consultation, psychotherapy, counseling, medication management, and referrals.
- Appointments have both virtual and in-person options.
- Services are free for all students and GME trainees, regardless of their insurance plan. There are no out-of-pocket costs such as co-pays, deductibles, and co-insurance.
- Insurance is billed directly; an explanation of benefits might be generated from the insurance carrier, but this is not a bill.
- If anyone is seeking long-term services or would prefer to see a provider outside of our institution, the program can perform an initial assessment and then provide suitable referrals.
- Any treatment outside of the mental health program will require payment according to the insurance plan or a fee negotiated with the outside provider.

BOX 14.4 Sample Policy: Resident and Fellow Wellness Days

To allow residents and fellows to attend to their personal health care, including medical, dental, and mental health appointments, residents and fellows will be provided with four (4) wellness days in addition to other leave time on an annual basis during each academic year. This is provided and structured with a goal of minimizing disruptions to both patient care and training while allowing residents and fellows sufficient time to appropriately attend to personal health maintenance.

- In addition to using this time for personal health maintenance, wellness days may also be used for the following:
- To care for the child of a resident/fellow who has a health condition requiring treatment or supervision.
- To care for an ill family member (e.g., parent, spouse, or child) or partner, including medical, dental, and mental health appointments where the resident/fellow's presence is needed.
- The four (4) days may be used in half-day (4-hour) increments to allow residents/fellows to attend to appointments and perform normal duties before and/or after the appointment in acknowledgment that many appointments do not require an entire duty period to be taken off.
- Departments will be required to make every effort to accommodate residents and fellows attending appointments during scheduled duties and are asked to establish policies and procedures for usage of this time.
- Departments will be given the latitude to allow for the use of this time for any additional wellness activities that they deem appropriate (example: a workshop on mindfulness or other stress reduction tools), however this is solely at the discretion of the Program Director.
- Departments will be asked to document and track this leave time separate from sick leave and may request documentation where appropriate.
- Prior to using a wellness day (or portion of a day), advance notice of at least 7 days wherever practicable should be provided to the resident's/fellow's Program Director to ensure adequate coverage.
- Programs are encouraged to implement a system of coverage to ensure that use of wellness days does not produce an undue burden on other residents and faculty and minimizes disruptions to patient care and resident/fellow learning.
- Residents/fellows are encouraged wherever possible to schedule appointments when not assigned to clinical duties, but should not be penalized by programs for use of a wellness day.
- Unlike sick leave, wellness days are earned quarterly, may not be accrued and carried over to subsequent training years, and may not be applied to a paid leave of absence.

Conclusion

Creating and implementing a comprehensive well-being program requires careful planning, inclusion of diverse stakeholders, and establishing institutional funding and support. Successful program development may involve a number of important initial steps, including developing mission and vision statements and choosing a well-being model. Establishing a governance and organizational structure that includes well-being leadership roles, an infrastructure of personnel, services, and supportive reporting lines are all highly useful to a successful well-being program. Developing well-being policies that both address regulation and meet local well-being needs requires a concerted effort involving numerous local stakeholders to help gather data, draft, implement, and monitor adherence to such policies.

Summary Points

- Establishing support and engaging key stakeholders are essential to developing a comprehensive GME well-being program.
- Developing a clear mission and vision for the well-being initiative is critical to its success and can serve to complement and enhance the mission of an institution.
- Creating a well-being model can help categorize drivers that promote well-being and organize the interventions that address these identified drivers.
- Developing a well thought out organizational structure for the well-being program can provide clarity of the roles for the individuals involved, as well as an element of accountability.
- Institutional policies should be developed to promote a culture of well-being in the learning environment.

Putting It into Practice

- *Establishing support*: *Create a planning committee.* The creation of a well-being program starts with representative stakeholders gathering to form a planning committee that can collect data, identify needs, set priorities, and present a compelling report to seek funding and support for the plan.
- *Organizational structure*: *Create a table to outline roles.* A comprehensive well-being program should consist of an organizational structure that includes clear delineation of well-being leadership roles that are created to enhance the well-being of medical students, GME trainees and faculty.
- *Mission and vision*: *Establish a mission and vision.* Establishing a mission and vision helps to tie employees to the meaning in their work while the development

of a model helps organize the many drivers and interventions that promote well-being and facilitates communications around what a well-being program is trying to accomplish.

- *Directors of Well-Being for UME/GME: Establish the roles of the Director of Well-Being for UME and Director of Well-Being for GME.* The establishment of the constituent-based well-being leader at the UME/GME level is a key feature of a comprehensive well-being program. These leaders can engage members of the organization and develop action plans for improving well-being at the medical school and GME trainee level.
- *Instituting policies: Establish policies.* Instituting well-being policies that both address regulation and ensure the meeting of local well-being needs requires a concerted effort involving numerous local stakeholders to help gather data, draft, implement, and monitor compliance of such policies.

References

1. National Academy of Medicine. *Taking Action Against Clinician Burnout: A Systems Approach to Professional Well-Being.* The National Academies Press; 2019. Accessed February 13, 2022. https://www.nap.edu/catalog/25521/taking-action-against-clinician-burnout-a-systems-approach-to-professional

2. Shanafelt T, Goh J, Sinsky C. The business case for investing in physician well-being. *JAMA Intern Med.* 2017;177(12):1826–1832. doi:10.1001/jamainternmed.2017.4340

3. Shanafelt T, Swensen SJ, Woody J, Levin J, Lillie J. Physician and nurse well-being: seven things hospital boards should know. *J Healthc Manag.* 2018;63(6):363–369. doi:10.1097/JHM-D-18-00209

4. Shanafelt T, Trockel M, Ripp J, Murphy ML, Sandborg C, Bohman B. Building a program on well-being: key design considerations to meet the unique needs of each organization. *Acad Med.* 2019;94(2):156–161. doi:10.1097/ACM.0000000000002415

5. Mari S, Meyen R, Kim B. Resident-led organizational initiatives to reduce burnout and improve wellness. *BMC Med Educ.* 2019;19(1):437. doi:10.1186/s12909-019-1756-y

6. Kenny G. Your company's purpose is not its vision, mission, or values. *Harv Bus Rev.* Published September 3, 2014. Accessed February 13, 2022. https://hbr.org/2014/09/your-companys-purpose-is-not-its-vision-mission-or-values

7. Disney Institute. Mission versus purpose: what's the difference? Published October 23, 2018. Accessed February 13, 2022. https://www.disneyinstitute.com/blog/mission-versus-purpose-whats-the-difference/

8. Amabile T, Kramer S. To give your employees meaning, start with mission. *Harv Bus Rev.* Published December 19, 2012. Accessed February 13, 2022. https://hbr.org/2012/12/to-give-your-employees-meaning.

9. Ripp J, Shanafelt T. The health care chief wellness officer: what the role is and is not. *Acad Med.* 2020;95(9):1354–1358. doi:10.1097/ACM.0000000000003433

Final Considerations

SECTION IV

Final Considerations

Novel Technology and Discoveries: The Future of Physician Well-Being

Keith A. Horvath and Anne J. Berry

Introduction

In its simplest form, technology is just a tool. As such, the technology used in health care should facilitate that care. However, like any tool, if misused or poorly designed, that same technology can impede care and, in its worst case, create harm. The prevention of harm has traditionally and appropriately been focused on the patient, but, as explored in earlier chapters, the challenges associated with health information technology (IT) also influence clinicians and are a major contributor to clinician burnout. Despite these challenges, innovation in the health care industry is occurring rapidly, and great potential exists for emerging technologies. As the medical profession adapts to these changes, it is important to understand how health technologies and innovations have been adopted over time. This chapter highlights three examples of health IT implementation: electronic health record (EHR) adoption through the Health Information Technology for Economic and Clinical Health (HITECH) Act, telehealth (TH) utilization during the COVID-19 pandemic, and the emerging area of artificial intelligence (AI) in health care—and examines how each change has introduced unintended consequences and new challenges to the medical profession. Considering the examples of these three technologies allows an evaluation of the past (arguably imperfect) EHR adoption, the present (rapid expansion during a crisis) use of TH, and the future (promise and threat) with AI. These cases illustrate how certain advances have both positive and negative impacts on the delivery of patient care and the importance of providing clinicians with a strong foundational knowledge of emerging technologies by offering ongoing training opportunities to medical students and graduate medical education (GME) trainees in areas related to digital health advancement.

Innovation as a Disruptor: How Technology Transforms Practice

Electronic Health Records: Wide Adoption, but Limited Utility

The HITECH Act of 2009 promoted the use of health IT and provided financial incentives to increase the adoption of EHRs that met "meaningful-use" criteria. The federal government provided these incentives based on the belief that health IT could improve health care delivery and that barriers, such as financial constraints and technical limitations, were limiting health professionals and health systems from adopting the use of this technology.[1] These incentives worked, driving a swift uptake of EHR adoption.[2] Between 2008 and 2015, there was a nine-fold increase in the percentage of US hospitals using a basic EHR, and 96% had adopted a certified EHR.[3]

Despite the rapid pace of EHR implementation and the promising outlook that EHRs would improve health care and create efficiencies, the technology had shortcomings. For example, instead of simplifying documentation and care delivery, EHRs have become a burdensome tool for clinicians. Much of the clinical documentation input in current EHRs does not add clinical value; the documentation does support enhanced billing capabilities; and it enables regulatory requirements to be met, rather than serving as a tool to support the clinician and patient.[4,5] These documentation requirements demand physicians spend more time entering data into an EHR. On average, EHR clinical notes in the United States are nearly four times longer than notes in other countries.[6] The need to complete documentation requirements creates an unnecessary burden for clinicians. Furthermore, time spent after hours in the EHR and the volume of inbox messages have both been associated with exhaustion among clinicians.[7]

The issues of design and usability also influence how EHRs contribute to clinician burnout.[8,9] Clinicians spend a significant amount of their time inputting electronic data, which takes away from time spent delivering direct patient care. One study found that clinicians spend over half of their workday using the EHR system.[10] Another study calculated that for each hour clinicians spend with patients, they spend 2 hours in the EHR and at their desk.[11] Even GME trainees report spending a significant amount of time during their day using EHRs, and, while it is important they be exposed to clinical documentation practices, it should be ensured that GME trainees do not lose valuable learning opportunities in direct patient care as a result of time spent on the EHRs.[12]

While the dramatic increase in clinician EHR use time has been problematic, the benefits of EHR implementation have not yet been fully realized. For example, the lack of ability to capture and share data across multiple settings (interoperability) limits the utility of EHRs.[13] Progress has been made to enhance the interoperability of EHRs over the past decade, but challenges still exist. In 2019, just over half of US hospitals met the four core domains of interoperability: the ability to send, receive, find, and integrate data.[14] EHR technology is also cumbersome to users. In a national survey of physicians, the usability of EHRs was ranked lower than other common technologies based on a standard technology usability scale. Physicians gave EHRs a grade of F, which falls in the "not acceptable" range on this particular scale (for reference, a microwave or an ATM received a B rating in the same scoring system).[15] Recognizing the challenges providers experience when using EHRs, health care organizations are implementing strategies—including work design approaches, in-basket management techniques, and EHR training—to optimize their health IT systems and in turn address clinician well-being.[16]

Telehealth

While EHR use in health care settings became standard fairly recently, largely as a result of federal mandates and funding, the technology and use of TH predates EHRs by decades. Fundamentally, TH involves providing care to a patient at a distance. Based on this definition, there have been some early niches in care delivery to remote settings. Over time, TH has shown particular utility in care delivery for mental health, for example, and for providing care that depends primarily on reviewing still images in specialties such as dermatology and radiology. TH can be performed either synchronously, with real-time interactions between provider and patient, or asynchronously, enabling patients and providers to connect when their schedules allow. It can be accomplished with audio and/or video linkage between participants, and, as these connections have become ubiquitous in our private lives, there has been a steady increase in their use in medicine. While the application of TH is still evolving, a recent systematic review of 93 randomized controlled trials that assessed the effectiveness of TH demonstrated similar outcomes with face-to-face visits in the management of chronic conditions such as congestive heart failure and diabetes.[17] TH also offers benefits beyond the traditional patient encounter in the physician's office. The technology allows clinicians to view a patient's home and identify what environmental or sociodemographic factors might be contributing to the individual's overall health. Studies that examined TH's capabilities have also documented the advantages of TH services (e.g., using remote ICUs that enable clinicians to monitor patients in other locations).[18]

There is little published research examining the association between TH use and clinician burnout. Additional well-being-focused studies are needed to better understand clinician attitudes toward TH, including feedback about its usability and recommendations for improvements.[8] One study reported that in a survey of 760 physicians, the utility of TH scored a 7.4 on a scale from 1 to 10.[19] Additional data from a survey of 15,000 physicians documented how TH might be able to alleviate burnout in three different ways. First, TH creates efficiencies by eliminating the down time clinicians experience in between treating patients during office visits and, more importantly, by adding flexibility to scheduling. TH also provides the opportunity for clinicians to deliver more consistent care to patients by eliminating travel times to and from physician offices which, for patients with chronic conditions and physical functional impairment, may lead to missed appointments due to the inherent frequency required. Finally, TH increases access to care and enables physicians to spend more time caring for patients.[20]

The recent surge in TH use in response to the COVID-19 pandemic provides an opportunity not only to study and learn from its implementation, but also to generate more evidence about what approaches are effective in order to inform its application.[18] To grasp the significance of this increase in TH use, health care claims data highlight the change. The number of Medicare fee-for-service beneficiaries receiving TH services dramatically increased from approximately 13,000 a week in the period just prior to the pandemic to nearly 1.7 million in the last week of April 2020, as depicted in Figure 15.1.[21] Using reports from an all-payer US database, there was an 8,000% increase in TH claims at the peak of the pandemic during the spring of 2020, compared with the same interval in the previous year.[22] The leading diagnosis category in the Spring 2020 claims analysis was mental health, which was also the most common pre-pandemic TH visit category.[22] Chronic conditions, such as hypertension and arthritis, rose to the top five TH diagnoses as the pandemic continued, which was previously unforeseen.[22] These findings likely underscore the circumstances of the pandemic, wherein many patients with chronic conditions avoided visiting emergency rooms, hospitals, and even doctors' offices for nonacute problems. As might be expected, TH provides an opportunity for those with nonurgent medical conditions to conveniently receive care through virtual appointments. Virtual

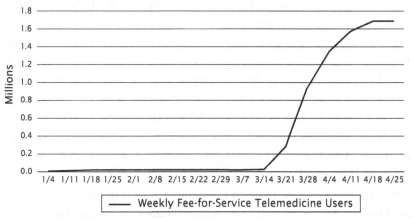

FIGURE 15.1 Telemedicine use among Medicare FFS beneficiaries during the early stages of the coronavirus pandemic. Telemedicine is defined as services on the Medicare telehealth list, including audio-only visits as well as virtual check-ins and e-visits. From internal CMS analysis of Medicare FFS claims data, March 17, 2020 through June 13, 2020 (using data processed through June, 19, 2020). Reproduced from Seema Verma, "Early Impact of CMS Expansion of Medicare Telehealth During COVID-19." Health Affairs Blog, July 15, 2020. doi:10.1377/hblog20200715.454789. Courtesy of Health Affairs/Project HOPE—The People-to-People Health Foundation, Inc.

patient visits also enabled individuals exhibiting nonemergent COVID-19 symptoms to receive care while remaining isolated at home, without the risk of potentially exposing others. This particular application of TH rapidly expanded out of necessity for patient and provider safety.

During the pandemic, health systems with a TH infrastructure already in place were able to respond to the changing environment immediately.[23] Other programs, however, were forced to accelerate their TH implementation plans to meet the needs of the community during a public health emergency. These systems with previous "stretch" goals of providing a few thousand TH visits in a year were able to achieve these metrics in a month or even a week in some instances.

Necessity being the mother of invention, TH enabled the technological means to provide necessary care during the pandemic. Clinicians not only stepped up their adoption and implementation of TH during the public health emergency but also recognized the need for medical students and GME trainees to understand how best to use TH.[24] This competency-based approach was welcomed across the continuum of medical education, which is in sharp contrast to the response EHRs have received. Given the opportunity to find a solution for delivering care, clinicians embraced TH as opposed to the dissatisfaction experienced with a different technology, EHRs. The difference in which these technologies were adopted exemplifies a critical takeaway when understanding the use of any technology and particularly when assessing its impact on clinician well-being: the past expansion of EHRs was largely done "to" clinicians with minimal input, while the present expansion of TH was done "with" clinicians. The recent TH expansion in response to the COVID-19 pandemic was a combined learning experience for both patients and clinicians and required a significant amount of clinician input to implement.

While TH's growth and acceptance were impressive, a key ingredient fostering this growth was outside of the technological realm. Specifically, the Centers for Medicare and Medicaid Services (CMS) waived critical TH regulations, an action that opened the door for wide TH expansion and put billing for TH visits on more equal footing with in-person visits.[25] Interestingly, many of the previous regulations that limited the use of telemedicine are now being reconsidered in light of the benefits seen during the crisis, and certain pandemic-related waivers could become permanent.[26,]One important lesson here is that policy shifts can have a significant impact on influencing the uptake of technology and, in so doing, influence clinician well-being. Given the role that legislation played in the past (EHRs) and present (TH) technologies under discussion, a newer innovation (AI) is now garnering the attention of regulators.

Artificial Intelligence

AI is an emerging technology with the potential to significantly impact the medical field. While AI in health care is still in its early stages, it is expected that every clinical specialty will be using the technology in the future.[27] AI tools provide both clinical and administrative applications and can perform functions to inform treatment decisions, predict

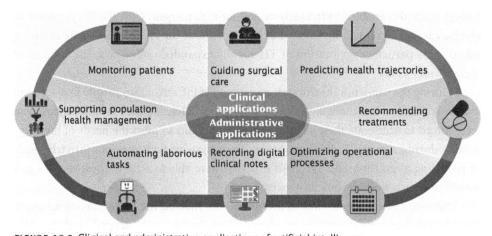

FIGURE 15.2 Clinical and administrative applications of artificial intelligence.

Source: US Government Accountability Office. *Artificial intelligence in health care: benefits and challenges of technologies to augment patient care.* Washington DC, Publication GAO-21-7SP. Published November 26, 2020. Accessed April 26, 2021. https://www.gao.gov/assets/gao-21-7sp.pdf Credit: Reproduced with permission from the US Government Accountability Office.

the onset of health conditions, optimize staffing and scheduling, and reduce burden on providers, as shown in Figure 15.2.[28] One promising use of AI could improve the EHR user experience. As clinicians continue to experience EHR documentation and usability challenges, natural language processing (NLP), a form of AI application, offers a solution to alleviate burden. NLP works to automate the note-taking process so clinicians can devote more time to direct patient care and less time to documentation.[29]

Despite studies documenting how AI can be applied to clinical care and how EHR data can be used to conduct analyses or make predictions, AI tools have not yet achieved widespread adoption in clinical practice. Of the research that has been published related to AI in health care, there are few randomized control trials, the gold standard for generating clinical evidence.[30,31] In 2017, funding for machine learning (ML) research through the National Institutes of Health accounted for a small amount (2.0%) of its total research budget, and a small subset of institutions received the majority of that funding.[32] Additionally, there was little support provided through grant-funding mechanisms to promote ML training and professional development among early-career investigators.[32]

This lack of evidence around AI performance can influence clinicians' enthusiasm for using AI tools. For this technology to be embraced by the medical profession, the uncertainties related to AI need to be addressed. For example, the lack of transparency about how the tools work causes concern. When a new treatment approach becomes available, physicians must ask questions of data and educate themselves about how the new method or device works, then use their clinical judgment to gauge the effectiveness of the tools and treatments.[33] AI will certainly play a major role with tasks such as automated imaging (e.g., radiology, ophthalmology, dermatology, and pathology) and signal processing (e.g., electrocardiogram, audiology, and electroencephalography). In addition to the interpretation of tests and images, AI will be used to integrate and arrange results with other clinical data to facilitate clinical workflow.

Looking back to the passage of the HITECH Act, when EHRs were championed as tools to improve health care delivery, it was likely not anticipated that EHR implementation would create additional burdens on clinicians. As the industry eyes AI adoption, it is important to reflect on the previous experience with EHRs and how the practice of medicine has changed since the introduction of electronic documentation. The technology that was expected to improve health care in our country ended up ushering in new requirements for clinicians, most of which were administrative in nature, and, a decade later, the technology has still not achieved interoperability or become user-friendly. At this early stage of AI research, development, and adoption, in order to ensure that AI alleviates rather than contributes to unnecessary burdens, clinicians, health educators, policymakers, regulators, patients, and the entire health care industry should all encourage a thorough and thoughtful assessment of what will be required of the health care professional when this new technology enters clinical practice.

Unintended Consequences of Innovation

Legal, Policy, and Regulatory Responses to New Technologies

Policymakers and regulators did not anticipate how the health IT implementation resulting from the HITECH Act would ultimately disrupt the medical profession and burden providers with EHR adoption.[34] The Department of Health and Human Services (HHS) identified five overarching goals when defining what would be considered meaningful use of health IT: improving care quality while reducing disparities, supporting patient engagement, promoting public and population health, improving care coordination, and enhancing privacy and security.[35] Missing from these specific aims was the functionality of this technology: namely, usability was not considered an initial priority. Federal efforts are now under way to improve clinician use of and satisfaction with health IT, specifically EHRs. The 21st Century Cures Act includes a provision requiring HHS to develop a plan to alleviate the burden related to health IT.[36,37] As the federal government approaches future policies and regulations around health IT, burden reduction should be a key consideration.

Health care professionals saw relief from numerous administrative burdens during the COVID-19 pandemic. Through regulatory changes, certain health care policies and practices shifted in response to the public health crisis.[38] For example, one factor contributing to the success of TH adoption during the COVID-19 pandemic was CMS's issuance of waivers and flexibilities which, among other changes, broadened TH eligibility to beneficiaries, expanded the services covered through TH, and paid for services at the same rate as if the service was conducted in-person.[21,25,39] Given the effectiveness of TH during the pandemic and the added value it brought to patients and providers, it is unlikely that the limited-reach, pre-COVID TH status quo will return. The pandemic forced fundamental changes to occur in the TH space.

Regulation is also on the horizon for AI in medicine. The Food and Drug Administration (FDA) is in early stages of developing a regulatory framework related to the consideration of AI/ML-based software as a medical device.[40] Developing such a framework will be a different process for the FDA because this medical technology is unlike others that are presently regulated; AI/ML tools can continuously learn, they can make recommendations, and the method by which they reach conclusions is not transparent.[41] Currently, it is unclear how medical liability applies to use of AI tools; therefore, using emerging technologies could contribute to added stress for clinicians.[8]

Ethical Considerations

The speed at which health technology evolves requires clinicians to be diligent in ensuring the platform is safe, confidential, and meets quality standards.[42] Before adopting a new technology, clinicians should consider the ethical implications of a new tool. Not only need it be safe and effective, but it must also be equitable. For example, while TH does expand access to services, it may also create disparities among patient populations that do not have the resources required to use the technology. Rural populations without reliable internet access or patients who lack the technical skills to effectively navigate the steps required to join a virtual visit are populations that may not embrace this innovation. Despite the rapid adoption of TH during the COVID-19 pandemic, disparities continue to exist for some patients in their ability to access virtual visits.[43] Therefore, simply because the technology is available does not mean that the general population benefits from it. Clinicians should recognize opportunities when health innovations can be utilized, but also identify limitations and ways to ensure that all members of society can receive quality care.

For example, clinicians should be familiar with the risks and limitations of AI/ML technologies. AI/ML tools can quickly analyze large amounts of data to make predictions, and the information generated from such technology has the potential to change the way that medicine is practiced. As the capabilities of AI/ML continue to evolve, there is a need to consider the ethical risks of AI. Racial and other biases have been found to exist in algorithmic design.[44] Because algorithms are trained using data, the data should represent the general population, and clinicians using the AI should be educated about the importance of including minority and underserved populations in datasets. Before AI tools are applied to health care decision-making, they must be monitored and evaluated in real-world settings to determine if they are effective.[45] And, on an ongoing basis, algorithms should be reviewed for bias and safety to confirm they are performing as intended.[46] The promise of AI is that it can automate simple tasks to free up time for the clinician to perform more complex functions. AI is designed to identify ways to streamline workflows, and, by achieving this through the management of repetitious administrative tasks, the technology has the potential to dramatically improve clinician well-being.[47] At the same time, however, it is critical that the medical field closely assesses and monitors the capabilities of new technologies to prevent any unintended consequences that may emerge as a result of their adoption.

The Role of the Clinician as Technology Evolves

There exists a perceived threat that AI is going to replace the clinician, but there are several reasons why this is unlikely to occur. First, there are many tasks that algorithms, even coupled with robots, cannot perform, which is particularly true when considering the very nonlinear working methods that clinicians routinely use. Additionally, it is not really about technology versus humans: both can learn, adapt, and support each other synergistically to achieve more together than either could alone.[48] The conventional wisdom, however, is that clinicians who can use AI may replace those who cannot. If technology realizes its promise of improving clinical efficiency, then the role of the clinician can appropriately shift from data entry clerk to empathetic caregiver.

Teaching Innovation: Including Students and GME Trainees in the Early Adoption of Technology

As health IT and digital health technologies continue to advance, it is critical to support all learners and provide them with adequate training and professional development to acquire new skills.[49] Modern medicine requires medical educators to introduce and integrate new knowledge and techniques into existing curricula. As more data become accessible and used in health care, clinicians need to understand how to locate and operationalize trusted information.[50] Emerging technologies expose clinicians to disciplines such as predictive analytics and data science, and clinicians should be familiar and comfortable with these concepts. Furthermore, as future technology introduces additional tools and methods for administering care, educators should recognize when it is necessary to incorporate new methods into medical training—from undergraduate and graduate medical education to continuing medical education (CME).

Beyond standard instruction, clinicians, medical students, and GME trainees should have opportunities to explore new innovations in a testing environment. This exposure enables them to be familiar with the tools and grow to become more efficient using them before applying them in a clinical environment. For example, simulation has been one method for ensuring that learners gain proficiency in using EHRs by replicating the system used while also ensuring that patient records remain private.[51]

The increased use of TH during the COVID-19 pandemic occurred at a rapid pace and emphasized the need for clinicians to develop skills for delivering care virtually.[52] The Telehealth Competencies Across the Learning Continuum report developed by the Association of American Medical Colleges and its Telehealth Advisory Committee, with input from medical education and clinical practice community leaders, helps inform medical educators of the key skills necessary for clinicians to deliver quality TH services to patients.[53] The six key domains for TH competencies are Patient Safety and Appropriate Use of TH; Access and Equity in TH; Communication via TH; Data Collection and Assessment via TH; Technology for TH; and Ethical Practices and Legal Requirements for TH.

Today's medical students and GME trainees should be introduced to AI and made aware of its applications in health care as well as the risks and uncertainties that exist when using this technology. A clinician with access to AI applications should be able to understand when it is clinically relevant for use and how to interpret and explain the results to patients and other health professionals. Additionally, clinicians must be aware of the potential for bias, error, and other limitations that may come with AI technology.[54] A biased national AI system is very dangerous, and the need for human override in AI is critical.

Strategies for Moving Forward

Training, collaboration, and resources are required to promote clinician well-being as the health care industry prepares for further innovation and health IT advancements. To aid clinicians in adapting to new technologies, educators must anticipate future needs and develop adequate training opportunities and methods to support clinicians, medical students, and GME trainees. Additionally, as these new tools and techniques are developed, clinicians have an important role in supporting innovation by collaborating across disciplines. The future of clinician well-being also depends on health systems providing the necessary resources to deliver training, enhance technology platforms, and support users of technology. Finally, the health care industry needs to advocate for an improved overall health IT infrastructure that supports interoperability of data across systems.

To support medical students and GME trainees and prepare them for work as practitioners, medical educators should provide exposure to health technologies and ensure learners have adequate growth opportunities to gain confidence in their abilities. Beyond medical students and GME trainees, the health system needs to prioritize training of all levels of clinicians as the industry responds to changing techniques for care delivery. For example, as TH has been further utilized, learners and educators will benefit from the Telehealth Competencies Across the Learning Continuum report developed by the Association of American Medical Colleges to help aid in the design of curricula and other professional development activities related to TH.[53]

Emerging technologies require multidisciplinary collaboration as new tools are developed, tested, and implemented.[55] For example, the expansion of AI is currently in its early stages, and AI governance processes are needed. Clinicians must play a role in developing and overseeing these plans and should recognize the importance of working with data scientists, information technologists, ethicists, and other key stakeholders as AI becomes more widely adopted.[47] Clinicians can make valuable recommendations to the design and implementation processes of new technologies given their clinical knowledge and understanding of the workflow.[28] Through techniques such as information extraction, NLP, automatic summarization, and deep learning, AI has the potential to synthesize multiple scientific manuscripts into patient-specific, interactive visualizations of clinical evidence that could then be easily accessed via the EHR. Potentially, this clinical evidence could be regularly updated with the results of new clinical trials, thus allowing EHRs to aid clinical decision-making and suggest changes to the treatment.[47]

Health systems that effectively implement health IT platforms could leverage the technology to improve health system and individual performance. For example, more advanced systems could use analytics to provide feedback, enhance the application of evidence-based medicine, and improve population health management. But, to realize these benefits, health systems must first make substantial foundational steps to enhance their health IT, which takes time and resources, and many health systems are at the early stages of this transformation.[56] Additionally, it is important to note that adopting new technology may not always simplify processes or procedures, and new tools could create unanticipated burdens and increased workloads for the users. As health systems adopt new technologies, it is critical to understand what is required of the users and provide them with adequate support.

Given the vast amount of health data available through EHRs, there are opportunities to apply these data for research purposes, and the health IT infrastructure should be improved to support research needs.[57] Additionally, there is a need to capture data related to the social determinants of health in EHRs. The adoption of data standards will help achieve the goal of interoperability and move the health care system in a direction that will use data from health IT to inform practice.[58] Achieving interoperability—with data exchanged between systems and linked across multiple data sources—could ultimately enable EHR technology to produce clear, user-friendly dashboard displays like the one depicted in Figure 15.3. In this example, a patient's health history, from immunizations and emergency care, to preventive screenings and medications, is captured on one screen that is easy to view and interpret by both the patient and the care team. There is much potential for the future design and function of electronic patient documentation platforms once the overall health care system reaches an interoperable state.

As the health industry responds to innovation, best practices should be developed to guide the design, implementation, and use of new advances in health care. These strategies (See Box 15.1) should be shared with educators and curriculum developers so that they may stay aware of the evolution of new technologies that ultimately will impact the next generation of health care providers.

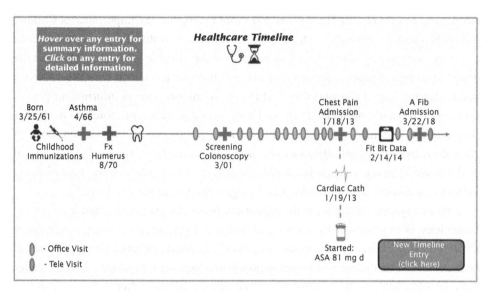

FIGURE 15.3 Dashboard display of a patient's health history linking interoperable patient data. Source: Horvath, K., P. Sengstack, F. Opelka, A. B. Kitts, P. Basch, D. Hoyt, A. Ommaya, P. Cipriano, K. Kawamoto, H. L. Paz, J. M. Overhage. 2018. A vision for a person-centered health information system. NAM Perspectives. Discussion Paper, National Academy of Medicine, Washington, DC. https://doi.org/10.31478/201810a

Credit: Reproduced with permission from the National Academy of Sciences, Courtesy of the National Academies Press, Washington, DC.

Conclusion

The introduction of technology to medicine is not a novel concept. The practice of medicine is built on foundational knowledge that expands as new conditions, treatments, and innovations are discovered. The medical profession is one of life-long learning; many clinicians are drawn to medicine for this very reason—they are inspired by the need to continuously learn and are dedicated to the call to help others. However, recent challenges brought forth by the convergence of technology and medicine require clinicians to spend more time and resources attending to administrative tasks, which diverts time

---

BOX 15.1 Strategies for Implementing New Advances in Health Care

- Integrate training about technologies into the education for clinicians, medical students, and GME trainees.
- Identify and address any unintended consequences or increased workload resulting from the adoption of new technologies.
- Involve clinicians and multidisciplinary stakeholder teams in the development of workflows and displays to enhance the patient and provider experience.

away from direct patient care. The introduction of new technologies offers great potential to improve health and health care, yet many burdens which have been attributed to health IT adoption and implementation, such as documentation requirements and usability constraints, are administrative and ultimately fall outside of the physician's clinical skillset. Because innovation is constant, it is the responsibility of educators to prepare learners for an evolving practice environment, and it is the responsibility of health leaders, the health care system, and society at large to continue to advocate for the well-being of clinicians and encourage the introduction of solutions to support clinicians as they adapt to new technologies.

Summary Points

- Technology is evolving rapidly, and clinicians must be prepared to adapt to changes. There is a role for education, training, and professional development in response to innovation.
- It is important to learn from past challenges related to EHR implementation and acknowledge that future emerging technologies—and the regulations that accompany them—could also unintentionally impact burnout.
- As new technologies are developed and implemented in health care, addressing the user experience is necessary.
- Despite usability difficulties, EHRs do offer promising capabilities to enable data analytics that drive research and health care improvement, and more emphasis should be placed on the potential to use EHR data for biomedical research and other purposes that improve health.
- Finally, any new technology should meet the following criteria without increasing the burden on clinicians. If faithful to these tenets, clinician well-being will be enhanced:
  o Supports clinical workflow and real-time decision making
  o Is interoperable, secure, evidence-based, and introspective
  o Supports management of acute, chronic, and preventative medical issues
  o Connects to all relevant health apps and devices
  o Facilitates use of data for analysis and research
  o Includes transparent and unbiased underlying algorithms

Putting It into Practice

- As new technologies are introduced in health care, clinicians need adequate training to enhance their awareness of the related tools, techniques, or treatments.
- Share best practices for identifying and incorporating new skills into curriculum development.

- Learn what peer institutions are developing so that educators can identify relevant curriculum models.
- Advocate for involving clinicians early and often in the design and implementation of innovations.
- Ensure that any new technology is well studied to determine its strengths and weaknesses, particularly its ability to improve or lessen well-being and disparities.

References

1. Blumenthal D. Wiring the health system: origins and provisions of a new federal program. *N Engl J Med.* 2011;*365*(24):2323–2329. doi:10.1056/NEJMsr1110507

2. Adler-Milstein J, Jha AK. HITECH act drove large gains in hospital electronic health record adoption. *Health Affairs.* 2017;*36*(8):1416–1422. doi:10.1377/hlthaff.2016.1651

3. Henry J, Pylypchuk Y, Searcy T, Patel V. Adoption of electronic health record systems among U.S. non-federal acute care hospitals: 2008–2015. ONC Data Brief, no. 35. Office of the National Coordinator for Health Information Technology. Published May 2016. Accessed April 26, 2021. https://dashboard.healt hit.gov/evaluations/data-briefs/non-federal-acute-care-hospital-ehr-adoption-2008-2015.php

4. Ommaya AK, Cipriano PF, Hoyt DB, et al. Care-centered clinical documentation in the digital environment: solutions to alleviate burnout. Discussion Paper, National Academy of Medicine. Published January 29, 2018. Accessed March 22, 2021. https://nam.edu/care-centered-clinical-documentation-digital-environment-solutions-alleviate-burnout

5. Johnson KB, Neuss MJ, Detmer DE. Electronic health records and clinician burnout: a story of three eras. *JAMIA.* 2021;*28*(5):967–973. doi:10.1093/jamia/ocaa274

6. Downing NL, Bates DW, Longhurst CA. Physician burnout in the electronic health record era: are we ignoring the real cause? *Ann Intern Med.* 2018 July;*169*(1):50–51. https://doi.org/10.7326/M18-0139

7. Adler-Milstein J, Zhao W, Willard-Grace R, Knox M, Grumbach K. Electronic health records and burnout: time spent on the electronic health record after hours and message volume associated with exhaustion but not with cynicism among primary care clinicians. *JAMIA.* 2020;*27*(4):531–538. doi:10.1093/jamia/ocz220

8. National Academies of Sciences, Engineering, and Medicine. *Taking Action Against Clinician Burnout: A Systems Approach to Professional Well-Being.* National Academies Press; 2019. Accessed March 22, 2021. https://doi.org/10.17226/25521

9. Shanafelt TD, Dyrbye LN, Sinsky C, et al. Relationship between clerical burden and characteristics of the electronic environment with physician burnout and professional satisfaction. *Mayo Clin Proc.* 2016;*91*(7),836–848. doi:10.1016/j.mayocp.2016.05.007

10. Arndt BG, Beasley JW, Watkinson MD, et al. Tethered to the EHR: primary care physician work-load assessment using EHR event log data and time-motion observations. *Ann Fam Med.* 2017;*15*(5):419–426. doi:10.1370/afm.2121

11. Sinsky C, Colligan L, Li L, et al. Allocation of physician time in ambulatory practice: a time and motion study in 4 specialties. *Ann Intern Med.* 2016;*165*(11):753–760. doi:10.7326/M16-0961.

12. Chen L, Guo U, Illipparambil LC, et al. Racing against the clock: internal medicine residents' time spent on electronic health records. *J Grad Med Educ.* 2016;*8*(1):39–44. https://doi.org/10.4300/JGME-D-15-00240.1

13. Gold M, McLaughlin C. Assessing HITECH implementation and lessons 5 years later. *Milbank Q.* 2016;*94*(3):654–687.

14. Johnson C, Pylypchuk Y. Use of certified health IT and methods to enable interoperability by U.S. non-federal acute care hospitals, 2019. ONC Data Brief, no.54. Office of the National Coordinator for Health Information Technology. Published January 2021. Accessed April 26, 2021. https://www.healthit.gov/sites/default/files/page/2021-02/Use-of-Certified-Health-IT-and-Methods-to-Enable-Interoperabil ity-by-U.S.-Non-Federal-Acute-Care-Hospitals-2019.pdf

15. Melnick ER, Dyrbye LN, Sinsky CA, et al. The association between perceived electronic health record usability and professional burnout among US physicians. *Mayo Clin Proc.* 2020;95(3):476–487. doi:10.1016/j.mayocp.2019.09.024

16. Shah T, Kitts AB, Gold JA, et al. EHR optimization and clinician well-being: a potential roadmap toward action. Discussion Paper, National Academy of Medicine. Published August 3, 2020. Accessed March 22, 2021. https://doi.org/10.31478/202008a

17. Flodgren G, Rachas A, Farmer AJ, Inzitari M, Shepperd S. Interactive telemedicine: effects on professional practice and health care outcomes. *Cochrane Database Syst Rev.* 2015;9:Cd002098. doi:10.1002/14651858.CD002098.pub2

18. Totten AM, McDonagh MS, Wagner JH. The evidence base for telehealth: reassurance in the face of rapid expansion during the COVID-19 pandemic. White paper commentary. AHRQ Publication No. 20-EHC015. Published May 14, 2020. Accessed March 22, 2021. https://doi.org/10.23970/AHRQEPC COVIDTELEHEALTH.

19. Ruiz Morilla MD, Sans M, Casasa A, Giménez N. Implementing technology in healthcare: insights from physicians. *BMC Med Inform Decis Mak.* 2017;17(1):92. doi:10.1186/s12911-017-0489-2

20. Sorenson G. 3 ways telemedicine reduces provider burnout. *Physicians Weekly.* July 20, 2018. Accessed March 22, 2020. https://www.physiciansweekly.com/3-ways-telemedicine-reduces-provider-burnout/

21. Verma, S. Early impact of CMS expansion of medicare telehealth during COVID-19. *Health Affairs.* Published July 15, 2020. Accessed March 22, 2021. doi:10.1377/hblog20200715.454789

22. FAIR Health. Monthly telehealth regional tracker completes full year of data. *FAIR Health Access.* Published March 18, 2021. Accessed March 22, 2021. https://www.fairhealth.org/article/monthly-tel ehealth-regional-tracker-completes-full-year-of-data

23. Hollander JE, Carr BG. 2020. Virtually perfect? Telemedicine for Covid-19. *N Engl J Med.* 2020;382(18):1679–1681. doi:10.1056/NEJMp2003539

24. Association of American Medical Colleges. Innovations in health technology: telehealth. 2021. Accessed March 22, 2021. https://www.aamc.org/news-insights/innovations-health-technology-telehealth

25. Centers for Medicare and Medicaid Services. Medicare telemedicine health care provider fact sheet. CMS. Published March 17, 2020. Accessed March 22, 2021. https://www.cms.gov/newsroom/fact-she ets/medicare-telemedicine-health-care-provider-fact-sheet

26. Cohen JK. House health panel chair says it's time to make Medicare telehealth permanent. *Modern Healthcare.* Published March 2, 2021. Accessed April 26, 2021. https://www.modernhealthcare.com/politics-policy/house-health-panel-chair-says-its-time-make-medicare-telehealth-permanent

27. Topol EJ. High-performance medicine: the convergence of human and artificial intelligence. *Nature Medicine.* 2019;25:44–56. https://doi.org/10.1038/s41591-018-0300-7

28. U.S. Government Accountability Office. *Artificial Intelligence in Health Care: Benefits and Challenges of Technologies to Augment Patient Care.* Publication GAO-21-7SP. Published November 26, 2020. Accessed April 26, 2021. https://www.gao.gov/assets/gao-21-7sp.pdf

29. Lin SY, Shanafelt DS, Asch SM. Reimagining clinical documentation with artificial intelligence. *Mayo Clin Proc,* 2018;93(5):563–565. https://doi.org/10.1016/j.mayocp.2018.02.016

30. Halamka J, Cerrato P. The digital reconstruction of healthcare. *NEJM Catalyst.* 2020;1(6). Accessed December 20, 2022. https://catalyst.nejm.org/doi/full/10.1056/CAT.20.0082

31. Kelly CJ, Karthikesalingam A, Suleyman M, Corrado G, King D. Key challenges for delivering clinical impact with artificial intelligence. *BMC Medicine.* 2019;17:195. https://doi.org/10.1186/s12 916-019-1426-2

32. Annapureddy AR, Angraal S, Caraballo C, et al. The National Institutes of Health funding for clinical research applying machine learning techniques in 2017. *NPJ Digit Med.* 2020;3:13. https://doi.org/10.1038/s41746-020-0223-9

33. Peterson ED. Machine learning, predictive analytics, and clinical practice, can the past inform the present? *JAMA.* 2019;322(23):2283–2284. doi:10.1001/jama.2019.17831

34. Gettinger A, Zayas-Caban T. HITECH to 21st century cures: clinical burden and evolving health IT policy. *JAMIA.* 2021;28(5):1022–1025. doi:10.1093/jamia/ocaa330

35. Blumenthal D. Launching HITECH. *N Engl J Med.* 2010;362(5):382–385. doi:10.1056/NEJMp0912825

36. 21st Century Cures Act, Pub. L. No. 114-255, 130 Stat. 1033.2016. Accessed December 20, 2022. https://www.congress.gov/114/plaws/publ255/PLAW-114publ255.pdf

37. Office of the National Coordinator for Health Information Technology. 2020. Strategy on reducing regulatory and administrative burden relating to the use of health IT and EHRs: final report. Published February 2020. Accessed April 26, 2021. https://www.healthit.gov/sites/default/files/page/2020-02/BurdenReport_0.pdf

38. Sinsky C, Linzer M. Practice and policy reset post-COVID-19: reversion, transition, or transformation? *Health Affairs.* 2020;*39*(8):1405–1411. doi:10.1377/hlthaff.2020.00612

39. Centers for Medicare and Medicaid Services. Telehealth: delivering care safely during COVID-19. HHS.gov Coronavirus website. Published July 15, 2020. Accessed March 22, 2021. https://www.hhs.gov/coronavirus/telehealth/index.html.

40. U.S. Food and Drug Administration. Artificial intelligence/machine learning (AI/ML)-based software as a medical device (SaMD) action plan. Published January 2021. Accessed March 22, 2021. https://www.fda.gov/medical-devices/software-medical-device-samd/artificial-intelligence-and-machine-learning-software-medical-device

41. Gerke S, Babic B, Evgeniou T, Cohen G. The need for a system view to regulate artificial intelligence/machine learning-based software as a medical device. *NPJ Digit Med.* 2020;*3*:53. https://doi.org/10.1038/s41746-020-0262-2

42. DeJong BA, Lucey CR, Adams Dudley R. Incorporating a new technology while doing no harm, virtually. *JAMA.* 2015;*314*(22):2351–2352. doi:10.1001/jama.2015.13572

43. Eberly LA, Kallan MJ, Julien HM, et al. Patient characteristics associated with telemedicine access for primary and specialty ambulatory care during the COVID-19 pandemic. *JAMA Network Open.* 2020;*3*(12):e2031640. doi:10.1001/jamanetworkopen.2020.31640

44. Obermeyer Z, Powers B, Vogeli C, Mullainathan S. Dissecting racial bias in an algorithm used to manage the health of populations. *Science.* 2019;*366*(6464):447–453. doi:10.1126/science.aax2342

45. Ganguli I, Gordon WJ, Lupo C, et al. Machine learning and the pursuit of high-value health care. *NEJM Catalyst.* 2020;*1*(6). Accessed December 20, 2022. https://catalyst.nejm.org/doi/full/10.1056/CAT.20.0094

46. Eaneff S, Obermeyer Z, Butte AJ. The case for algorithmic stewardship for artificial intelligence and machine learning technologies. *JAMA.* 2020;*324*(14):1397–1398. doi:10.1001/jama.2020.9371

47. Matheny M, Thadaney Israni S, Ahmed M, Whicher D, eds. *Artificial Intelligence in Health Care: The Hope, the Hype, the Promise, the Peril.* NAM Special Publication. National Academy of Medicine; 2019. Accessed April 26, 2021. https://nam.edu/wp-content/uploads/2019/12/AI-in-Health-Care-PREPUB-FINAL.pdf

48. Verghese A, Shah NH, Harrington RA. What this computer needs is a physician: humanism and artificial intelligence. *JAMA.* 2018;*319*(1):19–20. doi:10.1001/jama.2017.19198

49. Ripp JA, Privitera MR, West CP, et al. Well-being in graduate medical education: call to action. *Acad Med.* 2017;*92*(7):914–917. doi:10.1097/ACM.0000000000001735

50. Wartman SA. The empirical challenge of 21st-century medical education. *Acad Med.* 2019;*94*(10):1412–1415. doi:10.1097/ACM.0000000000002866

51. Mohan V, Scholl G, Gold JA. Intelligent simulation model to facilitate EHR training. *AMIA Annu Symp Proc.* 2015;*2015*: 925–932. PMID: 26958229; PMCID: PMC4765600. Accessed April 26, 2021. https://www.ncbi.nlm.nih.gov/pmc/articles/PMC4765600/.

52. Galpin K, Sikka N, King SL, Horvath KA, Shipman SA, AAMC Telehealth Advisory Committee. Expert consensus: telehealth skills for health care professionals. *Telemedicine and e-Health.* 2020. doi:10.1089/tmj.2020.0420. Epub ahead of print. PMID: 33236964.

53. Association of American Medical Colleges (AAMC). *Telehealth Competencies Across the Learning Continuum.* AAMC New and Emerging Areas in Medicine Series. 2021. Accessed April 26, 2021. https://store.aamc.org/telehealth-competencies-across-the-learning-continuum.html.

54. McCoy LG, Nagaraj S, Morgado F, Harish V, Das S, Celi LA. What do medical students actually need to know about artificial intelligence? *NJP Digit Med.* 2020;*3*:86. https://doi.org/10.1038/s41746-020-0294-7

55. Cutillo CM, Sharma KR, Foschini L, Kundu S, Mackintosh M, Mandl KD, MI in Healthcare Workshop Working Group. Machine intelligence in healthcare: perspectives on trustworthiness, explainability, usability, and transparency. *NJP Digit Med.* 2020;*3*:47. https://doi.org/10.1038/s41746-020-0254-2

56. Rudin RS, Fisher SH, Damberg CL, et al. Optimizing health IT to improve health system performance: a work in progress. *Healthcare*. 2020;8(4):100483. Accessed December 8, 2020. https://doi.org/10.1016/j.hjdsi.2020.100483.

57. Zayas-Cabán T, Wald JS. Opportunities for the use of health information technology to support research. *JAMIA Open*. 2020;3(3):321–325. https://doi.org/10.1093/jamiaopen/ooaa037

58. Horvath K, Sengstack P, Opelka F, et al. A vision for a person-centered health information system. Discussion paper, National Academy of Medicine. Published October 1, 2018. Accessed December 20, 2022. https://doi.org/10.31478/201810a

Institutional Responses and the Role of the Chief Wellness Officer

Jonathan A. Ripp, Sharon Kiely, and Amy Frieman

Introduction

Academic health centers are complex ecosystems with a broad array of diverse, interdependent, and specialized groups and entities that contribute to each organization's purpose and mission. In turn, these ecosystems influence the well-being of learners in their midst. As the complexity of these systems of care has increased over the past several decades, so, too, have the experiences of medical students and graduate medical education (GME) trainees become more complex. Consequently, institutional well-being efforts can significantly impact medical student and GME trainee well-being. Many organizations are beginning to address the well-being of these constituents through large-scale institutional commitments.

Historically, efforts to address medical student and GME trainee well-being have been organized within a traditional undergraduate/graduate medical education (UME/ GME) administrative leadership structure. However, as recognition of the importance of the well-being of the entire health care workforce has emerged, an increasing number of institutions have committed to larger institution-level well-being responses coordinated in partnership with UME/GME leadership. In the authors' experience, such institutional commitments to structural and operational change declare the importance of well-being and establish the expectation of a culture and strategy that broadly support well-being for the total enterprise. To be effective, the message of support needs to be coupled with resources, such as an institutional leader and a team with clear roles and responsibilities for the integration of well-being into the organization's vision, strategy, and operations. In this chapter, we discuss well-being within organizational decision-making, important institutional considerations for well-being, and the role of the institutional well-being leader, using the example of the emerging Chief Wellness Officer (CWO) position, based on the literature about this emerging role and experience of the authors.

The Importance of Including Well-Being in Strategic Planning

As described in Chapter 11, the aspirational state of organizational competency in well-being means that an institution integrates well-being considerations into all major organizational decisions and strategies. Institutional strategy can translate into institutional decisions that directly impact both medical students and GME trainees. Operational changes in staffing, support services, space considerations, and policy will impact the day-to-day and long-term experience and well-being of students and GME trainees. Including a well-being leader and expert within an institution's leadership structure may help guide the allocation of budgetary and operational resources in a way that optimizes employee, student, and GME trainee well-being. Implementation of major strategic initiatives without considering the effects on and needs of the health care workforce may exacerbate well-being challenges within an organization. An institutional leader who can view such changes through the lens of well-being can help mitigate the negative impacts and optimize the positive impacts of such strategic operational decisions.

The example below from one author's experience helps to illustrate the importance of consideration of simultaneous impacts of initiatives on well-being across the health system.

A health system planned and built a new replacement bed tower with an inadequate number of call rooms and no resident lounges within the structure. Workflows used to design the new space considered the location of emergency equipment, but did not factor in the travel time of house staff response teams. Existing call rooms, lounges, and workstations were 10–15 minutes away from the new care areas. Therefore, in order to be accessible at night, house staff resorted to using patient family lounges, nursing offices, and unoccupied nurse stations in the new building, often sleeping in chairs and leaving pillows, sheets, and trash behind. For GME trainees, this strategy of sleeping in spaces that were not intended for this purpose was a necessary measure to ensure the effectiveness of their role and responsibilities. However, this activity was perceived by administration as disrespectful and resulted in the need for extra cleaning staff time and unanticipated budgetary expenses. Ultimately, access to these areas was restricted for house staff, resulting in significant friction between GME trainees and hospital leadership.

It was not until some time later that the results of a house staff well-being survey revealed the impact and unintended consequences of these operational changes on the GME training experience. Ultimately, a resolution was achieved regarding space for residents to work closer to patient care areas. This particular challenge presented an opportunity for the institutional well-being leader to uncover the root cause of a problem, which enabled a solution to emerge.

Considerations for Institution-Level Well-Being Support for Medical Students and GME Trainees

A number of important considerations may inform an institution-level response to well-being and have an impact on the medical student and GME trainee experience.

First, the complexity and scope of the work needed to address medical student and GME trainee well-being requires effort and a leader with well-being expertise, especially in organizations with multiple care sites, levels of learners, and abundant educational and training programs. The CWO can provide advocacy and assess needs within programs while supporting and encouraging local program innovation and outcomes. As someone with a high-level view of the progress of individual programs over time, the CWO can expertly guide organizational performance.

Second, the CWO can help align medical student and GME trainee well-being with other professions and groups within an organization. For example, learners require a faculty supervisor as part of a care team. Faculty well-being, and the well-being of the entire care team, impact patient care, quality and safety, and the learner experience. Coherent alignment between the medical student and GME trainee well-being philosophy and that of the faculty, as well as other members of the health care professional team, can help drive the organization forward while modeling behaviors and skills to students and GME trainees. The CWO can serve as a go-between to ensure alignment of initiatives across professions and aim to avoid unintended consequences.

Third, the institutional leader for well-being can facilitate alignment between medical student and GME trainee environments and other operational areas. For example, a learner's experience of the adequacy of work space and lockers and lounges is an opportunity for collaboration. The CWO is familiar with the needs of the medical student and GME trainee as well as the process for resource allocation that might lead to addressing work space considerations. The CWO can serve as the liaison familiar with the intersection of these domains and thereby facilitate a smoother approach.

Institutional Resources to Support Well-Being

While there are a host of ways in which a hospital, school, or health system can commit to the well-being of a defined group of constituents, ultimately a commitment and dedication of resources will be necessary to have real impact. Perhaps what is most important is not necessarily the level of commitment, but rather the commitment itself. Institutions will have varying ability in terms of the scope of resources that can be dedicated to the well-being of their constituents. To ensure success, resources directed to the well-being effort must be commensurate with the size of the group for which the efforts are intended and, in turn, the expected deliverables of the well-being leader or team organizing the effort. Furthermore, the visibility and marketing of the dedicated resources themselves can have a salutary effect on the intended constituents, who may come to realize that their place of work or learning is truly serious about addressing their needs, essentially "putting money where their mouth is."

A school or hospital very likely will already have made some level of commitment to well-being, yet may be limited in its ability to make substantial further commitments for a host of reasons, including limited financial flexibility, lack of significant leadership prioritization, or competing interests of the organization. Barriers to greater levels of dedicated support will always exist. This reality is common to any institutional priority and not limited to well-being initiatives. Well-being stakeholders from small institutions may feel daunted or even defeated from the outset, especially when comparing their resources with the commitments they observe made at larger organizations. This comparison should not serve as a deterrent: what is most important is diagnosing the stage of commitment and readiness for change in one's own environment and creating a clear goal for the level of commitment needed to move further along the continuum from novice to expert, toward a more robust well-being program.[1]

Designating an Institutional Well-Being Leader

Should every school, hospital, or health system focus on the naming of a CWO as the example of the highest level of institutional commitment to well-being? While the naming of a CWO who is appropriately positioned and empowered to meet the well-being needs of an organization is a highly effective way to advance a systematic approach to promoting well-being and professional fulfillment of the intended constituents, establishing this role is not the only way for an institution to demonstrate real and intentional commitment. Furthermore, naming a CWO who is not enabled to do the work is, in many ways, a worse situation because the institution is saying that it is committed without actually creating a real opportunity for positive change. Such an approach potentially may lead to even more cynicism and an erosion of trust in the institution. While there are other models through which this work can be completed, tasking this volume of work to an individual CWO is an effective and efficient means to see the job done. If the institutional resources and will exist to establish a CWO, the role and responsibilities of this institutional leader will more likely be achievable. Should an institution decide to invest in a CWO, that individual can be highly effective in supporting other medical student and GME well-being leaders within the institution to positively impact learner well-being.

Role and Responsibilities of a Chief Wellness Officer

The system-level CWO executive is responsible for measuring, improving, and advocating for well-being in strategic and operational organizational decisions. The individual collaborates with system leadership and can amplify institutional initiatives that have the potential to optimize well-being. Most important is the unique expertise of operational impacts on well-being that the CWO brings to the executive leadership team. Since well-being is a relatively new emphasis in health care organizations, other executives can learn from the CWO as the subject matter expert. With day-to-day access, influence, and collaboration, the CWO can amplify and influence other executive-level work through the lens of well-being. The CWO, like the Chief Financial Officer (CFO) or Chief Nursing Officer (CNO), has a unique perspective on the differences between the impact and intent of key operational decisions on well-being and is the organization's visible commitment to the culture of well-being.

Necessary Skills and Authority

While the role of the CWO in health care organizations is relatively new, it has seen significant growth and attention since the appointment of the first health care CWO at Stanford in 2017. Organizations have clearly recognized the need for such a role, which aims to reduce burnout and increase professional fulfillment among clinicians while ideally creating a return on investment. The goal of the CWO is to facilitate "system-wide changes, including the implementation of evidence-based interventions that enable clinicians to effectively practice in a culture that prioritizes and promotes their well-being."[2]

Historically, the role of the non-health care corporate CWO has in part been to decrease organizational health insurance costs through the creation of well-being programs meant to improve the health of employees using initiatives like nutrition, physical fitness, and mindfulness. The role of the health care CWO role differs significantly from that paradigm. Rather than focusing on changing individuals, the CWO in health care focuses on improving the clinician experience by making structural changes to the organization. "The goal of this work is to address what is wrong with the practice environment, not to make individuals better able to tolerate a broken system."[3] The CWO role focuses less on individual-level self-care interventions and more on organizational-level interventions to improve the clinician experience.

As such, a CWO should be a senior C-suite level leader within the organization who has the power and authority to implement change and drive strategies that improve clinician well-being. The CWO should report to a top executive in the organization, typically a CEO, dean, or president, in order to be truly integrated into the leadership team and able to effect change. Additionally, in order to achieve success, it is necessary for the CWO to be provided with the budget and resources to perform the work. The broader the scope of responsibility, the greater the resources needed to allow for success.[2]

While expertise in well-being is important, to be successful the CWO must also have significant leadership experience, knowledge of quality improvement efforts, and an understanding of how organizations function.[4] These qualities and experience are critically important because the CWO must navigate the C-suite in order to truly effect change within an organization. The role requires strong communication skills and a high level of emotional intelligence to negotiate on behalf of the clinician experience and stand between the clinical teams and other members of the C-suite. This is a position that absolutely requires finesse and political acumen.

Collaborators and Stakeholder Relationships

Serving as a member of the senior executive leadership team, the CWO must collaborate closely with a host of stakeholders (Box 16.1), including executives such as the CEO, CNO, Chief Medical Officer (CMO), Chief Medical Information Officer (CMIO), Chief Quality Officer (CQO), Chief Human Resources Officer (CHRO), and others, in order to effectively implement change. Every high-level decision made by the organization should take into account the downstream effect that it might have on the experience of the clinical team. Working as an advocate for improving the clinician experience, the CWO must possess effective leadership skills. To achieve success at prioritizing engagement and professional fulfillment along with the mitigation of burnout, the CWO must align and collaborate with other organizational components that have ties to well-being.

As an example, the CWO must collaborate and work in a complementary fashion with human resources. Though the focus of the CWO is not on developing insurance benefits or individually focused self-care resources, it is important to consider these factors as potential elements of a robust well-being program. The human resources/benefits team within an organization often develops initiatives and programming focused on improving the physical and emotional health of employees, particularly as they relate to insurance claims and costs. The relationship between the benefits team and the CWO can be an area of complementarity in which partnership can be a strength for both parties. Behavioral health leaders within an organization also make excellent allies and

---

BOX 16.1 Example Institutional Stakeholders and Collaborators for the CWO

- Chief Executive Officer (CEO)
- Chief Medical Officer (CMO)
- Chief Medical Information Officer (CMIO)
- Chief Diversity Officer (CDO)
- Chief Nursing Officer (CNO)
- Chief Quality Officer (CQO)
- Chief Human Resources Officer (CHRO)
- Chief Experience Officer (CXO)
- Chief Information Officer (CIO)
- Chief Human Resources Officer (CHRO)
- Organizational Effectiveness and Operations Leaders
- Psychiatry/Behavioral Health Leaders

partners for the CWO, affording the ability to leverage existing resources and develop new programming aimed at improving clinician well-being, particularly as it pertains to emotional and psychological health. The destigmatization of mental health issues and care-seeking is more important than ever as the COVID pandemic has had clear psychological consequences on health care teams.[5] Organizational effectiveness and talent development teams are another group of potential collaborators for the CWO, with coaching and leadership development as key methods to improve clinician engagement. Information technology (IT) and quality improvement teams are also key strategic partners to make which, when leveraged, can assist the CWO in successfully implementing important operations-level change strategies.

Scope of Responsibility

The responsibilities of the CWO should be clearly established from the outset. Most importantly, the scope of constituents served through the intended role should be clearly defined. CWOs in different health care organizations oversee well-being efforts for different groups. A 2019 survey of 21 CWOs conducted through the Collaborative for Healing and Renewal in Medicine (CHARM) CWO Network demonstrated that 95.2% of CWOs were responsible for efforts to advance well-being that included practicing physicians, 76.2% included residents and fellows, 42.9% included medical students, and 42.9% included biomedical scientist faculty. With respect to non-physicians, 76.2% of surveyed CWOs were responsible for efforts to advance well-being for advanced practice providers (nurse practitioners and physician assistants), whereas fewer than half (38.1%), were responsible for nurses and other clinicians (e.g., pharmacists, physical therapists, and respiratory technicians) and 28.6% for nonclinical employees (information technology, administrative staff, and custodial staff).[6] It is necessary for the extent of constituent groups to be clearly defined to avoid scope creep over time and to determine the focus of the CWO's efforts from the start.

Important to note is that as the CWO raises the awareness of the well-being needs for one group, it is likely that members of other disciplines or segments of the workforce will begin to request an equal level of support. The CWO must be prepared for these requests and avoid increasing scope of work without a commensurate increase in the resources needed to accomplish the expanded responsibility. Whether the CWO focuses on physicians alone or includes other members of the clinical team or even nonclinical team members, to be successful, levels of resourcing and budget must match the scope of the role.

While it is tempting for the CWO to try to take on all aspects of well-being, it is important to specify focus areas, initiatives, and tactics for success. The strategy might include a limited number of long-term focus areas that will undergo minimal change year to year, even as the tactics to advance that dimension of the strategy change.[7] Prior to implementation of a strategic plan, it is advisable to undertake an assessment of the current state of well-being within an organization, determining where both best practices and gaps exist. The CWO will aim to coordinate, integrate, and support existing well-being initiatives while determining what pieces are missing that still need to be developed. This initial needs assessment and gap analysis can help inform a plan for moving forward, including specific areas of focus.

Key Responsibilities
Strategic Planning Responsibilities
The strategic plan of the CWO will likely include both operational and organizational interventions to advance a culture and environment of well-being. These initiatives might include improving practice efficiencies, optimizing workloads, addressing work–life integration, reviewing staffing practices to ensure multidisciplinary teamwork that decreases clerical burden, and collaborating with IT partners to improve the end-user experience of the electronic health record. Other initiatives might include working toward creating true community and collegiality between health care professionals, leadership development through coaching or other programs, and the development of support services for clinicians in distress.[3] The role that the CWO plays in supporting the emotional well-being of the team has been greatly amplified by the experience of the COVID-19 pandemic, which highlighted the immediate well-being needs of the workforce. As such, the CWO must work closely with behavioral health partners to ensure that emotional and psychological supports are in place and that the clinical team is aware of these services. Additionally, the CWO also often works with institutional partners to help break down the stigma associated with care-seeking.

Oversight of Measurement of Well-Being as an Organizational Metric
Often the role of the CWO includes well-being measurement. As described in detail in Chapter 2, a variety of dimensions of well-being can be assessed, including but not limited to burnout, engagement, professional fulfilment/satisfaction, fatigue, emotional health/stress, and various dimensions of well-being/quality of life.[8] Whether assessing well-being, burnout, engagement, or all of the above, the CWO often strives to make well-being one of the key performance indicators of interest to the organization. Measurements should be tracked over time and compared with national benchmarks. This tracking allows for the development of directed programming that addresses specific problem areas, locations, or constituents within an organization. In keeping with the role to capture these measurements, the CWO advocates for accountability of these outcomes. While the CWO is responsible for developing the strategy and plan for improving well-being across the organization, the CWO alone cannot be held solely responsible for well-being outcome. Achieving well-being requires input and action from leaders across all aspects of an organization.

Supporting Compliance with Regulatory Requirements for Well-Being

In academic settings, the CWO needs to collaborate with leaders of both undergraduate and graduate medical education, including designated institutional officials (DIOs), residency and fellowship program directors, and medical school leadership. Among other things, these relationships help facilitate the accreditation and regulatory process for educational programming. As described in detail in Chapter 10, both GME and UME have regulatory requirements related to well-being. According to Section VI of the Accreditation Council for Graduate Medical Education (ACGME) Common Program Requirements for all accredited residency and fellowship programs, "psychological, emotional, and physical well-being are critical in the development of the competent, caring, and resilient physician and require proactive attention to life inside and outside of medicine."[9] Furthermore, the Liaison Committee on Medical Education (LCME) requires that medical schools have "an effective system of personal counseling for its medical students that includes programs to promote their well-being and to facilitate their adjustment to the physical and emotional demands of medical education."[10] The CWO plays a key role in advocating for the well-being of students, GME trainees, and faculty by collaborating and coordinating with other senior leadership focused on these initiatives. As such, the CWO can serve as a strong voice for implementing, standardizing, and championing well-being programming to ensure that best practices are achieved at all levels.

Alignment Between the CWO and UME and GME Well-Being Leaders

Many academic institutions have designated UME and GME well-being leaders. These UME or GME well-being leaders and the CWO or institutional well-being leader need to coordinate their efforts. While the position of the CWO in the organization can support the UME or GME well-being leader to have greater effectiveness, the mandate of the UME or GME well-being leader can in turn support the CWO's. This synergy can manifest in a variety of ways. For instance, the CWO, often versed in the language of operational metrics, can help drive the development and implementation of assessment tools to measure well-being for use across constituencies, thereby alleviating the UME or GME leader from needing to specifically address these responsibilities themselves. Furthermore, the resources needed to analyze data and report out on collected well-being survey result metrics can be leveraged across multiple constituent groups beyond just GME and UME, even leading the organization to appreciate a cost savings. Each institution is structured slightly differently, so the exact organizational chart for these relationships and reporting structures will depend on those institutional structures. An example of the situation of GME well-being leadership within the context of the organization as a whole is illustrated in Figure 16.1.

Certain strategic initiatives promoted by the CWO's office may also benefit multiple constituent groups, thereby demonstrating a benefit for all. For example, an effort to

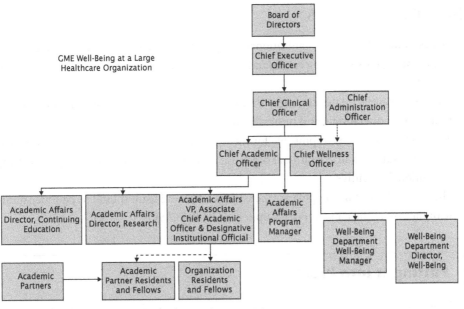

*Solid lines represent direct ACGME well-being compliance oversight
*Dotted lines represent indirect ACGME well-being compliance oversight

FIGURE 16.1 Example location of graduate medical education (GME) well-being within the organizational reporting structure of a large health care organization.

promote wellness-centered leadership training curricula for students and GME trainees may translate into trainings for other nursing and physician leaders.[11] Such a resource could easily be offered specifically to GME or UME leaders as well. In turn, the CWO also benefits from the work of the GME or UME well-being leader when the well-being needs of the UME and GME communities translate into benefits that can be experienced by other groups. In many institutions, for example, as a result of regulatory requirements, certain efforts or resources might already exist to address the well-being needs of GME and UME constituents. Often once the needs of a given group within a system are addressed, the effort serves to shine a light on the gap in attention directed at other constituencies within an organization. The CWO can leverage that attention to bring resources to other groups in need.

Conclusion

A talented and directed institutional well-being leader, such as a CWO, can lead a strong organizational effort to improve well-being. Initiatives that target and bolster the well-being needs of medical student and GME trainees have the ability to support and strengthen the mission of the CWO across an organization. Partnership with and between UME and GME leaders can result in a system that truly embraces well-being and greatly enhance the experience of students and GME trainees.

Summary Points

- The aspirational state of organizational competency in well-being means that an institution integrates well-being considerations into all major organizational decisions and strategies.
- The CWO can facilitate alignment between UME and GME trainee environments as well as other operational and professional domains.
- The CWO executive is responsible for measuring, improving, and advocating for well-being in strategic and operational organizational decisions and should report to a top institutional executive.
- The level of budgetary support for the CWO's office and team should be commensurate with the size of the constituent group served by the CWO.

Putting It into Practice

- Consider your organization's reporting structure. Is there a designated well-being leader? If one were established, consider where that person would sit within your organizational structure.
- Consider how your organization's structure facilitates or inhibits collaboration around important well-being initiatives and what changes to supports or structure may be helpful in reducing any barriers.
- Clearly define the scope of work and stakeholder populations for institutional well-being leaders.

References

1. Shanafelt T, Goh J, Sinsky C. The business case for investing in physician well-being. *JAMA Intern Med.* 2017;177(12):1826–1832. doi:10.1001/jamainternmed.2017.4340
2. Kishore S, Ripp J, Shanafelt T, et al. Making the case for the chief wellness officer in America's health systems: a call to action. *Health Affairs Blog.* Published October 26, 2018. Accessed February 28, 2021. doi:10.1377/hblog20181025.308059
3. Ripp J, Shanafelt T. The health care chief wellness officer: what the role is and is not. *Acad Med.* 2020 Sep;95(9):1354–1358. doi:10.1097/acm.0000000000003433.
4. Shanafelt, T, Sinsky, C. Establishing a chief wellness officer position: create the organizational groundwork for professional well-being. *AMA STEPS Forward.* Published June 25, 2020. Accessed February 28, 2021. https://edhub.ama-assn.org/steps-forward/module/2767739.
5. Feingold, Jordyn H., et al. Psychological impact of the COVID-19 pandemic on frontline health care workers during the pandemic surge in New York City. *Chronic Stress.* 2021;5: 2470547020977891.
6. Shanafelt, T, Farley, H, Wang, H, Ripp, J. Responsibilities and job characteristics of healthcare chief wellness officers in the United States. *Mayo Clin Proc.* 2020;95(11):2557–2572. doi:10.1016/j.mayocp.2020.09.004
7. Shanafelt, T, Sinsky, C. Chief wellness officer road map: implement a leadership strategy for professional well-being. *AMA STEPS Forward.* Published June 25, 2021. Accessed February 28, 2021.https://edhub.ama-assn.org/steps-forward/module/2767764.

8. Shanafelt, T, Noseworthy, J. Executive leadership and physician well-being: nine organizational strategies to promote engagement and reduce burnout. *Mayo Clin Proc.* 2017;92(1):129–146.

9. Accreditation Council for Graduate Medical Education. Common program requirements (residency). Published February 3, 2020. Accessed February 28, 2021. https://www.acgme.org/What-We-Do/Accreditation/Common-Program-Requirements

10. Liaison Committee on Medical Education. Functions and structure of a medical school: standards for accreditation of medical education programs leading to the MD degree. Published March 2020. Accessed February 28, 2021. https://lcme.org/publications/

11. Shanafelt T, Trockel M, Rodriguez A, Logan D. Wellness-centered leadership: equipping health care leaders to cultivate physician well-being and professional fulfillment. *Acad Med.* 2021;96(5):641–651. doi:10.1097/ACM.0000000000003907

Advocating for Physician Well-Being at the Societal Level

Christine A. Sinsky and Alexandra M. Ristow

Introduction

The Case for Advocacy

Physician burnout is a high-level metric that reflects the quality and stability of the US health care system, serving as both a leading and lagging indicator. One of the most important drivers of physician satisfaction is the ability to deliver high-quality care. When this ability is thwarted, physician burnout increases. Thus, a high level of physician burnout is a leading indicator of dysfunction within the health care system. Conversely, when physicians are burned out, access and quality of care are in turn diminished, and thus physician burnout is also a lagging indicator.[1-3]

Physician burnout is driven primarily by the external environment, rather than individual personal factors, and is influenced by the broader policy, regulatory, technological, and practice environments in which care is delivered.[4-8] Therefore, helping to create the conditions in which clinician burnout is diminished and where health care professional joy, purpose, and meaning in work are optimized is a shared responsibility among multiple stakeholders within the health care community, including policymakers, regulators, standard setters, measure developers, payers, technology vendors, and local institutional leaders.

What can be done to reduce burnout and increase joy? This question serves as the rallying cry for advocacy efforts at multiple levels within the medical community. There is cause for optimism, with accelerating activity among multiple stakeholders working within their spheres of influence to reduce burnout and increase joy in medicine.

The Role of Advocacy in Medical Student and GME Trainee Well-Being

A successful training program prepares physicians-in-training to meet the challenges of medical practice. Traditionally, this has meant arming physicians with medical knowledge, clinical reasoning acumen, and procedural skills. To combat the crisis of physician burnout, physicians must be equipped with a new set of tools: the knowledge of best practices for preventing burnout, a framework for critical thinking about practice environment and workflow, the skills to lead a multidisciplinary team, self-compassion, the ability to create a culture of vulnerability within work units, and "wellness-centered leadership."[9] Advocates for physician well-being at the societal level have been honing these tools for years.[10-12] Exposure to this advocacy work can prepare health care learners for joyful practice both during and after training through multiple mechanisms described below.

1. *Improving clinical experience during training.* Advocacy has informed best practices for creating an effective and nonchaotic clinical environment. By integrating these practices into training clinics,[13] leaders can promote professionally satisfying clinical practice during training.

2. *Improving clinical experience after training.* Medical students and GME trainees absorb the norms of the clinical practice in which they train, whether or not they are explicitly taught those norms. If they train in a "hero-model" system where the practice is chaotic and undersupported, where the physician is expected to compensate for a disorganized environment, and where physician well-being is neglected, this will influence heir expectations and habits. In contrast, medical students and GME trainees whose skills are honed in a high-functioning clinical environment learn how strong organizations can incorporate the quadruple aim[14] into their practice, developing skills such as team leadership and delegation while learning how to identify and proactively choose functional and supportive clinical environments when they enter the job market.

3. *Building community.* Exposure to the individuals and organizations working to improve physician well-being can provide learners with allies as they face challenges and frustrations, and it can engender a sense of community and optimism about the future of medicine.

4. *Providing resources.* Advocates have created educational resources[15] that learners can rely on both during and after training. From tips on leading team huddles, to suggestions for improving workflows, to inspirational stories about organizational efforts to improve physician satisfaction, these resources can teach important individual skills and institutional innovations that enhance well-being.

5. *Empowering trainees.* Understanding how advocacy works can empower medical students and GME trainees to become advocates themselves, whether during school and

GME training or after entry into the workforce. Participating in advocacy not only develops a new skill set which these trainees can bring into their workplaces; it also serves to enhance a sense of autonomy and optimism about medical practice.

The Levers of Advocacy

One can consider four levers to improve the US health care system's ability to care for its physician caregivers: research, activation, resources, and workforce demand (Figure 17.1). For each lever of advocacy, current activity is summarized below to offer aspirational directions for future efforts.

Research

Research serves as the foundation for effective advocacy. With a strong evidence base, advocates can better define an issue, more persuasively argue for change, and more confidently propose solutions. Since the year 2000, an explosion of research has shaped our understanding of the prevalence, drivers, and consequences of physician burnout. This growing body of knowledge informs policy and practice.

Studies have helped identify burnout as a true health care crisis: over the past decade research has demonstrated that approximately half of US physicians exhibit some sign of burnout. It is estimated that about 5,000 physicians leave medicine altogether for reasons other than retirement every 2 years. This is equivalent to the graduating medical school classes of 40 medical schools.[3]

Further research has identified drivers of burnout, informing our current understanding to suggest that it is primarily related to a dysfunctional practice environment[4-8] rather than personal deficiencies. For example, it has been shown that physicians in the top quartile of inbox volume (>300 messages per week) have a six-fold increase in odds of burnout compared to physicians in the lowest quartile (<150 messages per week).[12] Similarly, physicians in the top quartile for work outside of work (WOW) (>3 hours per week) have a 13-fold increase in the odds of burnout compared to physicians in the lowest quartile (<½ hour per week).[12] These measures have the potential to quantify the

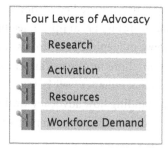

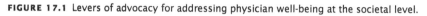

FIGURE 17.1 Levers of advocacy for addressing physician well-being at the societal level.

impact of interventions in the practice environment on outcomes such as documentation time, inbox time, WOW, and teamwork.

Studies showing the many downstream effects of burnout aid advocacy for change. Research contributes to a growing understanding that burnout affects not just physicians' and medical students' personal well-being, but also patient care. Despite beginning medical school with a stronger mental health profile than age-matched controls,[16] medical students and residents soon develop higher rates of burnout compared to their peers.[17] Residents with symptoms of burnout have higher rates of implicit and explicit racial bias[18] and are more likely to report unprofessional conduct and less altruistic professional values.[19]

Research on the financial costs of physician burnout also may influence policy and practice. For example, a health system of 1,000 physicians can expect to lose approximately 20 physicians a year due to burnout, at a total replacement cost more than $10 million.[20,21] Additional costs, unaccounted for in this estimate, are incurred by health systems related to medical error, higher malpractice claims, reduced patient satisfaction, and physicians reducing clinical effort. Available data suggest that if a health care system invested $1 million of the $10 million loss due to physician burnout-related turnover on interventions that would be expected to reduce burnout by 10%,[22,23] the return on investment (ROI)—that is, the cost savings achieved by reducing burnout and thus reducing turnover—would be more than 7%.[21] Furthermore it is estimated that physician burnout costs the US health care system $4.6 billion per year just in physician turnover and reduced clinical effort.[24]

Of even greater importance is research that identifies effective interventions to reduce burnout and increase professional fulfillment. Foundational to that goal is developing a science of physician practice: a research discipline devoted to more fully characterizing the current clinical work environment and measuring the impact of changes in that environment. Research could demonstrate how variables such as team structure, function, stability, co-location, and workflow affect outcomes such as capacity, access, quality, safety, physician recruitment and retention, burnout, and the financial stability of the practice. Teamwork is critical to achieve effective and efficient patient care as well as joy in the workplace.

The electronic health record (EHR) audit log data holds promise for the advancement of the science of practice by further characterizing the work environment, identifying the association between patterns of EHR use and burnout and demonstrating the efficacy of interventions intended to improve the work environment. For example, early work demonstrated that physicians spend 50% of their workday on the EHR, with almost as much time spent on security issues (i.e., logging in) as on reviewing the problem list.[25]

International comparisons of physician EHR activity point to opportunities for policy adjustments within the United States. For example, notes written by US physicians are more than four times longer than those written in other countries using the same EHR software.[26] Furthermore, when total time spent on the EHR is measured, the median physician in the United States spends the same amount of time as an international physician at the 99th percentile, using the same record.[27]

Aspirational Directions for Future Research

Research identifying EHR use and inbox volume as risk factors for burnout suggests that EHR use data can be used as a valuable tool for future research. Analysis of EHR use data has the potential to reveal details about the current state of the physician work environment, create a focus on interventions for improvement, and enable the assessment of efficacy of interventions.[28] In addition, by analyzing the relationships between EHR use data with other practice variables, such as staffing ratios, team stability, panel size, and quality outcomes, researchers can identify the practice characteristics associated with increased panel capacity[29] and quality of care.

Analysis of EHR use data also offers the possibility of scaling efforts directed at optimization. For example, a health system may find that physicians in the highest quartile for WOW and inbox time are also at the highest risk for burnout and turnover. Such local data, coupled with an understanding of the institutional costs of burnout, could trigger investment in interventions to reduce the documentation and inbox work required of physicians and thus reduce burnout and departure.

Much of the well-being research to date has focused on the drivers and consequences of burnout. Future research should equally focus on interventions to improve professional satisfaction. Observational research exists on innovations such as team-based documentation, team co-location, expanded rooming protocols, and nonphysician order entry;[10] further research defining the impact of these and other innovations on physician well-being could help target efforts and bolster the case for institutions to adopt successful methods. Additionally, more research is needed to better understand the prevalence and drivers of burnout stratified by race/ethnicity and gender as well as by specialty and setting. Measuring secondary outcomes—including physician WOW, inbox message volume, patient satisfaction, quality of care, medical errors, and clinic revenue and operating costs—would add to the understanding of feasibility and impact of efforts targeting physician professional satisfaction. Box 17.1 summarizes some actional strategies for starting to use research as a level for advocacy.

BOX 17.1 Research as a Lever for Advocacy

- Dedicate a journal club session to well-being research and practice science.
- Include measures of the impact on physician workflow and satisfaction when designing quality improvement projects.
- Compare the conditions of training clinics to the best practices defined in the literature.
- Explicitly teach skills such as efficient documentation and effective delegation.
- Consider creating a fellowship dedicated to practice science research.

Activation

Individuals, institutions, professional societies, national organizations, and government entities have been activated to improve professional fulfillment and joy in medicine. This activation manifests in diverse ways: calls to action, community-building, institutional initiatives, policy recommendations, and legislation. The ultimate goal is achievement of the quadruple aim[14]: better care for individuals, better health for the population, lower costs for society, and an improved experience for physicians and other health care workers.

Individual Level

Personal experience and reflection can be powerful calls to action. Physicians can voice their thoughts on professional well-being through an increasing variety of mediums, and many have found that their stories and ideas resonate with large audiences in both the medical and nonmedical community.

Opinion pieces regarding physician burnout and well-being appear regularly not only in medical journals, but also in national news outlets. These pieces have created and sustained a national conversation around physician well-being both *within* the medical community and among the general public.

Clinician-specific communities on social media can also amplify the voices of individual physicians, and these communities may allow physicians to air their collective frustrations, share lessons from their search for well-being, and foster communities dedicated to various aspects of physician well-being. Medical news and opinion sites such as Doximity, MedScape, and KevinMD provide platforms for physician writings on well-being and burnout. Through Facebook, physicians have created groups around well-being topics as general as "Healing the Practice of Medicine" and as specific as supporting breastfeeding and expressing milk for physician parents ("Dr. Milk" group). On Twitter, hashtags such as #medtwitter and #medstudenttwitter can facilitate conversations and connections between physicians and trainees worldwide, many centered around the themes of burnout and well-being. Social media use can entail significant downsides, including information spread via social media that is not fact-checked, and the relative anonymity of social media platforms which might encourage some users to harass others. Nevertheless, some physicians may find social media to be a valuable platform to hear others and be heard themselves.

The power of many of these platforms lies in their accessibility to individual physicians. Whether through op eds or by tagging teaching skills relevant for incoming resident physicians using #tipsfornewdocs on Twitter, a physician in any stage of training can learn from—and take part in—advocacy for physician well-being.

Institutional Level

In the face of mounting evidence about the causes and consequences of physician professional fulfillment and burnout, health systems have begun investing in well-being initiatives.[26-31] The American Medical Association (AMA)'s Joy in Medicine Health System Recognition provides one framework and roadmap for organizational action.[32] The program requires signature on the Charter on Physician Well-Being[33] and outlines criteria in six domains: commitment, assessment, leadership, practice efficiency, teamwork, and support, with three levels of achievement in each domain. For example, a bronze level of commitment is achieved by establishing a formalized well-being committee or office of well-being, separate from an employee assistance program. A silver level of commitment is achieved by establishing an executive leadership position, such as a Chief Wellness Officer, with at least 0.5 FTE. A silver level of assessment is met by a periodic survey of physician well-being using one of four validated tools (Mayo Well-Being Index, Stanford Professional Fulfillment Index, Maslach Burnout Inventory, or the Mini-Z Burnout Assessment) with review by the organizational leadership and/or board and targets for improvement identified. A gold level of achievement in the practice efficiency domain requires a demonstration of how the organization used EHR audit logs to capture WOW data to guide an intervention to improve practice efficiency.

As one example, Stanford Medicine has instituted a strategic plan to improve professional fulfillment among its physicians and PhD scientists.[34] This effort includes a holistic approach involving foundational programs, deliberate initiatives to foster change in the organizational culture, interactive experimentation, sustainability, and collaboration. Led by the WellMD Center, this strategy also involves several components: regularly measuring well-being and reporting to executive leadership; commissioning Well-Being Directors to lead improvement projects within each academic department; programming, such as "Story Rounds" where physicians, especially leaders, share experiences of failure and hardship to change the culture from one of unforgiving excellence to one of self-compassion and vulnerability; and focused task forces to investigate and make recommendations on key challenges such as decreasing the mistreatment of physicians by patients, families, or colleagues.

As another example, Hawaii Pacific Health has implemented a program entitled "Getting Rid of Stupid Stuff."[35,36] Physicians and other health care workers were invited to "look at their daily documentation experience and report anything in the EHR that they thought was poorly designed, unnecessary, or just plain stupid." Within months, 10 of the 12 most common alerts (aka "pebbles in the shoe") for clinicians were removed.

At Mt. Sinai Health System in New York City, the GME and faculty well-being champions are tasked with designing well-being plans at the program and departmental level to address well-being at the local level. These initiatives must address both individual- and system- level interventions, require approval of the department chair, and are reflected in the individual department budgets.

National Level

At the national level, professional societies and organizations have created resources to support physician and other health care worker well-being. The National Academy of

Medicine established the Action Collaborative on Clinician Well-Being in 2017, to raise visibility of clinician anxiety, burnout, depression, stress, and suicide; improve baseline understanding of these topics; and advance evidence-based solutions. Multiple publications have resulted, along with an online collection of knowledge resources and publications.[37] A related consensus study, Taking Action Against Clinician Burnout: A Systems Approach to Professional Well-Being, was published in 2019.[38] This study recommends a framework for balancing work demands with job resources, recognizing that the mismatch between physician workload and accountability, on the one hand, and infrastructure supports and control, on the other, plays a role in contributing to physician burnout.

Professional societies have become powerful advocates for physician well-being. The American College of Physicians (ACP) in 2017 published a bold set of recommendations for policymakers, payers, technology vendors, measure developers, regulators, and other accountability organizations in Putting Patients First by Reducing Administrative Tasks in Health Care: A Position Paper of the American College of Physicians.[39] The ACP recommends that stakeholders develop impact statements that quantify time, financial, quality, and burnout burden of the administrative tasks that result from their individual recommendations. The report also calls for a reorientation of EHRs to prioritize clinical care and prevent secondary administrative and monitoring functions from detracting the use of EHRs for clinical care.

Professional societies have also worked effectively with state and federal government agencies to advance professional well-being. For example, the American College of Emergency Physicians partnered with the Medical Society of Virginia to support passage of the 2020 SafeHaven emergency legislation.[40] This bill provides legal protections for a professional program which addresses issues related to burnout among physicians and physician assistants, ensuring that seeking help through this program will not jeopardize one's medical license except in the case of extraordinary circumstances. In related efforts, professional societies have worked to update the language in state medical licensure application forms to ask only about current impairment from mental illness, rather than asking about a history of mental illness.[41,42]

As another example, the AMA worked closely with the Centers for Medicare and Medicaid Services (CMS) to establish streamlined coding guidelines for evaluation and management services beginning in 2021.[43] It is anticipated that the simplified documentation requirements for billing level of service determination will reduce the time and effort physicians and others spend on low-value documentation and will decrease the "note bloat" that consumes time in both the creation of the note as well as later when the note is reviewed and found to be chock-full of clinically irrelevant text.

In 2017, the Collaborative for Healing and Renewal in Medicine, representing individual physician well-being advocates from multiple organizations, published the Charter on Physician Well-Being.[33] The purpose was to inspire collaborative action to support physician well-being among individuals, health systems, and the medical community. This document outlines commitments at the societal level, such as "Foster a trustworthy and supportive culture in medicine" and "Advocate for policies that enhance well-being"; at the organizational level, such as "Build supportive systems," "Develop engaged leadership," and "Optimize highly functional interprofessional teams"; and at the individual level, such as "Prioritize mental health care" and "practice and promote self-care."[33]

In early 2020, the CMS established the Office of Burden Reduction and Health Informatics to unify the agency's efforts to reduce administrative burden.[44] As part of CMS's overall COVID-19 efforts, emergency waivers[45] were announced early in the pandemic to provide relief from reporting requirements and offer new flexibilities.[45] For example, verbal orders were allowed in some settings where they had previously been disallowed or discouraged.

In 2021, the American Medical Informatics Association, the US National Library of Medicine, Columbia University's Department of Biomedical Informatics, and Vanderbilt University Medical Center collaborated on an initiative to reduce clinical documentation by 75% by 2025. Participants from industry, academia, clinical practice, and government contributed to the 6-week symposium.[46]

Aspirational Directions for Activation

An informed and activated workforce of practicing physicians, medical students, and GME trainees can influence change on the demand side. Physicians who have experienced highly functional teams and workflows will know what to look for in their first or next practice. They may also consider whether an organization takes the well-being of their physicians seriously, as evidenced by recognition in the AMA's Joy in Medicine Health System Recognition Program.[32] A prospective resident or practicing physician might ask if the practice they are considering has data on EHR WOW and inbox time.

A policy vision for the future includes an expectation for evidence-based policy, policy impact statements, and a regular practice of de-implementation of outdated policies. The medical community has come to expect evidence-based medical practice. A similar expectation for evidence-based policy, regulation, and information technology has not yet been established but is needed.[47] In addition, all stakeholders have a responsibility to consider the impact of policy in their arena on the physicians and other health care workers doing the work, akin to environmental impact statements. The ACP challenges each stakeholder to take a holistic view—to consider how actions in their domains affect physicians, their practices, and the patients and families they serve. Finally, individual delivery organizations, state and federal policymakers and federal standard setters have an opportunity to perform regular "sludge audits"[48] and de-implement outdated or non–evidence-based policies.[32] Box 17.2 provides some actional strategies for getting started with using activation as a lever for advocacy.

Resources for Taking Action

Advocates for clinician well-being have synthesized their research, recommendations, and success stories into accessible resources that can aid everyone from individual

---

BOX 17.2 Activation as a Lever for Advocacy

- Create a training clinic that reflects the best practices for wellness identified by organizations such as the American Medical Association, the National Academy of Medicine, and the American College of Physicians.
- Teach GME trainees to consider the quadruple aim when evaluating quality improvement projects or policy changes.
- Grant GME trainees access to any institutional structures or people that promote physician well-being, such as a wellness committee or Chief Wellness Officer.

---

physicians to institutional leaders and policymakers. These resources are presented in a variety of formats: as collections of research, conferences, how-to guides, assessment tools, and courses for well-being leaders.

Dissemination of Research: Knowledge Hubs and Conferences

The National Academy of Medicine has created a Clinician Well-Being Knowledge Hub[37] providing an organized resource on the causes and effects of and solutions to clinician burnout. Key peer-reviewed literature is highlighted, case studies of successful institutional interventions are presented, and recorded webinars are archived for on-demand access.

Mayo Clinic, Stanford Medicine, and the AMA co-sponsor the American Conference on Physician Health[49] every other year; on opposite years to when the International Conference on Physician Health[50] convenes, co-sponsored by the Canadian, British, and American Medical Associations. These conferences provide opportunities for researchers to share their work in abstract and poster sessions and for health system change agents to share their efforts in workshop settings. The Icahn School of Medicine at Mt. Sinai, in New York City, offers an annual GME Well-Being in the Learning Environment CHARM Course[51] for faculty of training programs seeking skills and knowledge to enhance their well-being initiatives.

Actionable Guidance: How-to Toolkits, Debunking Regulatory Myths, and Burnout Assessments

The AMA has developed resources and programming to support small practices as well as large health systems in advancing professional satisfaction. STEPS Forward[15] is a set of free, digital resources including more than 70 "how-to" toolkits providing practical, actionable guidance on the fundamentals of team-based care and efficient workflows such as team documentation,[52] inbox management,[53] pre-visit planning,[54] daily huddles,[55] team meetings,[56] and expanded roles for nurses and medical assistants.[57] There are also toolkits on improving organizational culture, including Creating the Organizational Foundation for Joy in Medicine,[21] establishing and performing in a Chief Wellness Officer role,[58,59] providing peer support,[60] Getting Rid of Stupid Stuff,[36] Building Bridges Between Practicing Physicians and Administrators,[61] and Caring for the Health Care Workforce During Crisis.[62] A toolkit, What to Look for in Your First or Next Practice,[63] helps physicians, especially those early in their career, ask appropriate questions to find a good practice fit. Modules on Medical Student Wellbeing[64] and Resident and Fellow Burnout[65] address needs during school and training.

Because some of the administrative burden experienced by physicians is the result of the misinterpretation of regulatory policies, the AMA has also established an initiative to clarify regulation and debunk myths around certain regulations.[66] For example, fact sheets that address common misunderstandings about who on the care team can document components of evaluation and management services and what is required to be performed by a physician are posted on a publicly available website. The AMA has also worked with the Joint Commission, a standards-setting organization, to clarify misunderstandings, for example, around food and drink in the workplace and appropriate use of verbal communication of orders delivered to a documentation assistant. For the latter, the Joint Commission has clarified, for example, that "All types of personnel performing documentation assistance may, at the direction of a physician or another LIP (licensed independent professional), enter orders into an EMR."[67]

The AMA also offers a survey instrument with basic analytics to help health systems assess and address burnout in their institution. Designed for practices and health systems that have more than 100 physicians, the Mini-Z and Organizational Biopsy provides leaders information about their physicians' perspectives on practice efficiency, including team structure, function, and stability; organizational culture, including leadership, control, meaning in work, and collegiality; and career plans for work effort and retention.[68] The surveys and accompanying analytics are provided at no cost as part of the mission work of the AMA.

Creating Well-Being Leaders

To develop the workforce of well-being leaders, Stanford Medicine hosts a Chief Wellness Officer course annually[69] as well as a companion Professional Well-Being Academic Consortium. Surveys deployed through the consortium provide benchmarking data for member organizations. Monthly CWO calls support networking and shared learning opportunities.

Aspirational Resource Goals

Additional resources that would advance well-being for trainees and practicing physicians alike include a single source of truth for state and federal regulations; additional

> ## BOX 17.3 Resources as a Lever for Advocacy
>
> - Introduce medical students and GME trainees to well-being resources early and in a variety of settings.
> - Encourage medical students GME trainees to engage in and present well-being research in a fashion that is equally important to other types of research commonly valued in medical training.
> - Encourage and fund medical students and GME trainees to attend well-being conferences.
> - Have open conversations with medical students and GME trainees about the well-being practices and performance of their training institution.
> - Use well-being resources to explicitly teach medical students and GME trainees skills such as pre-visit planning and team huddles.
> - Grant medical student and GME trainees access and exposure to well-being leaders in their institution.

training resources to upskill medical assistants and nurses in advanced models of team-based care; and mentorship programs for physicians and trainees with a particular interest in becoming well-being advocates through research, leadership, and/or innovation. Box 17.3 illustrates ways to get started with using resources as a lever for advocacy.

Leveraging Workforce Demand

One often-overlooked lever of advocacy available to the individual physician—and to newly trained doctors in particular—is the power of workplace demand. A June 2020 report from the Association of American Medical Colleges predicts a shortage of between 54,000 and 139,000 physicians by 2033.[70] This shortage suggests that most physicians will continue to have choices about where they practice. The ability to choose which practices to join—and which to leave—allows physicians to effectively vote with their feet for better well-being, thus impacting their own work satisfaction and, at a systemic level, pressuring organizations to adopt best practices to recruit and retain physicians.

This lever of advocacy requires physicians to recognize best practices for physician well-being, identify high-performing practices, and negotiate for wellness-promoting benefits in their contracts. Most physicians, especially those entering the workforce for the first time, have little experience or training in these areas. Thus, some recent advocacy efforts have focused on empowering physicians with the knowledge and skills needed to make their voice heard through their job selection.

In order to choose a practice that supports physician well-being, physicians must first know what to look for in terms of systems-level support. A physician who has never heard of inbox support or team-based care will not know to ask about—and thus advocate for—these best practices during an interview. Physicians who trained in an institution where the norm was long hours of WOW will not think to ask if an organization tracks WOW as a physician quality-of-life measure and makes efforts to mitigate it. A physician brought up in an "Iron Doc" culture through medical school and residency will not know to seek out an organization that promotes a culture of self-compassion and vulnerability.

Organizations such as the American Board of Internal Medicine Foundation and the Peterson Foundation support research[10,71] into the elements that create high-performing practices. Others, such as the AMA, have developed continuing medical education to disseminate knowledge around practice science as well as information on specific strategies for choosing a practice.[63] Awards such as the AMA's Joy in Medicine Health System Recognition Program[32] can guide job-seekers to high-performing practices and pressure organizations to meet higher standards of physician well-being in order to compete for candidates.

Ultimately, asking detailed questions about physician support and measurements of physician satisfaction will not only help an individual physician assess a practice; it also will signal to hiring organizations what physicians value in the job search. This eventually should lead organizations to compete for scarce physicians by meeting their well-being needs with strong systems and high-functioning practice environments.

Aspirational Directions for Leveraging Workforce Demand

When evaluating job options, physicians may find it difficult to get unbiased answers about the conditions of frontline physicians. Websites such as glassdoor.com and Indeed.com allow job seekers to read anonymous reviews of a company by its employees, but these sites are not tailored toward the needs of physicians. A similar resource focused on physician reviews of their practice could ask for more meaningful details and provide information for candidates to help pressure for improved practices amongst employers.

Physician employment opportunities vary significantly based on specialty, balance of inpatient and outpatient duties, and practice setting. Just as the Choosing Wisely Campaign[72] gathered recommendations from specialty societies to prevent medical waste, a campaign for joyful practice could gather recommendations about key systems-level support to look for in a job in each specialty. For example, for outpatient practices, the guidance could include standards for physician-to-nurse ratios, administrative time, inbox volume and support, and vacation coverage by specialty. National or regional data on average inbox volume, average WOW, and average patients seen per day could help physician job-seekers more objectively assess their prospective work environment. Box 17.4 introduces some initial strategies that can be helpful in levering workforce demands in advocacy efforts.

BOX 17.4 Leveraging Workforce Demand as a Lever of Advocacy

- Prepare medical students and GME trainees to learn how to advocate for their well-being through practice selection and negotiation when it comes time to apply for their first job position.
- Create a practice environment during training that models the high-functioning clinical practice that GME trainees should seek when their training is complete.
- Explicitly teach about well-being research and introduce medical students and GME trainees to resources on institutional best practices so that they know what to look for and what questions they should ask when looking for their first job.
- Normalize a job search strategy in which job-seekers ask detailed questions about all job criteria that impact physician well-being.

Conclusion

This chapter provided a framework for considering different levers of advocacy to benefit medical students and GME trainees and physicians in general (Box 17.5). While much work on well-being is being done by policy experts at the national level, local leaders have

---

BOX 17.5 Advocacy for Physician Well-Being

Benefits for GME trainees

    Improving clinical experience during training

    Improving clinical experience after training

    Building community

    Providing resources

    Empowering trainees

Four Levers of Advocacy

Research

Activation

    Individual level

    Institutional level

    National level

Resources

    Dissemination of research

    Actionable guidance

    Creating well-being leaders

Workforce Demand

---

the opportunity to influence their own work environment using these levers and some of the concrete strategies provided in this chapter.

Summary Points

- Advocacy for physician well-being can be accomplished using a variety of levers: research; activation of stakeholders at the individual, institutional, or national level; the creation and dissemination of resources; and the leverage of workforce demand.
- Research continues to refine the understanding of burnout and its effects. Research to advance the science of practice will help improve the practice environment and thus help to reduce physician burnout.
- Physician burnout is primarily driven by systems factors in the external environment, rather than by individual factors such as a lack of resiliency. Therefore, advocacy to reduce physician burnout must also be directed at systems levels, such as the levels of the clinical practice, the health care delivery organization, and, at the national level, stakeholders in technology, regulation, policy, payment, and health care delivery.
- Responsibility for improving physician well-being must be shared among multiple stakeholders within the medical community. Each stakeholder has the opportunity to hold up their decisions to the question: How will this decision, mandate, requirement, or policy impact the physicians and other health professionals who are closest to the patients?
- Physicians can advocate for well-being by "voting with their feet" and choosing to work at practices that value their professional satisfaction.
- Trainees can learn from and participate in all of these forms of advocacy.
- Changing the medical culture from one of solo perfectionism and the "Iron Doc" mentality to one of self-compassion, vulnerability, and shared responsibility for outcomes will be important to reducing burnout.

Putting It into Practice

- Focus on fixing the workplace, rather than fixing the worker. The system is broken, not the individuals within it.
- Measure burnout/well-being, along with drivers and consequences, regularly (every 1–2 years).
- Develop a "Getting Rid of Stupid Stuff" initiative to de-implement outdated or non–evidence-based policies and practices.
- Use EHR audit log data, such as WOW (aka "pajama time") to better understand physician work, identify targets for improvement, and assess whether interventions are effective.

- Expose medical students and GME trainees to practice science research, well-being resources, and institutional and national advocacy efforts to help prepare them to choose their medical practice carefully and, if they choose, engage in well-being advocacy of their own.

References

1. Friedberg MW. Relationships between physician professional satisfaction and patient safety. *Patient Safety Network*. Published February 16, 2016. Accessed March 30, 2021. https://psnet.ahrq.gov/perspective/relationships-between-physician-professional-satisfaction-and-patient-safety.
2. Tawfik DS, Scheid A, Profit J, et al. Evidence relating health care provider burnout and quality of care: a systematic review and meta-analysis. *Ann Intern Med*. 2019;171(8):555–567.
3. Sinsky CA, Dyrbye LN, West CP, Satele D, Tutty M, Shanafelt TD. Professional satisfaction and the career plans of US physicians. *Mayo Clin Proc*. 2017;92(11):1625–1635.
4. West CP, Dyrbye LN, Shanafelt TD. Physician burnout: contributors, consequences and solutions. *J Intern Med*. 2018;283(6):516–529.
5. Rassolian M, Peterson LE, Fang B, et al. Workplace factors associated with burnout of family physicians. *JAMA Intern Med*. 2017;177(7):1036–1038.
6. Shanafelt TD, Dyrbye LN, Sinsky C, et al. Relationship between clerical burden and characteristics of the electronic environment with physician burnout and professional satisfaction. *Mayo Clin Proc*. 2016;91(7):836–848.
7. Friedberg MW, Chen PG, Van Busum KR, et al. Factors affecting physician professional satisfaction and their implications for patient care, health systems, and health policy. *RAND Health Q*. 2014;3(4):1.
8. Olson K, Sinsky C, Rinne ST, et al. Cross-sectional survey of workplace stressors associated with physician burnout measured by the Mini-Z and the Maslach Burnout Inventory. *Stress Health*. 2019;35(2):157–175.
9. Shanafelt T, Trockel M, Rodriguez A, Logan D. Wellness-centered leadership: equipping health care leaders to cultivate physician well-being and professional fulfillment. *Acad Med*. 2021;96(5):641–651.
10. Sinsky CA, Willard-Grace R, Schutzbank AM, Sinsky TA, Margolius D, Bodenheimer T. In search of joy in practice: a report of 23 high-functioning primary care practices. *Ann Fam Med*. 2013;11(3):272–278.
11. National Academy of Medicine. Clinician well-being knowledge hub. 2020. Accessed September 16, 2020. https://nam.edu/clinicianwellbeing/.
12. Adler-Milstein J, Zhao W, Willard-Grace R, Knox M, Grumbach K. Electronic health records and burnout: time spent on the electronic health record after hours and message volume associated with exhaustion but not with cynicism among primary care clinicians. *JAMIA*. 2020;27(4):531–538.
13. Gupta R, Barnes K, Bodenheimer T. Clinic first: 6 actions to transform ambulatory residency training. *J Grad Med Educ*. 2016;8(4):500–503.
14. Bodenheimer T, Sinsky C. From triple to quadruple aim: care of the patient requires care of the provider. *Ann Fam Med*. 2014;12(6):573–576.
15. American Medical Association. Steps forward. 2020. Accessed September 9, 2020. www.stepsforward.org.
16. Brazeau CM, Shanafelt T, Durning SJ, et al. Distress among matriculating medical students relative to the general population. *Acad Med*. 2014;89(11):1520–1525.
17. Dyrbye LN, West CP, Satele D, et al. Burnout among U.S. medical students, residents, and early career physicians relative to the general U.S. population. *Acad Med*. 2014;89(3):443–451.
18. Dyrbye L, Herrin J, West CP, et al. Association of racial bias with burnout among resident physicians. *JAMA Netw Open*. 2019;2(7):e197457.
19. Dyrbye LN, Massie FS, Jr., Eacker A, et al. Relationship between burnout and professional conduct and attitudes among US medical students. *JAMA*. 2010;304(11):1173–1180.

20. Shanafelt T, Goh J, Sinsky C. The business case for investing in physician well-being. *JAMA Intern Med.* 2017;177(12):1826–1832.

21. Sinsky CA Shanafelt T, Murphy ML, et al. Creating the organizational foundation for joy in medicine. *AMA Steps Forward.* Published August 27, 2017. Accessed November 29, 2019. https://edhub.ama-assn.org/steps-forward/module/2702510.

22. West CP, Dyrbye LN, Erwin PJ, Shanafelt TD. Interventions to prevent and reduce physician burnout: a systematic review and meta-analysis. *Lancet.* 2016;388(10057):2272–2281.

23. West CP, Dyrbye LN, Rabatin JT, et al. Intervention to promote physician well-being, job satisfaction, and professionalism: a randomized clinical trial. *JAMA Intern Med.* 2014;174(4):527–533.

24. Han S, Shanafelt TD, Sinsky CA, et al. Estimating the attributable cost of physician burnout in the United States. *Ann Intern Med.* 2019;170(11):784–790.

25. Arndt BG, Beasley JW, Watkinson MD, et al. Tethered to the EHR: primary care physician workload assessment using EHR event log data and time-motion observations. *Ann Fam Med.* 2017;15(5):419–426.

26. Downing N, Bates DW, Longhurst CA. Physician burnout in the electronic health record era: Are we ignoring the real cause? *Ann Intern Med.* 2018;169(1):50–51.

27. Holmgren AJ, Downing NL, Bates DW, et al. Assessment of electronic health record use between US and non-US health systems. *JAMA Intern Med.* 2021;181(2):251–259.

28. Sinsky CA, Rule A, Cohen G, et al. Metrics for assessing physician activity using electronic health record log data. *JAMIA.* 2020;28(4):639–643.

29. Sinsky CA, Brown MT. Optimal Panel Size: Are We Asking the Right Question? *Ann Intern Med.* 2020;172(3):216-217.

30. Lucey, Catherine. Lecture presented at: American Board of Internal Medicine Foundation Forum, [Re]Building Trust: A Path Forward, August 6, 2019, Philadelphia, Pennsylvania.

31. Ofri D. The business of health care depends on exploiting doctors and nurses. *New York Times.* 2019. Accessed July 10, 2021. https://www.nytimes.com/2019/06/08/opinion/sunday/hospitals-doctors-nurses-burnout.html.

32. American Medical Association. Joy in medicine recognition program. Published 2021. Accessed July 10, 2021. https://wwwama-assn.org/practice-management/sustainability/joy-medicine-health-system-recognition-program.

33. Thomas LR, Ripp JA, West CP. Charter on physician well-being. *JAMA.* 2018;319(15):1541–1542.

34. Shanafelt T, Stolz S, Springer J, Murphy D, Bohman B, Trockel M. A blueprint for organizational strategies to promote the well-being of health care professionals. *NEJM Catalyst.* 1(6). Published October 21, 2020. Accessed July 10, 2021. https://catalyst.nejm.org/doi/full/10.1056/CAT.20.0266

35. Ashton M. Getting rid of stupid stuff. *N Engl J Med.* 2018;379(19):1789–1791.

36. Ashton M. Getting rid of stupid stuff. *AMA Steps Forward.* Published December 19, 2019. Accessed July 10, 2021. https://edhub.ama-assn.org/steps-forward/module/2757858.

37. National Academy of Medicine. What Is Clinician Burnout? Clinician well-being knowledge hub. 2021. Accessed July 10, 2021. https://nam.edu/clinicianwellbeing/about/.

38. National Academies of Sciences, Engineering, and Medicine. Taking action against clinician burnout: a systems approach to professional well-being. 2019. Accessed July 10, 2021. https://www.nap.edu/catalog/25521/taking-action-against-clinician-burnout-a-systems-approach-to-professional.

39. Erickson SM, Rockwern B, Koltov M, McLean RM. Putting patients first by reducing administrative tasks in health care: a position paper of the American College of Physicians. *Ann Intern Med.* 2017;166(9):659–661.

40. SafeHaven Confidential Support. Published 2020. Accessed September 7, 2020. https://wwwmsvorg/about-safehaven%E2%84%A2.

41. Dyrbye LN, West CP, Sinsky CA, Goeders LE, Satele DV, Shanafelt TD. Medical licensure questions and physician reluctance to seek care for mental health conditions. *Mayo Clin Proc.* 2017;92(10):1486–1493.

42. Saddawi-Konefka D, Brown A, Eisenhart I, Hicks K, Barrett E, Gold JA. Consistency between state medical license applications and recommendations regarding physician mental health. *JAMA.* 2021;325(19):2017–2018.

43. Centers for Medicare & Medicaid Services. CY 2021 physician fee schedule proposed rule. Published 2020. Accessed September 7, 2020. https://www.cms.gov/Medicare/Medicare-Fee-for-Service-Paym ent/PhysicianFeeSched.

44. Centers for Medicare & Medicaid Services. CMS unveils major organizational change to reduce provider and clinician burden and improve patient outcomes. Published June 23, 2020. Accessed September 7, 2020. https://www.cms.gov/newsroom/press-releases/cms-unveils-major-organizational-change-red uce-provider-and-clinician-burden-and-improve-patient.

45. CMS. COVID-19 emergency declaration blanket waivers for health care providers. Published 2020. Accessed April 11, 2020. https://www.cms.gov/newsroom/press-releases/cms-unveils-major-organiz ational-change-reduce-provider-and-clinician-burden-and-improve-patient.

46. American Medical Informatics Association. 25 × 5: symposium to reduce documentation burden on U.S. clinicians. Published 2021. Accessed March 3, 2021. https://www.dbmi.columbia.edu/25x5/.

47. Sinsky CA. Designing and regulating wisely: removing barriers to joy in practice. *Ann Intern Med*. 2017;166(9):677–678.

48. Sunstein C. Why is Trump gutting regulations that save lives? *New York Times*. Published 2020. Accessed April 19, 2020. https://www.nytimes.com/2020/04/17/opinion/coronavirus-trump-regulati ons.html?searchResultPosition=1.

49. American Conference on Physician Health. 2020. Accessed September 7, 2020. https://www.physician-wellbeing-conference.org/.

50. International Conference on Physician Health. 2020. Accessed September 7, 2020. https://www.ama-assn.org/practice-management/physician-health/international-conference-physician-health-reschedu led-2021.

51. Icahn School of Medicine at Mount Sinai. GME well-being in the learning environment CHARM course at Mount Sinai. Published 2021. Accessed March 3, 2021. https://mssm.cloud-cme.com/course/ courseoverview?P=3000&EID=4437.

52. Sinsky C. Team documentation. *AMA Steps Forward*. Published 2014. Accessed July 10, 2021. https:// edhub.ama-assn.org/steps-forward/module/2702598.

53. Jerzak J, Sinsky C. EHR in-basket restructuring for improved efficiency. *AMA Steps Forward*. Published 2017. Accessed July 10, 2021. https://edhub.ama-assn.org/steps-forward/module/2702694.

54. Sinsky C. Pre-visit planning. *AMA Steps Forward*. Published 2014. Accessed July 10, 2021. https:// edhub.ama-assn.org/steps-forward/module/2702514.

55. Yu E. Daily team huddles. *AMA Steps Forward*. Published 2015. Accessed September 7, 2020. https:// edhub.ama-assn.org/steps-forward/module/2702506.

56. Sinsky C. Team meetings. *AMA Steps Forward*. Published 2015. Accessed July 10, 2021. https://edhub. ama-assn.org/steps-forward/module/2702508.

57. Sinsky C. Expanded rooming and discharge protocols. *AMA Steps Forward*. Published 2014. Accessed July 10, 2021. https://edhub.ama-assn.org/steps-forward/module/2702600.

58. Shanafelt TD, Sinsky C. Establishing a chief wellness officer position. *AMA Steps Forward*. Published June 25, 2020. Accessed July 1, 2020. https://edhub.ama-assn.org/steps-forward/module/2767739.

59. Shanafelt TD, Sinsky C. Chief wellness officer road map. *AMA Steps Forward*. Published June 25, 2020. Accessed July 1, 2020. https://edhub.ama-assn.org/steps-forward/module/2767764.

60. Shapiro J. Peer support programs for physicians. *AMA Steps Forward*. Published June 25, 2020. Accessed July 1, 2020. https://edhub.ama-assn.org/steps-forward/module/2767766.

61. DeChant P. Building bridges between practicing physicians and administrators. *AMA Steps Forward*. Published 2021. Accessed July 10, 2021.

62. Shanafelt TD RJ, Brown MT, Sinsky CA. Caring for the health care workforce during crisis. *AMA Steps Forward*. Published July 23, 2020. Accessed September 7, 2020. https://edhub.ama-assn.org/steps-forw ard/module/2768609.

63. Ristow A. What to look for in your first or next practice. *AMA Steps Forward*. Published June 11, 2020. Accessed July 1, 2020. https://edhub.ama-assn.org/steps-forward/module/2767098.

64. Dyrbye L. Medical Student Well-Being. *AMA Steps Forward*. Published December 5, 2019. Accessed Septebmer 7, 2020. https://edhub.ama-assn.org/steps-forward/module/2757082.

65. Okanlawon, T. Resident and Fellow Burnout. *AMA Steps Forward*. Published October 7, 2015. Accessed September 7, 2020. https://edhub.ama-assn.org/steps-forward/module/2702511

66. American Medical Association. Debunking regulatory myths. 2021. Accessed July 10, 2021. https://www.ama-assn.org/amaone/debunking-regulatory-myths.

67. The Joint Commission. Documentation assistance provided by scribes: what guidelines should be followed when physicians or other licensed independent practitioners use scribes to assist with documentation? Published July 26, 2018. Accessed September 7, 2020. https://www.jointcommission.org/standards/standard-faqs/hospital-and-hospital-clinics/record-of-care-treatment-and-services-rc/000002210/.

68. American Medical Association. Practice transformation resources: measurement. Published 2021. Accessed March 3, 2021. https://wwwama-assnorg/practice-management/sustainability/practice-transformation.

69. Stanford University. Chief wellness officer course. 2020. Accessed September 7, 2020. https://wellmd stanfordedu/center1/cwocoursehtml.

70. Association of American Medical Colleges. The complexities of physician supply and demand: projections from 2018 to 2033. Published 2020. Accessed September 16, 2020. https://www.aamc.org/data-reports/workforce/data/complexities-physician-supply-and-demand-projections-2018-2033.

71. Milstein A.Uncovering America's most valuable care. Accessed November 18, 2019. https://petersonhealthcare.org/identification-uncovering-americas-most-valuable-care.

72. ABIM Foundation. Choosing wisely (home page). 2021. Accessed March 3, 2021. https://www.choosingwisely.org/.

Attending to Medical Student and GME Trainee Well-Being in the Midst of Crisis

The Example of the COVID-19 Pandemic

Jonathan DePierro, Lauren Peccoralo, Alicia Hurtado, Saadia Akhtar, and Jonathan A. Ripp

Introduction

A major institutional crisis creates special challenges for the well-being of the health care workforce. In late 2019 and early 2020, the COVID-19 pandemic swept across the globe, shaking our health care systems to their core and pushing health care workers (HCWs) to their limits. HCWs and staff worked long hours in layers of uncomfortable personal protective equipment (PPE), trying to care for patients with a highly contagious illness that had no cure while also working to avoid infecting themselves and their families. This unprecedented crisis created a highly stressful and challenging work and learning environment for graduate medical education (GME) trainees and medical students.[1] In areas experiencing the largest patient surges, GME trainees from fields such as psychiatry, medicine, surgery, and anesthesiology became front-line providers caring for COVID patients alongside nursing colleagues. In many circumstances, they were redeployed to clinical areas different from their training specialty and had little choice over which shifts or units they would cover, with no indication of when the pandemic surge would end. This uncertainty and lack of control, along with concern about infecting family and friends, fear of becoming infected oneself, and the moral distress of caring for COVID patients set the stage for a workplace in which the risk for mental health symptoms and burnout would be great.[2]

Medical students in their clinical years, on the other hand, were removed from the patient care environment to protect them from infection and conserve PPE. In addition, for preclinical students, classes were suspended, and all group activities were cancelled. Certain routine requirements, such as the board and licensing exams for which many had carefully planned, were cancelled at the last minute. Like so many others, medical students maintained social distancing, often in isolation in their dorms or apartments, away from friends and family members, thereby potentially compounding the risk for detrimental effects on well-being.

This chapter summarizes literature on crisis management and the effect of the COVID-19 pandemic on well-being, and uses case examples from one institution's experience to outline strategies to address well-being needs of medical students and GME trainees during a major crisis such as the COVID-19 pandemic. These strategies include attending to basic needs and safety, providing robust communications, ensuring adequate mental health and psychosocial support, providing on-the-ground support, and supporting leaders. A basic framework for responding to these well-being needs is shown in Box 18.1. Of note, these strategies also reflect the balance of an institutional ethical obligation to both trainees and the patients they may treat.[3]

BOX 18.1 Key Elements of Supporting Well-Being During Institutional Crisis

Each of the recommendations below corresponds to commonly cited requests of staff to their leaders. Leaders are encouraged to be transparent, unambiguous, and empathetic.

Hear me and respond to me: Use check-in and check-out routines with staff each day to hear concerns; ask open-ended questions; follow-up on reported concerns; consider appropriate self-disclosure as a leader.

Protect me: Ask about safety concerns and provide up-to-date information; acknowledge good safety culture (e.g., adherence to institutional guidelines and mandates).

Prepare me: Assure that staff have the resources to do their jobs and/or clearly acknowledge resource limitations.

Care for me: Support staff access to basic needs and mental health support; consider alternative work arrangements for staff with work–life integration challenges.

Honor me: Consider regular individual recognition and notes of appreciation, addressing specific things for which you are grateful.

Adapted from Shanafelt, Ripp, and Trockel.[44]

Meeting Basic Needs and Safety

Depending on the nature of the crisis, the types of resources needed to address basic needs and safety may vary substantially. The model of the physician wellness hierarchy proposed by Shapiro and colleagues illustrates that fulfillment of basic needs, which includes such areas as housing, transportation, nutrition, physical health, and safety, is the base on which all other needs sit.[4] Meeting basic needs should therefore be a top priority of a hospital or health care institution during a pandemic or other complex crisis. If people do not feel secure about how and when they might get their next meal or where they might sleep, attention to higher-order needs, such as feeling appreciated and respected, may be of a lower priority and, in fact, ring hollow. During a crisis such as the COVID-19 pandemic, the highly infectious and unknown nature of the disease caused mass closures of food services, hotels, public transportation, childcare programs, gyms, and recreational facilities. Moreover, the daily exposure of HCWs to the SARS CoV2 infectious agent raised considerable concern that HCWs themselves might be at risk for becoming infected and/or transmitting infection to their families, roommates, and close neighbors upon returning home from clinical work. Many of the needs of GME trainees mirror those of the health care workforce in general,[1] while the needs of students may differ when they are not on the front lines of clinical care.

Housing Accommodations, Transportation, and Caregiving Responsibilities

During noncrisis periods, medical students and GME trainees often count on receiving reduced housing rates near the hospital, free or subsidized meals, reduced parking rates, shuttle services, low-cost gym membership, and childcare options as benefits offered through their school or hospital employer. During a disaster or crisis such as COVID-19, the nature and availability of these services and programs may need to be rapidly reassessed and revised in ways that require removing traditional "red tape" or financial barriers to accessing services.[5] For example, during the early days of the pandemic, returning home to family or roommates after caring for COVID patients was a risk many HCWs preferred not to take. In such circumstances, the ability to provide HCWs with alternate housing arrangements, either on-site in the hospital or at local hotels providing a subsidized rate, was one potential solution.

Transportation for HCWs and trainees during a crisis or disaster can also be very challenging. In the case of New York City during the Spring 2020 COVID-19 surge, public transportation systems reduced the number of trains and buses and the hours of operation. Even when it was available, many feared taking public transportation. Similarly, rideshare or carpool services became less feasible due to social distancing restrictions, and single-rider taxis were cost-prohibitive for many. Some examples of ways to address these challenges during such periods include eliminating parking fees for all parking lots on and near hospital campuses, eliminating municipal parking fees and ticketing, increasing the availability and frequency of hospital-based shuttles and buses, and dedicating municipal public transportation programs for essential workers. In some cases, car and bike rental programs could be discounted by partnering with hospitals or municipalities to offset some of the cost.[5]

In an infectious pandemic crisis or major disaster, schools and childcare programs may be forced to close. A lack of available childcare can cause extreme stress and anxiety for HCWs and GME trainees who are required to be physically present at work (or could make it impossible for them to come to work). Examples of ways to address this challenge include municipality-run childcare centers open solely for HCW and essential workers, utilization of backup care programs subsidized by hospital systems, and the creation or utilization of existing childcare matching programs (which may be discounted or subsidized during the crisis) to link childcare workers to HCWs in need of urgent care for their children.[5]

Physical Health and Nutrition

Many HCWs and trainees during the initial COVID surge worked longer shifts than usual and were unable to return home to get food, while many local restaurants shuttered their doors. Such circumstances can also be expected for future natural disasters or crises. As such, providing regular healthy meals for HCWs and GME trainees may be critical during such a crisis. Potential solutions include pivoting hospital cafeterias to focus solely on feeding HCWs (since patient visitors were disallowed) and the solicitation of philanthropic funds for distribution of food to units or delivery points at common locations.[5] When possible and practical, hospitals may consider providing fresh produce to staff free of charge or establish "pop-up grocery stores" for essentials such as eggs, milk, and bread. Snack bins containing nutrient-dense foods such as fruits and nuts can be placed in staff break rooms. All these strategies require significant coordination and person-power to be successful. Health systems can consider reassigning certain staff and soliciting volunteers to assist in these logistical endeavors.

Regarding physical fitness and nutrition, during an infectious pandemic such as COVID-19 or a natural disaster, gyms may close and HCWs may be less able to exercise freely outdoors given the longer hours spent in the hospital, the need to wear masks in public spaces, and the potential restriction on outdoor activity. Notably, physical activity is one of the most common coping mechanisms in times of stress.[6] Hospitals can consider providing free or reduced-fee access to online gym and exercise programs, if available. In addition, given that many hospitals have in-house nutritionists, these experts can provide nutrition guidance, recipes, and tips for HCWs as well as free nutritional one-on-one or group consultations, especially for those with underlying conditions.

Personal Safety

Ensuring personal safety goes hand in hand with meeting basic needs for the medical students, GME trainee, and HCWs in the well-being hierarchy. Ensuring personal safety is critical to the well-being and mental health of the health care workforce, especially during a crisis such as the COVID-19 pandemic.[4] Early on in a public health emergency, when understanding about transmission, exposure, and effective prevention may be minimal or uncertain, having maximal adequate access to PPE is essential.[5] During such a time, perceived lack of PPE or guidelines for infection control can cause significant HCW distress.[6] In a study of New York City HCWs during the first COVID surge in April 2020, HCW perception of having insufficient access to PPE was associated with a higher likelihood of posttraumatic stress disorder (PTSD) and anxiety symptoms.[7] This suggests that pre-pandemic disaster preparations and efforts during a pandemic to secure an adequate PPE supply (e.g., gowns, gloves, respirators, face shields) are critical to ensuring the well-being of HCW. In addition, supplying hospital scrubs to be worn in the clinical setting so that HCWs need not wear their own clothing when treating patients may also alleviate HCW concerns around infection transmission. Finally, creating and continually updating evidence-based best practice protocols for infection control and prevention of spread within and outside the work setting is also critical to keeping HCWs and trainees safe and well during a pandemic. Well-being leaders can play a role in ensuring that such protocols and policies are shared with the workforce on a regular basis through clear and transparent communications and can, in turn, bring feedback to infection control team leaders when there are questions or concerns.

Furthermore, when uncertainty and anxiety around disease transmission are considerable, the ability for a hospital or health care system to provide access to testing, vaccination, and treatment (as available and applicable) for HCWs and GME trainees can have a significant impact on well-being. In a bivariate analysis, staff who believed there was insufficient access to testing were more likely to experience mental health symptoms (anxiety, stress, depression) and significant distress.[6,7] By creating access to rapid and frequent testing, vaccines when available, and the most current evidence-based treatment for pandemic-related infection, health care institutions may be able to reduce anxiety and stress in HCWs at the frontlines. In addition, on-site and easy access to medical care unrelated to the pandemic is also critical to maintaining the health and well-being of HCWs, GME trainees, and medical students both during and outside of pandemic periods.

Specific Needs of Medical Students

During the COVID-19 pandemic, medical students across the United States were pulled from in-person clinical activities to comply with infection prevention measures and preserve PPE. As a result, there may be different considerations regarding safety, housing, and nutrition for students during such times. Depending on the cost of living and student circumstances, students may experience challenges paying for housing, food, and transportation if they or their families are suddenly without paying employment. Additionally, it is important to consider the negative impact of the inability to meaningfully contribute during a time of crisis on the well-being of medical students. Therefore, it is important for medical education leaders to support student well-being by finding creative ways in which students can remain useful, since the medical student body is usually composed of capable, competent individuals with many kinds of skill sets that can be useful during a disaster or pandemic. At the authors' institution, medical student volunteers participated in a wide range of activities that, in non-pandemic times, were performed by hospital personnel who were pulled to fulfill other hospital needs.

At the authors' institution, for example, preclinical medical students staffed a triage support hotline, providing callers from the health system workforce with information about resources, such as in-person childcare or virtual tutoring for employees' children. Concurrently, clinical students telephonically assisted clinical ward teams with gathering patient history information from family members. Students' inability to participate in clinical rotations also paused their medical education, leading to increased anxiety in an already stressed student body. Whenever possible, students should be encouraged to carry out other elective activities that further their education. Medical students should also be reassured that the impact of a crisis or disaster on their education will be accounted for on their Medical Student Performance Evaluation.

It is critical that students feel autonomy, ownership, and the ability to contribute skills at the appropriate level during such crises. For example, all student volunteer activities at the authors' institution were student-initiated and supported by faculty and GME trainees. It is also concurrently important to ensure that safeguards are in place such that medical students do not practice beyond their level of training and that students and trainees do not face explicit or implicit pressure to participate in such volunteer activities. Schools need be cautious and careful about whether and how such activities are noted in the Medical Student Performance Evaluation, as overly highlighting such activities might reinforce competitiveness, in addition to disadvantaging medical students who are unable to volunteer due to not having a financial safety net or their need to care for dependents or other family members.

Promoting Robust and Supportive Communications

Even outside the context of a crisis, effective communications and a communications strategy are central to the promotion of well-being. Successfully communicating the availability of supportive resources both within and outside of a crisis can have multiple positive effects on well-being. First, resources intended to promote well-being, either at the individual or system level, are only as impactful as the extent to which the intended constituency knows about and can access them. In other words, a well-being program could be well-resourced, highly organized, and expertly managed, but if the group it serves is unaware of what is available the effort will fall flat. However, if the message does reach the intended audience, including medical students and GME trainees, raised awareness may lead to increased utilization and, in turn, enhanced well-being. This communication principle holds whether related to system-level (e.g., clerical/administrative burden reduction programs) or individual-level (e.g., psychosocial, and mental health support) efforts. Furthermore, the message itself may have a salutary effect, with the simple existence of such programs conveying a sentiment that the institution cares about and values its workforce and students. The effect of such a message can be further amplified by using a supportive tone and explicit verbiage that is characterized by authenticity and appreciation.

Disseminating Communication and Information

In terms of ensuring access to information during a crisis, besides ensuring that the resources available to specific learners are up-to-date and organized in an easy-to-navigate website, it may be necessary to set up a system, such as a resource navigation phone line that individuals can use to obtain assistance in navigating quickly-changing resources. During the COVID-19 crisis response, the authors' health system recognized the need to initiate a resource navigation phone line that would help its workforce and students identify and access the well-being resources available to them, including referrals to mental health treatment. Setting up and structuring a resource navigation phone line meant redeploying individuals with specific expertise from various areas of the hospital and recruiting volunteers, including medical students, GME trainees, and psychology postdoctoral fellows. During the peak of the pandemic, these volunteers not only triaged needs and guided individuals to helpful information, but also were empathic listeners during a moment of crisis who provided reassurance and comfort when needed.

Messaging sent from multiple sources can complicate the process of disseminating major communications or announcements. For example, the Designated Institutional Official (DIO) may send a message to all GME trainees on the same day that a similar message is sent to the entire health system, which may result in message fatigue and cause people to skip reading important messages. Conflicting messages or messages with differing tones can cause confusion, anxiety, fear, or anger. When available, a system-level well-being lead (e.g., Chief Well-Being Officer [CWO]) can help to coordinate messaging efforts that occur at the system versus constituent level. (e.g., GME and undergraduate [UME]).[8] One strategy to improve the likelihood that messages are complementary and not duplicative is to position the CWO or equivalent system well-being lead with a "seat at the table" on the institution's emergency operations command center in recognition of the importance of well-being as part of the emergency preparedness and management process.

The need for information and the extent to which a workforce may desire appreciation and recognition during times of crisis is likely to vary with the intensity of a crisis. As such, it is critical to have a means by which to gauge the informational needs of the community. This surveillance may best be accomplished through an organizational structure that funnels the informational needs through a well-being program apparatus. For example, a robust medical student or GME trainee well-being program ideally will have a network of "well-being leads" who can help solicit the needs of the community and bring that information back to the leaders responsible for crisis messaging. In effect, the well-being program can serve as an ad hoc "market research team" that gathers the informational content requested by students and GME trainees and provides feedback on the effectiveness, authenticity, and tone of communications. It is important that the well-being leads have regular access to GME and UME leadership (or others who will regularly be sending major institutional communications) to provide feedback on desired informational content.

Individual constituents within a community are likely to be heterogeneous in how they prefer to access information. Choosing the platform to deliver communications can be essential in optimizing the likelihood of reaching the intended audience. In fact, using existing well-being infrastructure for feedback or "market research" should also include a component that attempts to determine the preferred means by which the audience wishes to receive communications. While email is a valuable tool, it should not be the only means to extend communications reach because email inboxes are often overloaded with unread messages. Town halls are an important adjunct and may be a preferable way for some constituents to receive information. Medical students and GME trainees also prefer text-based information or messages posted to social media platforms. Posted paper flyers with resource links may also be a way to connect with the community. Some combination of all these tools will likely be most effective. Repeated messaging on multiple platforms does run the risk of overmessaging, such that the audience may "stop listening"; however, the benefit of providing the community with the information needed to unload uncertainty-related anxiety is almost certainly worth the risk of "overcommunication."

Messaging for Psychological Well-Being

In addition to addressing uncertainty-related anxiety through robust, supportive, regular, and authentic communications, messages specifically acknowledging and validating common emotions experienced during crisis may be helpful in normalizing a shared experience. During times of crisis, it is important to validate difficult emotions such as anger, disappointment, grief, and anxiety. It is also common for those in a crisis to experience multiple emotions at the same time or in cycles, which can feel overwhelming and exhausting. Validating emotions, which communicates to the community that an individual's emotional response makes sense and is valid and appropriate for the situation at hand, is a well-established technique used in many psychotherapies. Validation has been shown to help soothe emotional discomfort and allows the individual to feel understood and comforted.[9] Messaging should encourage self-compassion and patience with ourselves. During times of crisis, it may be helpful for leaders to acknowledge the difficulty of a situation and that it is okay to take care of ourselves as we take care of our patients. While inspiring hope, leaders can choose to share how they are practicing self-compassion, such as self-forgiveness when making a mistake or seeking more self-care.

When crafting messaging, it is important to recognize the communal response to trauma that includes a sense of disillusionment following an acute crisis.[10] Similarly, though a pandemic creates a different traumatic exposure than a more time-limited event, after the peak waves of intensity, the community will process, grieve, and experience a psychological toll. It can be helpful during the acute phase itself, but more importantly in the weeks and months that follow, to "name" common emotional reactions to minimize the secondary burden of isolation that may occur in not recognizing the universality of these emotional responses. Critical times to deliver messages that normalize the experience and promote help-seeking behavior are often during the acute and prolonged aftermath of a crisis. For example, during a crisis, difficult emotions may be tempered by feelings of heroism and comradery, but, as the crisis wanes on or begins to dissipate, a period of disillusionment may set in.[10,11] During this time, strong emotions compounded by disengagement can make it difficult to cope. Supportive and compassionate messaging can not only fold in common emotions, but also refer to specific mental health conditions (e.g., depression, anxiety) which commonly may flare or result from the experience. Highlighting the common prevalence of these diagnoses and the highly effective treatments for them can be another essential element of communication. In addition, suggestions for how to care for members of the workforce and community who may be struggling, coupled with information for easily accessible resources, should also be included. An example email for crisis communication is shown in Box 18.2

Ensuring Adequate Psychosocial and Mental Health Support

Multiple studies have documented the adverse effect of the pandemic on the emotional well-being of HCWs, including medical students, residents, and fellows. One survey of frontline HCWs conducted in New York City during the first peak of the pandemic in 2020 found that 39% of respondents ($n = 2,579$) endorsed symptoms consistent with depression, generalized anxiety, and/or PTSD.[7] At Icahn School of Medicine at Mount Sinai, of 108 third-year medical students who responded to a prospective well-being survey during the summer of the pandemic in 2020, 40% screened positive for symptoms of either major depressive disorder, generalized anxiety disorder, or PTSD.[12] In addition, emergency medicine providers in the United States who worked in areas that were not impacted considerably during the first wave of COVID also experienced increased levels of burnout and a significant increase in levels of stress related to anticipated COVID exposure.[13]

Already a concern within medical schools and GME programs, mental health began to worsen as the pandemic unfolded and conferred risk for persistent distress. Saali et al.[12] found that among third-year medical students surveyed during the pandemic in the summer of 2020, factors associated with greater overall symptom severity included

---

BOX 18.2 Example Email for Crisis Communication

In the midst of this pandemic, many of us are exhausted, even before we process the news about [new stressor]. If you're feeling anxiety, frustration, and discouragement, you're not alone. Here are a number of ways to take care of ourselves as we face more uncertainty together:

- Remember that it is normal to react with emotion or numbness during these difficult times. Be kind and patient with yourself and each other.
- Keep in mind the progress we've made since the beginning of the pandemic, including vaccines and new treatments. It can help us stay hopeful.
- Leaning on your support system—a friend, family member, spiritual leader, mentor, or leader—is vital.
- Continue to address your physical wellness. Pay attention to your diet, exercise, and sleep. Limit time on social media, especially before bed.
- Check in with each other. Share the resources here with a colleague or co-worker, including those who may not regularly use email.

And please remember that we are here for you. We are invested in your well-being. Make use of the support resources available to you. Click here for a summary of well-being and mental health resources, including the [system-wide behavioral health resource].

The past [timeframe] have proven our collective strength, creativity, and teamwork. And no matter what lies ahead, that strength, creativity, and teamwork will help us get through it, just as we have before. I believe in you, and I hope you believe in each other. Together, we will meet the challenges to come.

---

more avoidant coping, more traumatic events witnessed, lower trait emotional stability, and lower social support. It became clear to experts in the field of resilience and traumatic stress[5,14] that a multipronged approach was needed to meet the complex psychosocial needs of HCWs. As part of broader strategies to enhance the resilience and address the mental health needs of the health care workforce, numerous health care systems created new support structures to "care for their own." For example, the Mount Sinai Health System founded the Center for Stress, Resilience and Personal Growth (CSRPG) in the summer of 2020,[15] Columbia University Irving Medical Center's established CopeColumbia,[16] and Northwell Health created its Center for Traumatic Stress, Resilience and Recovery. Approaches to address mental health needs during a pandemic or crisis can be designed to boost modifiable non-pandemic factors associated with resilience, including positive emotionality, perceived emotional support, and active and adaptive coping skills.[17] Some factors associated with resilience during a crisis are shown in Box 18.3.

BOX 18.3 Factors Associated with Psychological Resilience

Social support: Make time for giving and providing support to others.

Realistic optimism: Connect to small moments of joy and focus on aspects of the situation within one's control.

Facing fears and active coping: Use humor, cognitive reframing, and creative problem-solving to address challenging situations; minimize use of emotional avoidance strategies such as substance use or denial; leverage trusted sources of information, including from leaders, to manage uncertainty.

Meaning and Purpose: Connect to a sense of something greater than yourself through spiritual practices or a sense of a shared mission.

Self-Care: Engage in regular exercise and maintain a balanced diet, recognize and respond to bodily signs of stress, and take "breaks" from social media to manage exposure to stressful content.

Adapted from Southwick and Charney.[20]

Supportive and Psychoeducational Interventions

Low-intensity interventions that may be effective during and after pandemic crisis periods include meditation, self-assessment, and psychoeducation. Given the considerable evidence supporting the benefits of mindfulness practice in stress reduction, many institutions opted to expand these services. Indeed, preliminary evidence suggests that virtual mindfulness programs may reduce burnout and increase resilience in HCWs, including learners.[18] One institution offered workshops that focused on five evidence-based factors related to resilience: (1) social support, (2) facing fears and active coping, (3) meaning and purpose, (4) self-care, and (5) realistic optimism. Each workshop included components of psychoeducation, group discussion, and practical suggestions for improving resilience in these areas.[15,19,20]

For those who benefit from spiritual support, the support provided by hospital chaplains can be enormously helpful, particularly if the chaplains had preexisting relationships with medical units and service lines. Prior to the pandemic, research with medical students found that lower spiritual well-being and daily spiritual practice were associated with greater distress and burnout.[21] During the pandemic, further work found that positive religious coping, including connecting to a higher power through prayer, was associated with lower anxiety and depression in HCWs more broadly.[22] Chaplains are also critical in helping the workforce to grieve, and they can play an important role in conducting memorial services following staff losses and leading support groups. At one institution, a beloved and highly utilized pre-pandemic cart-based ritualized tea service organized by the chaplains and including calming music and aromatherapy[23,24] was modified during the pandemic to take into account infection prevention while continuing to serve as an "oasis" and respite for staff across the health system. As learners continue to process loss, manage moral distress and burnout, and grapple with existential concerns, the supportive presence of a chaplain can remain useful for recovery and growth.

Unique Supports for Medical Students and GME Trainees

For medical students and GME trainees who already may already experience isolation due to separation from loved ones during training, pandemics and disasters may amplify those feelings. For example, during the COVID-19 pandemic, medical students who observed social distancing and a shift to remote learning sometimes never met their peers in person and had few opportunities to develop a friend support network. In a pandemic, due to infection prevention restrictions, students and GME trainees may have limited ability to physically see and socialize with peers. Community-building opportunities can be helpful to address this sense of isolation, celebrate joyous moments, and process difficult events (e.g., moments of silence/commemoration for lives lost during a pandemic).

When in-person activities are not possible, virtual events can substitute to provide support in coping with pandemic challenges, although such virtual events should be small enough or composed of smaller groups to enable meaningful discussions. Including trained facilitators is optimal in case challenging emotions or conflicts come up in these sessions. Finally, creating a buddy system for regularly checking in on at-risk or vulnerable medical students and GME trainees can also be helpful to maintain a sense of community and support.[25] In addition to facilitating a buddy system, medical school and GME training program leadership should check in with medical students and trainees through frequent meetings. Larger group town halls hosted by institution-wide leadership can also be effective in maintaining a sense of community connection. It can be particularly important to focus on community-building activities during holiday periods, when some students or GME trainees with poor social support may feel more alienated, and to involve peer-run groups in the development of such events.

Regular Assessment of Psychological Well-Being

Students and GME trainees with less social support, a history of psychiatric hospitalizations, or academic difficulties may experience increased difficulty with navigating the extra challenges encountered during a disaster or crisis. Being proactive to leverage advisors and mentors who know their advisees well can help better identify those who may be struggling. Developing individualized academic and learning plans may be necessary, and it can be helpful to normalize the option of stepping back from responsibilities to take care of themselves and resume obligations only when they are feeling better. This option can be particularly challenging given that medical students and GME trainees have a tendency toward perfectionism, often making it more challenging to accept relinquishing responsibility. It may be helpful to involve the Offices of Student Affairs (or equivalent team) to enhance outreach and well-being checks on students deemed at elevated risk. Even with best efforts, identifying those at elevated risk can be challenging for numerous reasons, including stigma around reporting distress, self-selection of those who present for care, and the need for a trained clinician to respond to positive screens. Some of these concerns can be addressed through robust self-screening programs initiated during non-crisis times. As described in Chapters 6 and 9, many medical schools and GME programs across the country have invested in confidential web- or app-based tools to monitor and respond to distress in students and trainees. Other confidential self-administered surveys have also been developed for students and GME trainees through app-based formats including examples developed specifically during the pandemic.[15,26] Investing in resources prior to a crisis will allow these resources to be more effectively deployed when a crisis need arises.

Providing Access to Mental Health Care

As described above, throughout the pandemic, mental health providers experienced a high level of referrals above baseline needs, corresponding to rising levels of emotional distress, including symptoms of depression, anxiety, and PTSD.[7] As further described in Chapters 2 and 9, even outside of pandemic times, mental health symptoms in medical students and GME trainees are common.[27] It is therefore critical for medical schools, hospitals, and health care institutions to provide easy access to mental health services during non-crisis periods, and even more so during and following a crisis. Depending on the capacity of the institution, these services could be provided by the organization itself or through contracts/partnerships with other mental health providers or vendors that provide such support services (see Chapter 9). For example, during the acute phase of the pandemic, at the Mount Sinai Health System in New York City, a triage hub for employees and students in distress was established with a number to reach a clinician from 9 AM to 9 PM, with overnight emergency coverage routed to on-call trained nurses available to field calls. This hub enabled triage and either direct mental health services or referral to the institution's employee treatment service. Additionally, many of the institution-based medical student and GME mental health treatment programs diverted their efforts to providing crisis services during the acute surge periods. Additionally, employee assistance programs (EAPs) also functioned to provide frontline support in responding to a host of upticks in verbal and physical workplace disputes, patient- or visitor-perpetrated assaults, substance misuse, and domestic violence concerns observed during the pandemic.[28]

Providing "On the Ground" Support

During a crisis such as the COVID-19 pandemic, it may be essential to provide on-the-ground support to HCWs in the work environment. This type of support can be offered through a variety of platforms including mental health rounding teams, snack and well-being stations, and frontline respite and well-being centers.

Psychological First Aid with "Mental Health Rounding"

Drawing on principles of psychological first aid,[29] on-the-ground mental health support promotes (1) calmness, by actively listening to others in a nonjudgmental stance; (2) connectedness, by helping folks to connect with their support systems that include family and friends; and (3) self-efficacy. It further serves to link those reached to resources. Unit leaders should be reminded of these services and should be encouraged to remind their staff of these services. Those units with HCWs facing the greatest challenges, in this example, those directly working in dedicated COVID-19 units, should be prioritized. When possible, a space that allows mental health rounding teams to debrief should also be provided.

As experienced in other community-level traumas, like the September 11, 2001, terrorist attacks,[14] initial strategies to provide on-the-ground support in COVID included deploying trained clinical personnel to provide psychosocial support for frontline workers.[16,30,31] Within Mount Sinai, as part of a broader program termed "Mental Health PPE," a team of 129 mental health liaisons (MHLs) had 973 individual staff support and 117 group encounters.[31] There is a compelling case for preserving proactive rounding by trusted and supportive mental health clinicians. Mental health rounding teams can provide a process for individuals to obtain the assistance they need in real time by providing experienced mental health providers who can go to where individuals are working. These teams have a dual purpose: providing immediate, brief support, and serving as a liaison for future care. This outreach captures those individuals who may be apprehensive about reaching out for help and emphasizes the important message that caring for those providing care is also a priority.

Break Spaces and "Recharge Rooms"

Frontline relief and well-being centers, known as "recharge rooms,"[32] offer an opportunity for HCWs to step away from the chaos and stress of the workplace into an environment offering a space to nourish the mind, body, and spirit. The science of relaxation, which utilizes technology to boost human performance, can be applied to develop a place for an immersive, multisensory experience that is designed to change an individual's physiology. Even brief exposure to natural environments, such as those recreated by recharge rooms, can have a stress-relieving effect.[32] Using screen projections of beautiful high-definition images of natural scenes, such as waterfalls and campfires can lead to a reduction in heart rate, blood pressure, and stress hormones within the body of the observer.[33] An auditory element can amplify the experience and reduce stress by utilizing specific timbres, tempo, and intervals of music.[34] Intervention with the use of music therapy can have a positive effect on clinicians who are exposed to highly stressful situations. The addition of an olfactory element utilizing aromatherapy can also decrease stress.[35] Last, recharge room lighting can also impact the mood of the user. In Japan and South Korea,

> ## BOX 18.4 Examples of Elements for a Recharge Room
>
> Consider using converted laboratory space and underutilized family waiting rooms.
> User-selected, projected natural landscapes
> Lounge chairs
> Silk imitation plants
> Low lighting
> Nature sounds
> Soothing aromas (essential oil diffusor)
>
> Adapted from Putrino et al.[32]

"forest bathing" is known to be a powerful natural way of creating daily stress relief by lowering stress hormones.[36] Examples of elements to consider including in a "recharge room" are shown in Box 18.4.

Support from and for Leaders During Times of Crisis

Previous well-being literature points to the relationship between interpersonal leadership behaviors and the well-being of the physicians they supervise. For example, with every 1-point increase in the ratings of leaders on the Mayo Leadership Index, their faculty report 3.3% lower burnout and 9% increase in professional satisfaction.[37] Workers who feel respected by their immediate supervisors report 56% better overall health and well-being and 83% higher job satisfaction, and they are less likely to leave their roles.[38] In addition, during a pandemic, feeling valued and supported by leaders has been associated with a lower risk of developing mental health–related symptoms[7] and with improved overall well-being.[39] Therefore, leaders play an important role in supporting the well-being and engagement of clinicians, especially during a pandemic, and they may have a significant impact on the workforce when creating a supportive approach to crisis management.

Leadership Strategies to Support Well-Being During a Crisis

Studies during the COVID pandemic and other crises have shown that several core leadership qualities and behaviors can help the workforce feel truly supported during times of crisis. A recent qualitative study of hospital systems in Connecticut found that HCWs most valued several behaviors or strategies from their leadership: (1) effective and transparent communication; (2) placing value on HCW health and safety; (3) showing appreciation; (4) being present and listening; (5) enabling schedule flexibility, autonomy, and rest-time; and (6) providing necessary resources.[40] Another hospital system in West

Virginia outlined a process for health care leadership during the pandemic that modeled their response after Kotter's eight steps for organizational change (introduced in Chapter 11): namely, (1) establishment of a sense of urgency, (2) formation of a powerful guiding coalition, (3) creation of a vision, (4) communication of that vision, (5) empowerment of others to act on the vision, (6) planning for and creation of short-term wins, (7) consolidation of improvements and production of more changes, and (8) institutionalization of new approaches.[41,42] In addition, adopting a resilient leadership approach can be effective, as outlined by Everly et al.,[43] in which four principles are adopted: vision for the future, decisiveness, effective communication, and following a moral compass. This approach also highlights the importance of developing structure, listening first, delivering information, being transparent in communications, placing importance on behaviors over words, enabling group cohesion, and providing leadership support.[43] These approaches can be utilized in part or in combination to establish an effective leadership strategy during a crisis such as the COVID-19 pandemic.

Health care institutions should consider providing resources to help guide leaders to support the well-being of their constituents during challenging times. The previously mentioned approach described by Shanafelt, Ripp, and Trockel[44] to leadership interaction with their teams was based on six core causes of anxiety during a pandemic (see Box 18.1), and this approach can be helpful to create leadership-rounding guides.[44] Leaders can also be given training in psychological first aid to better identify struggling HCWs and trainees, create safe spaces for reporting, encourage trusting relationships, connect with supportive and needed resources, and promote resilience and growth through challenges.[45] This training can be provided through digital learning platforms, virtual workshops, or prerecorded videos.[43,46] Finally, institutions can offer additional training or workshops to help with skills-building, particularly around interpersonal leadership behaviors such as appreciation, coaching, implicit bias, conflict resolution, and communication. Some useful tools are summarized in Table 18.1.

Support for Leader Well-Being

Because much of the burden of organizing the response to a crisis or disaster and the challenges that follow in its wake falls on the shoulders of leaders, they, too, need support and time for self-care during a crisis. Self-care should be a valued and encouraged practice for leaders themselves, based on their individual needs and interests. Examples of coping and self-care programs include meditation, physical activity, and psychological support. In addition, health care institutional wellness and mental health programs can provide group-facilitated discussions that cater to groups of leaders and are expertly led by appropriately selected social workers, mental health professionals, or spiritual care leaders. Individual programs such as stress management consultations, coaching, and psychological support should also be offered to leaders (see Table 18.1).

As described throughout the chapter, leaders who oversee medical students and GME trainees have a unique set of challenges and needs to contend with given their

TABLE 18.1 Potential tools for leaders supporting well-being during a crisis

Tool	Purpose
Rounding guide	Guide for leaders to structure frequent in-person rounding to demonstrate caring and compassion for their teams.
Leadership workshops	Learning programs for leaders to practice skills such as appreciation, coaching, giving feedback, and leading through crises.
Psychological first-aid training	Training for leaders to better identify and respond to trainees, students, or team members in emotional crisis with tools for action.
Guide for employees in distress	Guide for identification of employees, students, or trainees in distress, with appropriate responses and resources.
Guide for coping with grief in team members	Guide for leaders to help their teams through grief and loss.
Stress management consults	Consults with a stress management specialist who can help identify and teach potential coping tools.
Coaching during a crisis	Coaches can help leaders identify goals and approaches to reach them, particularly during a crisis.
Discussion groups	Groups led by a mental health professional that provide emotional and peer support

responsibility for managing a crisis within the context of overseeing a training program. As such, they may benefit from additional support, such as through peer connections outside of their institution to share best practices.

Conclusion

Throughout this chapter, we argued for a multipronged approach to supporting medical student and GME trainee well-being during the COVID-19 pandemic and future public health emergencies. These efforts, particularly in large health systems, require close coordination of key stakeholders, including GME and UME leadership, experts in mental health, and human resource professionals. The sustainability of these programs will also require ongoing institutional prioritization and budgetary support for well-being endeavors. UME and GME leaders may benefit from structured support around identifying mental health distress in their trainees and providing clear communications in times of crisis. On a final note, where possible, research investment is needed to evaluate the efficacy of basic needs, leadership, and psychosocial support efforts detailed above

Summary Points

- The COVID-19 pandemic was disruptive and disorienting for medical students and GME trainees, adversely impacting their educational trajectories and emotional well-being.

- A variety of resources that were brought to bear during the first wave of the COVID-19 pandemic (acute phase of disaster) may prove helpful for managing the complex needs of medical students and GME trainees in future large-scale disasters. These resources include accessible and evidence-based individual and group-level structured psychological interventions, acute crisis support lines, and the provision of food and temporary housing.
- Clear, coordinated and responsive messaging from leadership has been shown to be protective to emotional well-being during the COVID-19 pandemic and will be essential to the response to future disasters impacting medical students and GME trainees.

Putting It into Practice

- Consider drafting a template for a crisis communication email, including how to access supportive resources, as preparation for supporting medical student and GME trainee well-being during a crisis.
- Devise plans to provide for basic needs around food, safety, transportation and housing during a crisis.
- Identify gaps in existing psychoeducational interventions, including individual and group counseling, mindfulness training, resilience building, and facilitated reflection groups, that can be successfully integrated into the curricula of medical schools and GME programs during a crisis.

References

1. Akhtar S, Dua S, Rosenfield PJ, et al. Graduate medical education on the frontlines during the COVID-19 Pandemic in New York City-A response to promote well-being. *J Wellness.* 2021;3(2):9.
2. Kaplan CA, Chan CC, Feingold JH, et al. Psychological consequences among residents and fellows during the COVID-19 Pandemic in New York City: implications for targeted interventions. *Acad Med.* 2021;96(12):1722.
3. Barach P, Ahmed R, Nadel ES, Hafferty F, Philibert I. COVID-19 and medical education: a four-part model to assess risks, benefits, and institutional obligations during a global pandemic. *Mayo Clin Proc.* 2021; 96(1): 20–28.
4. Shapiro DE, Duquette C, Abbott LM, Babineau T, Pearl A, Haidet P. Beyond burnout: a physician wellness hierarchy designed to prioritize interventions at the systems level. *Am J Med.* 2019;132(5):556–563.
5. Ripp J, Peccoralo L, Charney D. Attending to the emotional well-being of the health care workforce in a New York City health system during the COVID-19 pandemic. *Acad Med.* 2020;95(8):1136–1139.
6. Shechter A, Diaz F, Moise N, et al. Psychological distress, coping behaviors, and preferences for support among New York healthcare workers during the COVID-19 pandemic. *Gen Hosp Psychiatry.* 2020;66:1–8.
7. Feingold JH, Peccoralo L, Chan CC, et al. Psychological impact of the COVID-19 Pandemic on frontline health care workers during the pandemic surge in New York City. *Chronic Stress.* 2021;5:2470547020977891. doi:10.1177/2470547020977891
8. Brower KJ, Brazeau CM, Kiely SC, et al. The evolving role of the chief wellness officer in the management of crises by health care systems: lessons from the Covid-19 pandemic. *NEJM Catalyst Innovations*

in Care Delivery. 2021;2(5). Accessed December 22, 2022. https://catalyst.nejm.org/doi/full/10.1056/CAT.20.0612

9. Fruzzetti AE, Ruork AK. Validation principles and practices in dialectical behaviour therapy. In: Swales MA, ed. *The Oxford Handbook of Dialectical Behaviour Therapy.* Oxford University Press; 2019:325–344.

10. DeWolfe DJ. Training manual for mental health and human service workers in major disasters. 2000. Accessed Deccember 22, 2022. https://www.hsdl.org/?view&did=4017.

11. Stowe A, Upshaw K, Estep C, Lanzi RG. Getting to the sandbar: understanding the emotional phases of COVID-19 among college and university students. *Psychol Rep.* 2022;125(6):2956–2980.

12. Saali A, Stanislawski ER, Kumar V, et al. The psychiatric burden on medical students in New York City entering clinical clerkships during the COVID-19 Pandemic. *Psychiatr Q.* 2022;93(2):419–434.

13. Rodriguez RM, Medak AJ, Baumann BM, et al. Academic emergency medicine physicians' anxiety levels, stressors, and potential stress mitigation measures during the acceleration phase of the COVID-19 pandemic. *Acad Emerg Med.* 2020;27(8):700–707.

14. DePierro J, Lowe S, Katz C. Lessons learned from 9/11: mental health perspectives on the COVID-19 pandemic. *Psychiatr Res.* 2020;288:113024. doi:10.1016/j.psychres.2020.113024

15. DePierro J, Katz CL, Marin D, et al. Mount Sinai's Center for Stress, Resilience and Personal Growth as a model for responding to the impact of COVID-19 on health care workers. *Psychiatr Res.* 2020;293:113426. doi:10.1016/j.psychres.2020.113426

16. Mellins CA, Mayer LE, Glasofer DR, et al. Supporting the well-being of health care providers during the COVID-19 pandemic: the CopeColumbia response. *Gen Hosp Psychiatry.* 2020;67:62–69.

17. Pietrzak RH, Feingold JH, Feder A, et al. Psychological resilience in frontline health care workers during the acute phase of the COVID-19 pandemic in New York City. *J Clin Psychiatry.* 2020;82(1):20I13749. doi:10.4088/JCP.20I13749

18. Klatt MD, Bawa R, Gabram O, et al. Embracing change: a mindful medical center meets COVID-19. *Glob Adv Health Med.* 2020;9:2164956120975369.

19. DePierro J, Marin DB, Sharma V, et al. Developments in the first year of a resilience-focused program for health care workers. *Psychiatr Res.* 2021;306:114280. doi:10.1016/j.psychres.2021.114280

20. Southwick SM, Charney DS. Resilience for frontline health care workers: evidence-based recommendations. *Am J Med.* 2021;134(7):829–830.

21. Wachholtz A, Rogoff M. The relationship between spirituality and burnout among medical students. *J Contemp Med Educ.* 2013;1(2):83.

22. Chow SK, Francis B, Ng YH, et al. Religious coping, depression and anxiety among healthcare workers during the COVID-19 pandemic: a Malaysian perspective. *Healthcare.* 2021;9(1):79.

23. Keogh M, Marin DB, Jandorf L, Wetmore JB, Sharma V. Chi time: expanding a novel approach for hospital employee engagement. *Nurs Manage.* 2020;51(4):32–38.

24. Keogh M, Sharma V, Myerson SL, Marin DB. The Chi cart ministry. *Nurs Manage.* 2017;48(8):32–38.

25. Albott CS, Wozniak JR, McGlinch BP, Wall MH, Gold BS, Vinogradov S. Battle buddies: rapid deployment of a psychological resilience intervention for health care workers during the coronavirus disease 2019 pandemic. *Anesth Analg.* 2020;131(1):43–54.

26. Golden EA, Zweig M, Danieletto M, et al. A resilience-building app to support the mental health of health care workers in the COVID-19 era: design process, distribution, and evaluation. *JMIR Form Res.* 2021;5(5):e26590. doi:10.2196/26590

27. Rotenstein LS, Ramos MA, Torre M, et al. Prevalence of depression, depressive symptoms, and suicidal ideation among medical students: a systematic review and meta-analysis. *JAMA.* 2016;316(21):2214–2236.

28. Hughes D, Fairley A. The COVID chronicles: an employee assistance program's observations and responses to the pandemic. *J Workplace Behav Health.* 2021;36(3):177–196.

29. Hobfoll SE, Watson P, Bell CC, et al. Five essential elements of immediate and mid-term mass trauma intervention: empirical evidence. *Psychiatry.* 2007;70(4):283–315.

30. Bernstein CA, Bhattacharyya S, Adler S, Alpert JE. Staff emotional support at Montefiore Medical Center during the covid-19 pandemic. *Jt Comm J Qual Patient Saf.* 2021;47(3):185–189.

31. Gray M, Monti K, Katz C, Klipstein K, Lim S. A "Mental Health PPE" model of proactive mental health support for frontline health care workers during the COVID-19 pandemic. *Psychiatr Res.* 2021;299:113878.

32. Putrino D, Ripp J, Herrera JE, et al. Multisensory, nature-inspired recharge rooms yield short-term reductions in perceived stress among frontline healthcare workers. *Front Psychol.* 2020;11. doi:10.3389/fpsyg.2020.560833

33. i Badia SB, Quintero LV, Cameirao MS, et al. Toward emotionally adaptive virtual reality for mental health applications. *IEEE J Biomed Health Inform.* 2018;23(5):1877–1887.

34. de Witte M, Spruit A, van Hooren S, Moonen X, Stams GJ. Effects of music interventions on stress-related outcomes: a systematic review and two meta-analyses. *Health Psychol Rev.* 2020;14(2):294–324.

35. Maxwell S, Lovell R. Evidence statement on the links between natural environments and human health. Department for Environment, Food and Rural Affairs. March 9, 2017. Accessed December 22, 2022. https://beyondgreenspace.files.wordpress.com/ 2017/03/evidence-statement-on-the-links-between-natural-environments-and-human-health1.pdf.

36. Hansen MM, Jones R, Tocchini K. Shinrin-yoku (forest bathing) and nature therapy: astate-of-the-art review. *Int J Environ Res Public Health.* 2017;14(8):851.

37. Shanafelt TD, Gorringe G, Menaker R, et al. Impact of organizational leadership on physician burnout and satisfaction. *Mayo Clin Proc.* 2015;90(4):432–440.

38. Porath C. Half of employees don't feel respected by their bosses. *Harv Bus Rev.* November 19, 2014. Accessed December 22, 2022. https://hbr.org/2014/11/half-of-employees-dont-feel-respected-by-their-bosses.

39. Simard K, Parent-Lamarche A. Abusive leadership, psychological well-being, and intention to quit during the COVID-19 pandemic: a moderated mediation analysis among Quebec's healthcare system workers. *Int Arch Occup Environ Health.* 2022;95:437–450.

40. Adeyemo OO, Tu S, Keene D. How to lead health care workers during unprecedented crises: a qualitative study of the COVID-19 pandemic in Connecticut, USA. *PloS One.* 2021;16(9):e0257423.

41. Kotter JP. *Leading Change.* Harvard Business Press; 2012.

42. Crain MA, Bush AL, Hayanga H, et al. Healthcare leadership in the COVID-19 Pandemic: from innovative preparation to evolutionary transformation. *J Healthc Leadersh.* 2021;13:199.

43. Everly GS, Wu AW, Cumpsty-Fowler CJ, Dang D, Potash JB. Leadership principles to decrease psychological casualties in COVID-19 and other disasters of uncertainty. *Disaster Med Public Health Prep.* Published online 2020:1–3. doi:https://doi.org/10.1017/dmp.2020.395

44. Shanafelt T, Ripp J, Trockel M. Understanding and addressing sources of anxiety among health care professionals during the COVID-19 pandemic. *JAMA.* 2020;323(21):2133–2134.

45. Owen RD, Schimmels J. Leadership after a crisis: the application of psychological first aid. *JONA: J Nurs Adm.* 2020;50(10):505–507.

46. Blake H, Bermingham F, Johnson G, Tabner A. Mitigating the psychological impact of COVID-19 on healthcare workers: digital learning package. *Int J Environ Res Public Health.* 2020;17(9):2997. doi:10.3390/ijerph17092997

Index

For the benefit of digital users, indexed terms that span two pages (e.g., 52–53) may, on occasion, appear on only one of those pages.

Tables, figures, and boxes are indicated by *t*, *f*, and *b* following the page number

AAMC (Association of American Medical
    Colleges), 1–2, 175, 181–82, 222, 224, 225,
    313–14, 345
accomplishment and efficacy, 88–89. *See also*
    fulfillment and satisfaction; meaning and
    purpose
  autonomy and, 65–66
  decreased, as component of burnout, 12–13, 26,
    40, 88–89, 197
  decreased, prevalence of in GME globally, 48–49
  decreased, prevalence of in GME in US, 46–47
  decreased, prevalence of in UME globally, 45, 46
  decreased, prevalence of in UME in US, 43–44
  dropping out and, 90–91
  effects of poor patient outcome or patient death
    on self-efficacy, 200
  mindfulness and, 110–11
  minority populations, 96–97
  personality traits and, 72–73
  premedical students, 44
  professional fulfillment and self-efficacy, 26
  promotion of self-efficacy through mental health
    support, 366
  safety risks and, 87
  supportive relationships and, 65–66, 70
  workload balance and self-efficacy, 117
Accreditation Council for Graduate Medical
    Education (ACGME), 229–36, 247, 260

Action Collaborative on Clinician Well-Being,
    1–2
  challenges of compliance with, 235
  Chief Wellness Officers and compliance, 330
  Common Program Requirements (CPRs), 3,
    121, 184, 210, 230–35, 298, 330
  data gathering, 287
  learning communities, 182
  measuring program success, 249
  retreats, 185
  Review Committee for Internal Medicine, 229
  Section 1.D, Institutional and Program
    Resources, 231
  Section VI.B, Learning and Working
    Environment: Professionalism, 232
  Section VI.C, Well-Being, 232–33, 298
  Section VI.D, Fatigue Mitigation, 233–34
  Section VI.E, Clinical Responsibilities,
    Teamwork, and Transition of Care, 234
  Section VI.F, Clinical Experience, Education,
    and Work Hours, 234–35
  self-screening, 208–9
  supervision and oversight, 119
  Symposia in Physician Well-being, 1–2, 3
  time provisions for treatment, 203
  work-hour limitations, 62–63, 64, 115, 138, 172–
    73, 229–30, 260
ACEs (adverse childhood experiences), 55

ACE Scale, 55
ACP (American College of Physicians), 341, 342
activation for advocacy, 339–42, 343b
  aspirational directions for, 342
  individual level, 339
  institutional level, 339–40
  national level, 340–42
adaptability. *See* flexibility and adaptability
adverse childhood experiences (ACEs), 55
affect regulation model, 200–1, 202
AI (artificial intelligence), 305–6, 309–11, 310f, 312–13, 314–15
alcohol and substance use
  adverse childhood experiences and, 55
  burnout cascade, 84
  as consequence of burnout, 86
  decline in self-care, 59
  impacts of wellness programs and curricula, 184–85
  questions of impairment and drug screening, 203–4
allostatic load ("wear and tear" effect), 175–77
altruism
  bias and erosion of, 177
  burnout and, 88, 337
  cultural shift toward healthy altruism, 135–36
  growth mindset, 146–47
  pathologic altruism, 135–36
AMA. *See* American Medical Association
Amabile, T., 280
American Academy of Sleep Medicine, 137–38
American Board of Family Medicine, 89
American College of Emergency Physicians, 341
American College of Physicians (ACP), 341, 342
American Conference on Physician Health, 1–2
American Foundation for Suicide Prevention, 122, 211
American Medical Association (AMA), 224, 263, 341, 343–44, 346
  American Conference on Physician Health, 343
  Health System Recognition, 18
  Joy in Medicine Health System Recognition, 18, 339–40, 342
  Physician Master File, 43–44
American Medical Informatics Association, 342
American Medical Student Association (AMSA), 224
anxiety, 26
  bias and discrimination, 175–77
  burnout cascade, 84
  cognitive restructuring, 111
  coping with, as individual driver of well-being, 71–72
  COVID-19 pandemic, 98, 211–12
  curricular changes to reduce, 56–57
  debt and, 60
  equilibrium of survival anxiety and learning anxiety, 260, 261f
  exercise, 139
  impacts of wellness programs and curricula, 184–85
  impostor syndrome and perfectionism, 142
  individual-level stress, 200
  mind-body practices, 140
  prevalence of, 42–43, 123
  stress continuum, 197
  women and, 47
Aristotle, 274–75
art-based interventions, 140–41, 148, 152–54
artificial intelligence (AI), 305–6, 309–11, 310f, 312–13, 314–15
arts and humanities programs, 111–12, 140–41, 148
Association of American Medical Colleges (AAMC), 1–2, 175, 181–82, 222, 224, 225, 313–14, 345
autogenic training, 140
autonomy
  advocacy, 335–36
  autonomy-supervision balance, 65–66, 117, 119–20
  importance of, 358
  learning environment, 24
  low levels of, 46, 63–64, 71, 200, 257
  predictor of high performance, 280
behavior change plans, 57
Bell Commission, 229
belonging, connectivity, and community, 144, 199, 207, 220–21
  advocacy for well-being, 335
  art-based interventions, 140–41
  curricular adjustments to promote, 144–45, 146, 147–48
  definition of well-being, 23–24
  learning communities, 56–57, 118, 182
  self-care strategies, 144
  team culture and community, 118–19
  "wellness infrastructure," 185–86
bias and discrimination, 175–77, 179, 223–24, 259, 288, 312–13. *See also* diversity and inclusion
Big Five personality traits, 72–73
Bloom's Taxonomy, 272–74, 279–80
Bodenheimer, T., 10, 14
Brief Fatigue Inventory, 27–28
burnout, 40–53
  advocacy for well-being, 334
  career satisfaction, 85t
  components of, 12–13, 26, 28–29, 40, 197
  consequences of, 41–42, 82–103
  COVID-19 pandemic, 211–12

definition of, 12–13, 40–41
diversity and inclusion, 96–97
evolution of understanding about, 11–14, 12*f*
increase in reference to in medical literature, 3, 40–41
latent profiles, 28–29
learning environment, 94–96
measures of, 28–30, 31*t*
mental and physical health, 84–87, 85*t*
origin of term and concept, 40
overview of, 26
prevalence of among health care professionals, 41, 336
prevalence of by specialty, 47–49
prevalence of globally, 45–46, 47–50
prevalence of in graduate medical education, 46–50
prevalence of in premedical students, 44–45
prevalence of in undergraduate medical education, 42–46
prevalence of in United States, 42–44, 46–47
professional behavior, 85*t*, 87–88
professional efficacy, 85*t*
relationship between depression and, 35, 41, 42, 44, 198–99
relationship between learning environment and, 43
relationship between stress and, 198
relationship between suicidality and, 42
relationship between well-being and, 35
relationship between work environment and, 41
research into consequences of, 83–84, 98
societal consequences of, 91*b*, 91–94
stress continuum and, 197–99
stressors leading to, vii, 42, 43*f*
suicidality, 42
burnout cascade, 83–84
business case for commitment to well-being, 258*t*, 263–65, 264*t*, 265*b*

care-seeking behavior. *See* help-seeking behavior
CBCT (cognitive-based compassion training), 145
CBI (Copenhagen Burnout Inventory), 29, 31*t*, 93
CCT (compassion cultivation training), 145
Center for Stress, Resilience and Personal Growth (CSRPG), 361–62
Center for Traumatic Stress, Resilience and Recovery, 361–62
Centers for Medicare and Medicaid Services (CMS), 309, 311–12, 341, 342
CG-CAHPS (Clinician and Group Consumer Assessment of Healthcare Providers and Systems) survey, 262
CHANGE (Medical Student Cognitive Habits and Growth Evaluation) Study, 59

change management, 243–56
  communication, 252
  creating quick wins, 250*f*, 250
  general principles of, 245–46
  metrics, 249–50, 253–54
  participatory leadership, 252
  pausing and reflecting, 254
  pilot tests, 253
  pitfalls and roadblocks, 253
  scaling up, 253
  stakeholders and alliances, 248*f*, 248–49
  theories of, 243–45
  timing, 247
  zero-sum traps, 251*f*, 251–52
CHARM (Collaborative for Healing and Renewal in Medicine), 1–2, 328, 341–42
Charter on Physician Well-Being (social-ecological model), 12*f*, 16*f*, 16–17, 18, 24, 135–36, 339–40, 341–42
Chief Wellness Officers (CWOs), 294*f*, 322–23, 325–31, 343–44
  alignment with well-being leaders, 330–31, 331*f*
  benefits of, 324
  collaborators and stakeholder relationships, 327*b*, 327–28
  compliance with regulatory requirements, 330
  designating, 325
  disseminating information during crises, 359
  institution-wide reporting structures, 294
  oversight of well-being metrics, 329
  role and responsibilities of, 325–31
  scope of responsibility, 328–29
  skills and authority of, 326–27
  strategic planning responsibilities, 329
childcare, 356
Choosing Wisely Campaign, 346
Clinical Learning Environment Review (CLER) reports, 287
Clinician and Group Consumer Assessment of Healthcare Providers and Systems (CG-CAHPS) survey, 262
CME (continuing medical education), 87–88, 89, 313, 346
CMS (Centers for Medicare and Medicaid Services), 309, 311–12, 341, 342
coaching
  leadership, 327–28, 329, 368
  learning community, 182
  positive psychology, 143
  in well-being programs, 112
  "wellness infrastructure," 186
cognitive-based compassion training (CBCT), 145
cognitive behavioral therapy, 111, 168–69
cognitive distortions and restructuring, 111, 142, 154

cognitive strategies
  healthy emotion processing, 152–54
  resilience training, 141–42
Collaborative for Healing and Renewal in
    Medicine (CHARM), 1–2, 328, 341–42
Columbia University
  CopeColumbia, 361–62
  Department of Biomedical Informatics, 342
  Irving Medical Center, 361–62
community. *See* belonging, connectivity, and
    community
compassion
  compassionate medical practice, 134–35
  enhancing, 145
  healthy emotion processing, 141
  messaging, 360–61
  self-compassion, 145–46, 360
compassion cultivation training (CCT), 145
complex adaptive systems, 9–10, 13–14, 171,
    245–46, 249–50
connectivity. *See* belonging, connectivity, and
    community
consequences validity, 22*t*, 23
construct validity, 21–22
content validity, 21–22, 22*t*
continuing medical education (CME), 87–88, 89,
    313, 346
Copenhagen Burnout Inventory (CBI), 29, 31*t*, 93
Coping with Work and Family Stress intervention,
    184–85
costs
  as barrier to treatment, 203
  of burnout, 93
  as motivation for institutional commitment to
    well-being, 258*t*, 263–65, 264*t*
COVID-19 pandemic, 328, 353–54, 355, 361
  burnout, 98
  changes in discussion of mental health, 211–12
  classroom attendance, 58
  disseminating information during, 359
  on-the-ground support, 365–66
  housing needs, 355
  leadership, 367–68
  model of well-being developed during, 17
  needs of medical students, 357–58, 364
  peer support programs, 124
  personal safety, 356–57
  physical health and nutrition, 356
  regulatory responses, 311–12
  Step 2 Clinical Skills examination, 172
  telehealth, 207, 305–6, 308*f*, 308–9, 311–12,
    313–14
  transportation needs, 355–56
  work-hour limitations, 260
creative self-expression, 140–41, 152–54

crises. *See* disasters, crises, and tragedies
criterion validity, 21–22
Csikszentmihalyi, Mihaly, 280
CSRPG (Center for Stress, Resilience and Personal
    Growth), 361–62
culture
  diversity and inclusion, 175
  environment vs., 180
  GME culture and learning environment, 182–86
  learning environment, 108*b*, 117–20
  organizational culture, 12*f*, 14–15, 25, 132–34,
    340, 343–44
  team culture and community, 118–19
  UME culture and learning environment,
    180–82
curricula
  ACGME Common Program Requirements, 3,
    121, 184, 210, 230–35, 298, 330
  avoiding pitfalls, 146–47
  content themes, 150–55
  design of, 113–15
  hidden curriculum, 174, 177, 180, 224–25
  LCME standards, 226*t*, 227
  longitudinal wellness curricula, 146–55, 151*t*
  multimodal techniques and activities, 147–49
  system impacts of, 184–85
CWOs. *See* Chief Wellness Officers

Data Collection Instrument (DCI), 224–25
debt
  as barrier to treatment, 203
  burnout and, 71
  as individual driver of well-being, 60
Demands-Resources model. *See* Job
    Demands-Resources model
Department of Health and Human Services
    (HHS), 311
depersonalization
  alcohol and substance use, 86
  art-based interventions, 140–41
  autonomy-supervision balance, 65–66
  as component of burnout, 12–13, 26, 40, 197
  coping strategies, 71–72
  definition of, 26
  dropping out and, 90–91
  emotional intelligence, 72
  empathy, 87
  impacts of wellness programs and curricula,
    184–85
  job turnover, 90
  learning environment, 65
  measures of burnout, 28–29
  minority populations, 96–97
  pass-fail grading and, 56
  patient satisfaction, 93

personality styles and personal characteristics, 72–73

prevalence of, 43–44, 45, 46–47, 48–49

quality of care, 92

social support, 70

support from faculty, 68

support from peers, 67

unprofessional behaviors, 87–88

workload and, 62

depression, 26, 55, 98, 123, 196–99, 206, 212, 220

ACGME Common Program Requirements, 230–31, 232, 233, 235

alcohol and substance use, 86

bias and discrimination, 175–77

burnout vs., 41, 197

cognitive restructuring, 111

as consequence of burnout, 83, 84–86

COVID-19 pandemic, 98, 211–12, 361

diversity and inclusion, 59, 120

dropping out and, 90–91

exercise, 139

faculty professionalism, 181

fatigue and, 26

health care system-related stress, 202–3

hours worked, 63–64

impostor syndrome and perfectionism, 142

individual-level stress, 200–1

job turnover, 90

measures of, 28, 31t, 34

medico-legal risk, 92–93

mental health screening, 122

mindfulness and meditation, 140, 145

moral imperative to support well-being, 258–59

occupational health and safety risks, 87

pass-fail grading, 56–57

positive psychology, 142

prevalence of, 42–43, 44

quality of care, 92

relationship between burnout and, 35, 41–42, 198–99

relationship between stress and, 198

sleep, 137–38

spiritual/religious practice, 363–64

suicidal ideation and suicide, 86, 210

terminology, 35

unprofessional behaviors, 88

"wellness infrastructure," 186

wellness programs and mental health care, 180, 184–85, 365

Designated Institutional Officials (DIOs), 297–98, 330, 359

developmental psychology, 11

disasters, crises, and tragedies, 353–72. See also COVID-19 pandemic

childcare, 356

communications, 358–61, 362b

crisis planning, 124

disseminating information during, 359–60, 362b

framework for responding to, 354b

"on the ground" support, 365–67

housing needs, 355

leadership and leader well-being, 367–69, 369t

meeting basic needs, 355–58

mental health care access, 365

"mental health rounding," 366

mental health support, 361–65

messaging for psychological well-being, 360–61

models of well-being for, 17

as motivation for institutional commitment to well-being, 258t, 259–60

personal safety, 356–57

physical health and nutrition, 356

psychoeducational interventions, 363–64

psychological assessments, 364–65

recharge rooms, 366–67, 367b

resilience, 363b

response to tragedies, 210–11

specific needs of students, 357–58, 364

tragedy response, 210–11

transportation needs, 355–56

discussion groups, 112, 369t

distress, 180, 196–97, 221–22

bias and discrimination, 177

burnout cascade, 83–84

cognitive restructuring, 111

COVID-19 pandemic, 211

definition of, 197

discussion groups, 112

dropping out and, 90–91

empathy, 87, 262

healthy emotion processing, 141

individual-level stress, 200

learning environment, 117–18

leaving the medical field, 263

meaning and purpose, 120

medical errors, 92

mental health support, 121–22, 207, 364–65

mindfulness and meditation, 143

moral imperative to support well-being, 258–59

occupational health and safety risks, 356–57

pass-fail grading, 172

peer support, 112

personal events and characteristics, 60–61

premedical students, 44

prevalence of, 42–43

quality of care, 262

spiritual/religious practice, 363–64

stress continuum and burnout, 197–99

team culture and community, 118–19

terminology, 35

distress (*cont.*)
    well-being assessments, 112–13, 122, 364–65
    women, 97
diversity and inclusion, 175
    artificial intelligence, 312–13
    bias and discrimination, 175–77, 179, 223–24,
        259, 288, 312–13
    burnout in minority populations, 96–97
    consequences of burnout, 96–97
    "isms," 175
    learning environment, 120
    support for, 59, 67–68, 73*t*
    terminology, 175, 176*t*
    trauma-informed medical education, 177–79
    well-being programs, 120, 288
domains of well-being. *See also names of specific*
    domains
    burnout, 26
    engagement, 26
    fatigue, 26
    joy in the workplace, 26
    mental health, 26
    professional fulfillment, 26
    quality of life, 26
    stress, 25–26
Doximity, 339
drivers of well-being, 54–81
    individual, in GME, 69–73
    individual, in UME, 59–61
    institutional, in GME, 61–69
    institutional, in UME, 55–59
dropping out of medical training, 90–91
drug use. *See* alcohol and substance use
dual-role responsibilities, 71
Dunn, Halbert L., 196–97
Dupuy General Well-Being Schedule, 56–57
durability, in models of well-being, 11
Dweck, Carol, 279
Dyrbye, Liselotte, 42–44, 46–47

EAPs (employee assistance programs), 122, 179,
    207–8, 339–40, 365
educational attainment, consequences of burnout, 89
efficacy. *See* accomplishment and efficacy;
    fulfillment and satisfaction; meaning and
    purpose
effort-impact analysis ("Pick" charts), 250*f*, 250
EHRs. *See* electronic health records
Eight-Step Change Model, 244–45
    avoiding zero-sum traps, 251–52
    communication, 252
    short-term wins, 250
    stakeholders and alliances, 248–49
electronic health records (EHRs), 305–7, 311, 315
    adoption and utility of, 306–7

artificial intelligence, 309–10
audit log data, 337
burnout and, 90, 171
dashboard displays, 315, 316*f*
data for research, 315, 338
improving end-user experience, 329
metrics, 249
reorientation of, 341
workload and, 62, 116, 306
elevator speeches, 270–72, 271*b*, 281
emotional exhaustion
    alcohol and substance use, 86
    coaching, 112
    as component of burnout, 12–13, 26, 40, 197
    coping strategies, 71–72
    creative self-expression, 140–41
    dropping out and, 90–91
    educational attainment, 89
    emotional intelligence, 72
    exercise, 139
    hours worked, 63
    job turnover, 90
    learning environment, 65
    measures of burnout, 28–29, 30, 31
    mindfulness and meditation, 140
    minority populations, 96–97
    pass-fail grading, 56
    personality styles and personal characteristics,
        72–73
    positive psychology, 143
    prevalence of, 43–44, 45, 46–47, 48–49
    quality of care, 90–91
    reduction in hours worked, 90
    social support, 70
    support from faculty, 68, 183
    supportive team and professional relationships, 67
    "wellness infrastructure," 186
    wellness programs, 184–85
    workload, 62
emotional intelligence
    Chief Wellness Officers, 326–27
    communication theory, 274–75
    healthy emotion processing, 141, 152, 153*b*
    as individual driver of well-being, 72
    learning environment, 115, 117
empathy
    arts and humanities programs, 111–12
    bias and discrimination, 177, 179
    cognitive and emotive, 72
    communication theory, 274–75
    consequences of burnout, 82–83, 87
    empathic concern, 87
    as individual driver of well-being, 72
    listening, 359
    medical student experience, 221–22

narrative medicine, 140–41
patient satisfaction, 93
personal distress, 87
quality of care, 262
retreats, 185
risk of burnout, 47
sleep, 137–38
systems-level wellness interventions, 169
team dynamics, 183
wellness curricula, 146
employee assistance programs (EAPs), 122, 179,
207–8, 339–40, 365
engagement
as antithesis of burnout, 15, 55
burnout cascade, 84
Chief Wellness Officers, 327, 329
consequences of burnout, 83
job turnover, 90
learning environment, 183
meaning and purpose, 120, 171
measures of, 30, 31t
overview of, 26
patient satisfaction, 93–94
in professional development, 89
Epworth Sleepiness Scale, 27–28
ethos, 274–76
evidence-based instruments, 27–32
burnout, 28–30
engagement, 30
fatigue, 27–28
joy, 30–31
limitations of, 32
mental health, 28
professional fulfillment, satisfaction, and
meaning, 30
quality of life, 27
stress, 27
evidence-based self-care practices, 137–46
belonging and connectivity, 144
creative self-expression, 140–41
exercise, 139
health care utilization, 139–40
healthy emotion processing, 141
humanism and compassion, 145
meaning in work, 144–45
mind-body practices, 140
mindfulness and meditation, 143
nutrition, 138–39
positive psychology, 142–43
resilience training, 141–42
self-compassion, 145–46
sleep, 137–38
spiritual/religious practice, 144
strategies to address impostor syndrome and
perfectionism, 142

exercise
strategic self-care, 139
in well-being programs, 109
exhaustion. See emotional exhaustion; fatigue and
exhaustion
expectation alignment, as driver of well-being,
66–67, 73t
expert trap, 278
Ey, Sydney, 123–24

Facebook, 339
faculty
role of faculty professionalism in learning
environment, 181
support from, 58, 68–69, 73t
Family Educational Rights and Privacy Act
(FERPA), 203
fatigue and exhaustion, 150. See also emotional
exhaustion
ACGME Common Program Requirements, 233–34
burnout cascade, 84
as consequence of burnout, 84–86
depression, 198
hours worked, 172–73, 229–30
learning environment, 113
measures of, 27–28, 29, 31
medical errors, 92, 262
overview of, 26
patient outcomes, 200
quality of care, 232
sleep, 109–10, 137–38
strategic sleep training, 150
FDA (Food and Drug Administration), 312
Federation of State Medical Boards, 204
female population. See women
FERPA (Family Educational Rights and Privacy
Act), 203
FIRST (Flexibility in Duty Hour Requirements for
Surgical Trainees) trial, 138–72, 173–74
flexibility and adaptability
in models of well-being, 10, 15, 25
scheduling and work-hour control and
flexibility, 57, 66, 73t, 172–73, 185–86, 200,
232, 307–8, 367–68
Flexibility in Duty Hour Requirements for Surgical
Trainees (FIRST) trial, 138–72, 173–74
Flexner Report, 2
Food and Drug Administration (FDA), 312
food insecurity, 109
forest bathing, 366–67
Freudenberger, Herbert J., 40
fulfillment and satisfaction. See also accomplishment
and efficacy; meaning and purpose
career satisfaction-related consequences of
burnout, 85t, 90–91

fulfillment and satisfaction (*cont.*)
  job turnover, 90
  learning environment in GME, 182–84
  leaving clinical practice, 90
  leaving medical field, 90–91
  measures of, 30, 31*t*
  overview of, 26
  reducing clinical hours, 90
  regretting choice of specialty, 90–91

generational differences, 135–36, 201, 209
"Getting Rid of Stupid Stuff" program, 340, 343–44
Gladwell, Malcolm, 280
Goldman, M. L., 232–33
grading methods, 56–57, 114–15, 117–18, 172
Graduation Questionnaire (GQ), 222, 225
growth mindset, 141–42, 146–47, 152–54, 228, 279
gyms and gym membership, 109, 184, 355, 356

Happiness Practice, The, 184–85
Harvard Business Review, 280
Harvard Negotiation Project (HNP), 275–76, 278–79
Hawaii Pacific Health, 340
Healer's Art Curriculum, 144–45
health information technology (IT). *See* technology and innovation
Health Information Technology for Economic and Clinical Health (HITECH) Act, 305–6, 311
Health Insurance Portability and Accountability Act (HIPAA), 203
health-related consequences of burnout, 84–87, 85*t*
  alcohol and substance use, 86
  general mental and physical health, 84–86
  occupational health and safety risks, 87
  suicidal ideation and suicide, 86
healthy altruism, 135–36. *See also* altruism
healthy emotion processing, 141, 152–54
help-seeking (care-seeking) behavior
  barriers to, 24, 123, 174, 203–5
  education, awareness, and promotion, 118, 121, 123–24, 168–69, 207, 209, 295–96, 327–28, 329, 361
  personal characteristics and, 61
HHS (Department of Health and Human Services), 311
hidden curriculum, 174, 177, 180, 224–25
Higher Education Mental Health Alliance, 211
HIPAA (Health Insurance Portability and Accountability Act), 203
HITECH (Health Information Technology for Economic and Clinical Health) Act, 305–6, 311
HNP (Harvard Negotiation Project), 275–76, 278–79

hours worked
  as institutional driver of well-being, 62–64, 73*t*
  reduced, as consequence of burnout, 90, 93–94
  residency training, 229
  scheduling and work-hour control and flexibility, 57, 66, 73*t*, 172–73, 185–86, 200, 232, 307–8, 367–68
  sleep deprivation, 138
  societal consequences of, 93–94
  well-being and, 173–74
  work-hour limitations, 62–63, 64, 115, 138, 172–73, 229–30, 234–35
housing, during crises, 355
humanism, 145

Icahn School of Medicine, 343
iCOMPARE (Individualized Comparative Effectiveness of Models Optimizing Patient Safety and Resident Education), 63, 138, 172–73
Implicit Association Test (IAT), 179
impostor syndrome
  cognitive restructuring, 111
  feedback, 117–18
  prevalence of, 142
  self-compassion, 145–46
  strategies to address, 142, 154
Indiana University, 59
individual drivers of well-being, 59–61, 69–73
  coping with stress and anxiety, 71–72
  debt, 60
  empathy and emotional intelligence, 72
  in graduate medical education, 69–73
  personal events and characteristics, 60–61
  personality styles, 72–73
  self-care, 59–60, 69–70
  social support, 70–71
  in undergraduate medical education, 59–61
Individualized Comparative Effectiveness of Models Optimizing Patient Safety and Resident Education (iCOMPARE), 63, 138, 172–73
individually-focused self-care practices and well-being interventions, 132–67
  cultural shift toward healthy altruism, 135–36
  evidence-based practices, 137–46
  longitudinal curricula, 146–55, 151*t*
  physical health practices, 137–40
  psychological health practices, 140–43
  relational/spiritual health practices, 144–46
  shared responsibility for, 135–36
  strategic self-care, 136*f*, 136–37
  timing of interventions, 135
Institute for Healthcare Improvement
  Joy in Work initiative, 30–31
  Triple Aim, 10, 14

institutional commitment to well-being, 257–69
    costs, 258t, 263–65, 264t
    moral imperative, 258–59, 258t
    quality and safety of care, 258t, 262–63
    regulatory requirements, 258t, 260
    tragedy as imperative, 258t, 259–60
institutional drivers of well-being, 55–59, 61–69
    autonomy-supervision balance, 65–66
    demands of providing clinical care, 64–65, 73t
    expectation alignment and well-being mindset,
        66–67, 73t
    in graduate medical education, 61–69
    hours worked, 62–64, 73t
    learning environment, 65–66, 73t
    making errors, 64–65, 73t
    mentorship, 68–69
    program- and system-level demands, 62–65
    program- and system-level resources, 65–69
    scheduling control and flexibility, 57, 66, 73t
    support for diversity and inclusion, 59, 67–68,
        73t
    support for learning, 56–57, 73t
    support for personal development, 57–58, 73t
    support for self-care, 57–58
    support from faculty, 58, 68–69, 73t
    supportive peers, team, and professional
        relationships, 58, 67, 73t
    in undergraduate medical education, 55–59
    work compression, 64, 73t
    workload, 62, 73t
instrument validity, 21–23, 22t
    consequences validity, 23
    content validity, 21–22
    definition of, 21
    historical classifications of validity, 21–22
    internal structure validity, 23
    relationships with other variables validity, 23
    response process validity, 22–23
intentional relaxation, 140
internal structure validity, 22t, 23
International Conference on Physician Health, 1–2
in-training examination (ITE), 89, 172–73, 183–84
IT (health information technology). See technology
    and innovation

Jackson, Susan, 40
Jed Foundation, 207
Jefferson Scale of Empathy (JSE), 93
Job Demands-Resources model, 12f, 13–14, 24,
    25–26, 170, 183
job turnover
    burnout cascade, 84
    as consequence of burnout, 82–83, 90, 93–94
    operational costs of, 263, 264t, 337
    societal consequences of, 93–94

Journal of the American Medical Association, 4
joy in the workplace, 26, 30–32, 113, 232, 334,
    337, 339
JSE (Jefferson Scale of Empathy), 93

Kabat-Zinn, Jon, 143
KevinMD, 339
Kotter, John, 244–45
Kramer, S., 280
Krasner, Michael, 4

LASAs (linear analog scale assessments), 27–28
latent profiles, 28–29, 98
LCME. See Liaison Committee on Medical
    Education
leadership
    Chief Wellness Officers, 294f, 322–23, 325–31,
        343–44
    crisis situations, 367–68
    participatory, 252
    role of faculty professionalism in learning
        environment, 181
    support for leaders, 368–69, 369t
    support from faculty, 58, 68–69, 73t
    well-being champions/directors, 295–96, 330–31
    well-being committees, 246, 287–88, 294, 296–
        98, 339–40
learning conversations, 273–74, 275, 278, 279–80
learning environment, 180–86
    ACGME Common Program Requirements, 232
    assessment strategies, 114–15
    autonomy-supervision balance, 119–20
    consequences of burnout, 89, 94–96
    culture and climate of, 108b, 117–20
    culture vs., 180
    curriculum design, 113–15
    dissatisfaction with, 95–96
    diversity and inclusion, 120
    efficiency and function of, 113–17, 114f
    feedback, 117–18
    grades, 117–18
    hidden curriculum and formation of
        professional identity, 180
    impact of bias and discrimination on, 175–77
    as institutional driver of well-being, 65–66, 73t
    interpersonal-level stress, 201–2
    LCME standards, 225–27, 226t
    meaning and purpose, 120
    meeting educational needs of team members,
        115–16
    mentorship, 68–69, 182
    mistreatment and neglect, 181–82
    role of faculty professionalism in, 181
    role of GME trainees in UME environment, 181
    structure of, 115–17

learning environment (*cont.*)
   support for learning, 56–57, 73*t*
   support from faculty, 58, 68–69, 73*t*
   system impacts of wellness programs and
      curricula, 184–85
   team culture and community, 118–19
   team dynamics and, 183
   well-being curricula and advising systems, 118
   well-being programs, 113–20
   "wellness infrastructure," 185–86
   workload, 116–17
Leiter, M. P., 12–13
Lewin, Kurt, 244, 245*t*
LGBTQ+ population, 97
Liaison Committee on Medical Education (LCME),
   224–28, 247, 260
   challenges of compliance with, 228
   Chief Wellness Officers and compliance, 330
   current standards, 224–25, 225*b*
   Functions and Structure of a Medical School, 224,
      225–27
   measuring program success, 249
   mistreatment, 222
   Standard 3, Academic and Learning
      Environment, 225–27, 226*t*
   Standard 8, Curricular Management, Evaluation
      and Enhancement, 226*t*, 227
   Standard 12, Medical Student Health Services,
      Personal Counseling, and Financial Aid
      Services, 226*t*, 227
   well-being programs and services, 221–22
Lian Rong Survey (LRS), 45
linear analog scale assessments (LASAs), 27–28
Logic Model, 273*f*, 273–74, 279–80, 281–83
logos, 274–75, 276, 282

machine learning (ML), 310, 312–13
maladaptive perfectionism. *See* perfectionism
malpractice, 202, 263, 264, 289, 337
Maslach, Christina, 12*f*, 12–13, 13*t*, 15, 35, 40, 73, 73*t*
Maslach Burnout Inventory (MBI), 22*t*, 28–29, 30,
   31*t*, 33–34, 339–40
   consequences of burnout, 86, 87–90, 92–94,
      95–97, 98
   depression, 198–99
   domains of burnout, 28–29, 30, 43–44
   drivers of well-being, 61, 72–73
   MBI-HSS (Human Services Survey), 28–29
   MBI-SS (Student Survey), 44
   prevalence of burnout, 40, 43–44, 45, 46–47, 48
Maslow, A. H., 11
Maslow's Hierarchy of Needs, 11, 280
Mayo (Shanafelt-Noseworthy) Model, 12*f*, 13*t*, 15, 25
Mayo Clinic and Medical School, 56, 343
Mayo Well-Being Index, 31, 31*t*, 112–13, 339–40

MBI. *See* Maslach Burnout Inventory
MBSR (Mindfulness-Based Stress Reduction)
   course, 143
MCAT (Medical College Admissions Test), 220
McManus, I. C., 29
meaning and purpose, 1. *See also* accomplishment
   and efficacy; fulfillment and satisfaction
   culture and, 14
   finding in work, 144–45, 154–55
   learning environment, 113, 120
   measures of, 30, 31*t*
   mission and vision statements, 290–91
   MVPs of well-being, 24–25
   professional fulfillment, 26
   self-care, 136–37
   tasks and, 171
   workload and, 171
measures of well-being, 21–39
   domains of well-being, 25–26
   evidence-based instruments, 27–32
   instrument validity, 21–23, 22*t*
   models of well-being, 23–25
   survey design, 32–34
   terminology, 35–36
Medical College Admissions Test (MCAT), 220
medical errors
   alcohol and substance use, 86
   burnout, 41–42, 64–65, 73*t*, 92, 262
   burnout cascade, 84
   fatigue, 137–38, 229–30, 262
   stress, 200
Medical Society of Virginia, 341
Medical Student Cognitive Habits and Growth
   Evaluation (CHANGE) Study, 59
Medical Student Learning Environment Survey
   (MLES), 121
medico-legal risk. *See* malpractice
meditation. *See* mind-body practices
MedScape, 339
mental health, 196–218, 361–65
   access to care, 206–9, 365
   assessment and screening, 122–23
   awareness and education, 121–22, 209–10
   barriers to treatment-seeking, 203–5
   consequences of burnout, 84–86
   counseling services, 123–24
   COVID-19 pandemic, 211–12
   crisis planning, 124
   destigmatization, 209–10
   measures of, 28
   mental health care for GME trainees, 207–9
   mental health care for UME trainees, 206–7
   mental health disorders, defined, 197
   "mental health rounding," 366
   models of mental health care, 206–9

overview of, 26
peer support programs, 124
psychiatric services, 123–24
psychological first-aid training, 122
stress continuum and burnout, 197–99
stressors, 199–203
tragedy response, 210–11
well-being program components, 108b, 121–24
mental health liaisons (MHLs), 366
mentorship
learning environment, 68–69, 118
personal development, 57–58
pitch for change, 280
positive psychology, 143
well-being and, 182
MHLs (mental health liaisons), 366
MI (motivational interviewing), 275–76, 278
microaggressions, 96, 120, 174, 175–77, 176t, 179, 222–23, 259
mind-body practices, 140, 143
art-based interventions, 140–41
calming practices, 149
healthy emotion processing, 141, 152
hidden curriculum, 180
impostor syndrome and perfectionism, 154
mindfulness and meditation, 4, 56–57, 60, 69, 71–72, 108–9, 110–11, 140, 145, 149, 152–54, 184, 197, 202–3, 232–33, 287–88, 326, 363, 368
resilience training, 141–42
strategic sleep training, 150
training, 4, 56–57, 60
Mindfulness-Based Stress Reduction (MBSR) course, 143
Mindset (Dweck), 279
Mini Z tool, 30, 31, 31t, 112–13, 339–40, 344
minority populations. See also diversity and inclusion
access to treatments, 206–7
AI/ML tools, 312–13
belonging and connectivity, 144
burnout in, 44, 96–97, 338
conscripted curricula, 96
metrics and, 35–36
mistreatment and neglect, 181–82, 259, 288
support for diversity and inclusion, 59, 120, 179
underrepresentation of mental health treatment providers, 204
mission statements, 290–91, 292b
mistreatment and neglect, 181–82, 222–24, 226t, 227, 259, 288. See also diversity and inclusion
ML (machine learning), 310, 312–13
MLES (Medical Student Learning Environment Survey), 121
models of well-being, 9–20, 291–93

commonly used, 14–17, 24–25
considerations in selecting, 10–11
contributions to current models, 11–12, 12f
process for selecting, 11
reasons for selecting, 9–10, 292–93
selecting, 9–11
for specific needs, 17
moral injury, 35
motivational interviewing (MI), 275–76, 278
Mount Sinai Health System, 340, 343, 361–62, 365, 366
Mount Sinai Model, 12f, 16
Myers-Briggs Type Indicator, 72–73

narrative medicine, 111–12, 119, 140–41, 148
NASA Task-Load Index, 170
National Academy of Medicine (NAM)
Action Collaborative on Clinician Well-Being, 1–2, 15, 18, 27, 340–41
Clinician Well-Being Knowledge Hub, 343
commitment statement, 18
model of well-being, 12f, 15, 24–25
"Systems Approaches to Improve Patient Care by Supporting Clinician Well-Being" Consensus Study, 3
Taking Action Against Clinician Burnout, 83, 340–41
Neff, Kristin, 145–46
neuroplasticity, 142, 146
Northwell Health, 361–62
Northwestern University Feinberg School of Medicine (NUFSM), 57
Noseworthy, J. H., 15, 73, 73t
nutrition
crisis situations, 356
strategic self-care, 138–39
in well-being programs, 109

Oath to Self-Care and Well-Being (Oath of Geneva), 135–36, 220–21, 259
occupational health and safety risks, 87
Office of Burden Reduction and Health Informatics, 342
Oldenburg Burnout Inventory (OLBI), 29, 31t
Organizational Biopsy, 344
organizational commitment statements, 18
AMA Joy in Medicine Health System Recognition, 18
NAM commitment statement, 18
purpose of, 18
organizational competency continuum, 246, 246t, 249, 254, 323
organizational psychology, 11–14
overnight call, 71, 172, 180
"oxygen mask principle," 210

parental leave, 235–36
pass-fail grading, 56–57, 117–18, 172, 180
pathologic altruism, 135–36
pathos, 274–76
patient-centered communication, 87
Patient Health Questionnaire (PHQ)
    burnout, 44
    mental health, 28, 31t
Patient-Reported Outcomes Measurement
        Information System (PROMIS)
    fatigue, 27–28
    mental health, 28
    professional fulfillment, satisfaction, and
        meaning, 30
patient satisfaction, 83, 92, 93, 262, 337, 338
peers, support from. See also belonging,
        connectivity, and community
    drivers of well-being, 58, 67, 73t
    peer support programs, 124
    in well-being programs, 112
Perceived Cohesion Scale, 56–57
Perceived Stress Scale (PSS), 27, 31t, 56
perfectionism
    assessment of psychological well-being,
        364–65
    as barrier to treatment, 205
    cognitive restructuring, 111
    growth mindset, 279
    individual-level stress, 200
    maladaptive perfectionism, 111
    prevalence of, 142
    self-compassion, 145–46
    strategies to address, 142, 154
PERMA (Positive Emotions, Engagement,
        Relationships, Meaning and Purpose, and
        Accomplishment) model, 111
personal accomplishment. See accomplishment
        and efficacy
personal and professional development, 314
    ACGME Common Program Requirements, 231
    consequences of burnout, 89
    expectation alignment and well-being mindset,
        66–67
    support for, 57–58, 68, 73t, 118
    technology skills, 310, 313
personal events
    adverse childhood experiences, 55
    as individual drivers of well-being, 60–61
personality styles and personal characteristics
    as barrier to treatment, 205
    as individual drivers of well-being, 60–61, 72–73
personal protective equipment (PPE), 353–54,
        356–58
PFI (Stanford Professional Fulfillment Index). See
        Stanford Professional Fulfillment Index

PHQ (Patient Health Questionnaire). See Patient
        Health Questionnaire
Physician Job Satisfaction Scale, 30, 31t
Physician Task Load Index, 116, 170f, 170
"Pick" charts (effort-impact analysis), 250f, 250
Pink, Daniel, 280
Positive Emotions, Engagement, Relationships,
        Meaning and Purpose, and Accomplishment
        (PERMA) model, 111
positive psychology, 111, 142–43, 148–49, 154–55,
        182, 278
PPE (personal protective equipment), 353–54,
        356–58
premature closure, 276
premedical students
    adverse childhood experiences, 55
    career interest, 94
    competitive nature of entering medicine, 220
    holistic review in admissions, 220
    journey of, 219–20
    prevalence of burnout in, 44–45, 46, 220
    prevalence of depression in, 220
PRIME-MD, 28, 31t, 34
Prins, J. T., 47–48
professional behavior-related consequences of
        burnout, 85t, 87–88
    professional behaviors, 87–88
    reduced empathy, 87
    reduced patient-centered communication, 87
professional efficacy-related consequences of
        burnout, 85t
    educational attainment, 89
    engagement in professional development, 89
    impact on learning environment, 89
    reduced personal achievement, 88–89
    suboptimal role modeling, 89
Professional Fulfillment Index (PFI). See Stanford
        Professional Fulfillment Index
professional identities
    autonomy-supervision balance, 119–20
    hidden curriculum and formation of, 180
    meaning and purpose, 120
    mentorship, 182
    social support, 71
professionalism. See also personal and professional
        development; unprofessional behaviors
    ACGME Common Program Requirements, 232,
        237t
    integrating well-being into professional ethos, 210
    LCME standards, 226t, 227
    role of faculty professionalism in learning
        environment, 181
Professional Quality of Life (ProQOL) Scale, 27
professional relationships, support from, 58, 67,
        73t, See also faculty

professional satisfaction. *See* accomplishment and efficacy; fulfillment and satisfaction; meaning and purpose
PROMIS. *See* Patient-Reported Outcomes Measurement Information System
ProQOL (Professional Quality of Life) Scale, 27
PSS (Perceived Stress Scale), 27, 31*t*, 56
Psychological Empowerment at Work Scale, 30, 31*t*
psychological first-aid training, 122
psychological safety, 118–19, 132–34, 140–41, 177, 178
purpose. *See* accomplishment and efficacy; fulfillment and satisfaction; meaning and purpose

Quadruple Aim, 10, 12*f*, 14, 134–35, 246, 257–58, 335, 339
quality of care
  consequences of burnout, 88, 92, 334
  future research, 338
  as motivation for institutional commitment to well-being, 258*t*, 262–63
  Quadruple Aim, 14
quality of life
  alcohol and substance use, 86
  Chief Wellness Officers, 329
  diversity and inclusion, 67–68
  drivers of well-being, 60
  dropping out and, 90–91
  educational attainment, 89
  exercise, 139
  measures of, 27
  medical errors, 92
  mindfulness and meditation, 143
  moral imperative to support well-being, 258–59
  overview of, 26
  premedical students, 55
  self-care, 136

race and ethnicity. *See* minority populations
RAFTs (resident assessment facilitation teams), 186
recharge rooms, 366–67, 367*b*
regulatory requirements, 219–40
  ACGME Common Program Requirements, 229–36
  Chief Wellness Officers, 330
  COVID-19 pandemic, 311–12
  graduate medical education, 228–36
  LCME standards, 224–28, 225*b*, 226*t*
  medical student experience, 220–22
  mistreatment, 222–24
  as motivation for institutional commitment to well-being, 258*t*, 260
  premedical journey, 219–20
  residency training and work hours, 228–29

technology, 311–12
undergraduate medical education, 219–28
relationships with other variables validity, 22*t*, 23
religious/spiritual practices, 144, 363–64
resident assessment facilitation teams (RAFTs), 186
resilience, 4
  adverse childhood experiences and, 55
  belonging and connectivity, 144
  crisis situations, 361–63, 363*b*
  education and training, 56–57, 141–42
  growth mindset, 154
  medical students, 221–22
  minority populations, 59, 96–97
  models of well-being, 15–16, 25
  negative connotation, 135
  stress and, 65
  support from faculty and staff, 95
  wellness curricula, 146, 183–84
response process validity, 22–23, 22*t*
retreats, 185, 249
righting reflex, 278
role modeling
  consequences of burnout, 82–83, 89, 262–63
  diversity and inclusion, 177, 178
  faculty professionalism, 181
  hidden curriculum, 180
  learning environment, 180
  perfectionism, 154
  well-being champions/directors, 295–96

Saali, A., 361–62
SafeHaven emergency legislation, 341
safety
  consequences of burnout, 87, 92
  crisis situations, 356–57
  as motivation for institutional commitment to well-being, 258*t*, 262–63
  occupational safety risks, 87
  psychological safety, 118–19, 132–34, 140–41, 177, 178
sanctuary spaces, 147
satisfaction. *See* accomplishment and efficacy; fulfillment and satisfaction; meaning and purpose
scheduling and work-hour control and flexibility, 57, 66, 73*t*, 172–73, 185–86, 200, 232, 307–8, 367–68
Schein, Edgar, 12*f*, 14, 15
self-affirmation, 144–45
self-care
  ACGME Common Program Requirements, 232
  exercise, 109
  help-seeking behavior, 61
  importance of, 4
  as individual driver of well-being, 59–60, 69–70

self-care (*cont.*)
  individually-focused self-care practices, 132–67
  as institutional driver of well-being, 57–58
  negative connotation, 135
  nutrition, 109
  promotion of, 108–9
  sleep, 109–10
  strategic, 136*f*, 136–46, 150
  "wellness infrastructure," 185–86
self-compassion, 145–46, 340, 345–46, 360
self-reflection, 111–12
self-screening, 208–9, 230–31, 233, 364–65
Seligman, Martin, 111
semantic framing, 276–78
SF (Short Form) Survey, 27
Shanafelt, T. D., 15, 73, 73*t*, 246, 260
Shanafelt-Noseworthy (Mayo) Model, 12*f*, 13*t*, 15, 25
Shapiro, D. E., 355
shared responsibility model, 9, 25, 70, 132–36, 133*f*, 137, 146–47, 207
Short Form (SF) Survey, 27
simplicity, in models of well-being, 10, 13–14, 15
Sinsky, C., 10, 14
Slavin, Stuart, 222
sleep. *See* fatigue and exhaustion
SMART (specific, measurable, achievable, relevant, and timebound) goals, 150
social-ecological model (Charter on Physician Well-Being), 12*f*, 16*f*, 16–17, 18, 24, 135–36, 339–40, 341–42
social support, 70–71. *See also* belonging, connectivity, and community
  faculty, 58, 68–69, 73*t*
  peers, 58, 67, 73*t*, 112, 124
  teams, 67, 73*t*
societal consequences of burnout, 91*b*, 91–94
  cost of care, 93
  job turnover, 93–94
  medico-legal risk, 92–93
  patient satisfaction, 93
  quality and safety of care, 92
  reduced clinical hours, 93–94
societal-level advocacy for well-being, 334–52, 336*f*, 347*b*
  activation as lever for, 339–42, 343*b*
  benefits of, 335–36
  leveraging workforce demand as lever for, 345–46, 347*b*
  research as lever for, 336–38, 338*b*
  resources as lever for, 342–45, 345*b*
specialties
  prevalence of burnout by specialty, 47–49
  regretting choice of, as consequence of burnout, 90–91
specific, measurable, achievable, relevant, and timebound (SMART) goals, 150

spiritual/religious practices, 144, 363–64
stakeholders, 248*f*, 248–49, 285–87, 327*b*, 327–28
Stanford Medicine, 340, 343, 344
Stanford Model for Professional Fulfillment, 12*f*, 15, 25
Stanford Professional Fulfillment Index (PFI), 31*t*, 97, 112–13, 339–40
  burnout, 29
  joy in the workplace, 31
  professional fulfillment, satisfaction, and meaning, 30
Stanford University, 263
Step 1 examination, 56–57
Step 2 examination, 172
STEPS Forward, 343–44
stigma and destigmatization, 121, 123–24, 199, 204, 207, 209, 327–28, 329, 364–65
strategic self-care, 136*f*, 136–37. *See also* self-care
  longitudinal curricula, 150
  physical health practices, 137–40
  psychological health practices, 140–43
  relational/spiritual health practices, 144–46
stress
  coping with as individual driver of well-being, 71–72
  definition of, 197
  health care system-related stress, 202–3
  individual-level stress, 200–1
  interpersonal-level stress, 201–2
  measures of, 27, 31*t*
  overview of, 25–26
  recharge rooms, 366–67
  relationship between burnout and, 198
  relationship between depression and, 198
  stress continuum and burnout, 197–99
stress continuum model, 17, 197–98
stress-diathesis model, 202, 205, 210
student debt. *See* debt
student wellness committees, 57–58
substance use. *See* alcohol and substance use
suicidal ideation and suicide, 3, 210–11
  burnout and, 42, 86, 92
  burnout cascade, 84
  help-seeking behavior, 206–7
  hidden curriculum, 180
  LGBTQ+ population, 97
  measures of, 28, 34
  mental health screening, 122
  rates of, 123, 210, 230, 258–59, 263
  responding to, 210–11
  student debt, 60
  suicide contagion, 211
  suicide risk reduction programs, 168–69, 207
survey design, 32–34
  aligning data analysis plans with survey items, 33–34

human subjects protection issues, 34
item development, 32–33
maximizing response rate, 33
question types, 33
system-level well-being interventions, 168–95, 187*f*
culture, 180–86
individual needs aligned with, 169*t*
need for, 169
overview of, 168–69
workload, 170–74
systems science, 12–14

tactical breathing, 140, 149, 152–54
teaching kitchens, 109
teams
ACGME Common Program Requirements, 234
distributing work across, 116
meeting educational needs of members, 115–16
support from, 67, 73*t*
team culture and community, 118–19
team dynamics in GME, 183
tensions related to individual vs. team goals, 201–2
workload and team-based care, 171
technology and innovation, 305–21
artificial intelligence, 305–6, 309–11, 310*f*, 312–13, 314–15
Chief Wellness Officers and, 327–28, 329
early adoption of, 313–14
electronic health records, 62, 90, 116, 171, 249, 305–7, 309–10, 311, 315, 316*f*, 329, 337
ethical considerations, 312–13
legal, policy, and regulatory responses to, 311–12
role of clinician in evolution of, 313
strategies for including students and trainees in, 314–15
telehealth, 207, 305–6, 307–9, 308*f*, 311–12, 313–14
telehealth (TH), 207, 305–6, 307–9, 308*f*, 311–12, 313–14
Telehealth Competencies Across the Learning Continuum report, 313–14
Theory of Planned Change ("Unfreeze-Change-Refreeze" model), 244, 245*t*
changing, 252–54
refreezing, 254
unfreezing, 247–52
"three good things" strategy, 111, 148–49, 154–55
time constraints, as barrier to treatment, 203
"To Err is Human" report, 15
tragedies. *See* disasters, crises, and tragedies
transportation, during crises, 355–56
trauma-informed medical education (TIME), 177–79, 178*f*
Realize, 177–78
Recognize, 178

Resist, 179
Respond, 179
Triple Aim, 10, 14, 257
21st Century Cures Act, 311
Twitter, 339

"Unfreeze-Change-Refreeze" model. *See* Theory of Planned Change
University of Pennsylvania, 111
University of Toronto, 60
University of Virginia, 56
unprofessional behaviors
acceptance/tolerance of, 4
burnout and, 41–42, 87–88
burnout cascade, 84
cost of remediation, 263, 264
US Medical Licensing Examination (USMLE), 56–57, 172, 221
US National Library of Medicine, 342
utilization of health care services, 123, 139–40, 206–7, 209, 249–50, 358–59. *See also* help-seeking behavior
Utrecht Work Engagement Scale (UWES), 30, 31*t*

Vanderbilt University Medical Center, 342
Vanderbilt University School of Medicine (VMS), 57–58
VIA Survey of Character Strengths, 148–49
vision statements, 290, 292*b*

Washington University School of Medicine, 56–57
"wear and tear" effect (allostatic load), 175–77
well-being, 232. *See also* models of well-being
ACGME Common Program Requirements, 232–33
adverse childhood experiences and, 55
assessments of, 112–13
contributors/obstacles to, 24
crises, 353–72
definition of, 23–24
drivers of, 54–81
drivers of increased attention to, 2–4
evolution of understanding about, 11–14
importance of self-care, 4
increase in reference to burnout in medical literature, 3
individually-focused interventions, 132–67
influence of workplace on, 12–14
institutional commitment to, 257–69
measures of, 21–39
organizational commitment statements, 18
origin of term and concept, 196–97
preventing well-being from becoming performance metric, 209–10
relationship of burnout to, 35
stressors, vii, 3, 42, 43*f*, 55–56

well-being (*cont.*)
    system-level interventions, 168–95
    technology and innovation, 305–21
    well-being mindset as institutional driver of
        well-being, 66–67, 73*t*
    work-life integration, 4
well-being champions/directors, 295–96
    Chief Wellness Officers and, 330–31
    graduate medical education, 295–96
    undergraduate medical education, 296
well-being committees, 246, 287–88, 294, 296–98,
    339–40
Well-Being Index, 31, 31*t*
well-being program components, 107–31, 108*b*
    culture and climate of learning environment,
        108*b*, 117–20
    efficiency and function of learning environment,
        108*b*, 113–17
    individual factors and health, 108*b*, 108–13
    individually-focused self-care practices, 132–67
    mental health support, 108*b*, 121–24
    Shared Responsibility Framework, 132–34, 133*f*
well-being program development, 285–301
    data gathering, 287
    engaging stakeholders, 286–87
    governance and organizational structure, 293–
        97, 294*f*
    independent constituent group reporting
        structures, 295
    initial planning, 285–86
    institution-wide reporting structures, 294
    mission statements, 290–91, 292*b*
    models of well-being, 291–93
    needs assessment, 287
    oversight, 288–89
    policies and guidelines, 297*f*, 297–98, 298*b*, 299*b*
    prioritizing efforts, 287–88
    proposal generation, 289
    purpose, 290
    vision statements, 290, 292*b*
    well-being champions, 295–96
    well-being committees, 296–97
well-being program motivations, 257–69
    costs, 258*t*, 263–65, 264*t*
    moral imperative, 258–59, 258*t*
    quality and safety of care, 258*t*, 262–63
    regulatory requirements, 258*t*, 260
    tragedy as imperative, 258*t*, 259–60
well-being program promotion and
    communication, 270–84
    Bloom's Taxonomy, 272–74
    communication frameworks, 275–76

    communication theory, 274–75
    elevator speeches, 270–72, 271*b*
    growth mindset, 279–80
    listening, 275–76
    Logic Model, 273*f*, 273–74, 281–83
    semantic framing, 276–78
well-being programs at institutional level, 207
    Chief Wellness Officers, 322–23, 324, 325–31, 331*f*
    considerations for, 324
    including well-being in strategic planning, 323
    resources to support well-being, 324–31
WellMD Center, 340
Western Sydney University, 57
White Coat Ceremony, 220–21
WHO (World Health Organization), 11, 35, 134–35,
    196–97, 198
women
    alcohol and substance use, 86
    belonging and connectivity, 144
    burnout, 32, 35–36, 47, 49–50, 97
    diversity and inclusion, 67–68
    dual-role responsibilities, 71
    parental leave, 235–36
    self-care, 60
    social support, 67, 70
    suicidal ideation and suicide, 42, 259
work compression and intensity, 64, 73*t*, 173–74,
    230, 233, 251, 287–88, 294
work hours. *See* hours worked; workload
work-life integration and balance, 4, 25, 65, 71, 90,
    115, 136–37, 235–36, 329
workload, 116–17, 170–74
    balance of education and, 117
    electronic health records, 62, 116, 306
    inconsistent relationship between workload
        measures and well-being measures, 173–74
    as institutional driver of well-being, 62, 73*t*
    meaning in work and, 171
    measuring and defining, 170–71
    overall student workload, 116
    work-load interventions in GME, 172–73
    work-load interventions in UME, 172
work outside of work (WOW), 336–37, 345–46
work-sharing, 116
World Health Organization (WHO), 11, 35, 134–35,
    196–97, 198
World Medical Association, 135–36

Yale University, 61

zero-sum traps, 11, 13–14, 171, 251*f*, 251–52
Zion, Libby, 2, 138, 229